Pro

To Jon and Sara

Commissioning Editor: Mairi McCubbin
Development Editor: Sally Davies
Project Manager: Elouise Ball
Designer: Kirsteen Wright
Illustration Manager: Merlyn Harvey

Promoting Health

A Practical Guide

Angela Scriven BA(Hons) MEd CertEd FRSPH MIUHPE
Reader in Health Promotion, Brunel University, London, UK

Forewords by
Linda Ewles BSc MSc MA

Ina Simnett MA(Oxon) DPhil CertEd
Bristol, UK

Richard Parish BSc Med PDHEd CBiol MIBiol FRSPH FFPH CMIPR HonMAPHA
Chief Executive, Royal Society for Public Health, London, UK

SIXTH EDITION

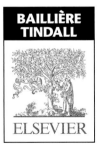

BAILLIÈRE
TINDALL

ELSEVIER

EDINBURGH LONDON NEW YORK OXFORD PHILADELPHIA ST LOUIS SYDNEY TORONTO 2010

BAILLIÈRE
TINDALL
ELSEVIER

First edition 1985
Second edition 1992
Third edition 1995
Fourth edition 1999
Fifth edition 2003
Sixth edition 2010

ISBN: 978 0 7020 3139 7

British Library Cataloguing in Publication Data
A catalogue record for this book is available from the British Library

Library of Congress Cataloging in Publication Data
A catalog record for this book is available from the Library of Congress

Notices
Knowledge and best practice in this field are constantly changing. As new research and experience broaden our understanding, changes in research methods, professional practices, or medical treatment may become necessary.

Practitioners and researchers must always rely on their own experience and knowledge in evaluating and using any information, methods, compounds, or experiments described herein. In using such information or methods they should be mindful of their own safety and the safety of others, including parties for whom they have a professional responsibility.

With respect to any drug or pharmaceutical products identified, readers are advised to check the most current information provided (i) on procedures featured or (ii) by the manufacturer of each product to be administered, to verify the recommended dose or formula, the method and duration of administration, and contraindications. It is the responsibility of practitioners, relying on their own experience and knowledge of their patients, to make diagnoses, to determine dosages and the best treatment for each individual patient, and to take all appropriate safety precautions.

To the fullest extent of the law, neither the Publisher nor the author assumes any liability for any injury and/or damage to persons or property as a matter of products liability, negligence or otherwise, or from any use or operation of any methods, products, instructions, or ideas contained in the material herein.

Working together to grow
libraries in developing countries

www.elsevier.com | www.bookaid.org | www.sabre.org

ELSEVIER   BOOK AID International   Sabre Foundation

ELSEVIER   your source for books, journals and multimedia in the health sciences

www.elsevierhealth.com

The publisher's policy is to use paper manufactured from sustainable forests

Printed in China

Contents

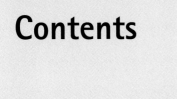

Foreword

We are delighted that *Promoting Health* is now in its sixth edition.

We embarked on writing the first edition back in the early 1980s. One of us (Linda Ewles) was then working at Bristol Polytechnic (now the University of the West of England) running one of the three postgraduate Diploma courses in health education which existed in the UK at that time. The other (Ina Simnett) had recently moved to Bristol and was working in health education in the NHS. We had each independently recognised the need for a health education textbook; amazing as it seems now, at the time there were none in the UK. We were put in touch with each other by Jane Randell who did much to develop education and training at the national Health Education Council. It was the start of our long collaboration and friendship.

We put together an outline of the book's proposed content, drawing heavily on our combined experience and training. We typed the chapters on a manual typewriter (no word processors then) and laboriously looked up all the references in libraries (no Internet). Our first publisher was John Wiley, and *Promoting Health: A Practical Guide To Health Education* was launched in May 1985 at a nursing conference in Harrogate.

We fully expected that the book would have a shelf life of a few years, and then be superseded by many others. Indeed, more textbooks on health education and health promotion (when that new term started to be used) did appear – but ours continued to be well used. We had met a need. Every few years from then on, our publisher (who changed several times as publishing companies were sold and amalgamated) approached us for an updated edition.

But the last request for a new edition came at the stage in our lives when we had both retired from work in health promotion. We felt that the update should be done by someone in closer touch with current professional thinking and practice. We are delighted that Angela Scriven undertook the task and has given the book a new lease of life with a thoroughly updated version which still retains the style and scope of its predecessors. We are very grateful to her for her excellent work.

Twenty-five years after the first edition was written, we can look back and see that some themes we wrote about then are still totally relevant today. Health promoters still need to explore what 'health' means, understand the underlying values and approaches in health promotion, think about ethical issues, base their work on evidence of effectiveness and learn skills of communicating and managing, planning and evaluating. A surprising amount of the sixth edition has scarcely changed since the first one.

But of course a great deal *has* changed, and this is reflected in the current edition. We are struck by the huge expansion of the evidence base of 'what works' and how much research and information is now available on the Internet. In terms of delivering health promotion, the rise of partnership working between sectors and agencies and the integration of health promotion specialist work in the NHS into mainstream public health (rather than remaining a Cinderella 'add-on' service) are also remarkable. Health promotion has become an integral part of basic training for health workers and there has been a massive growth in specialist training opportunities.

Some health education acorns undoubtedly failed to take root, but others have become sturdy oak trees. For example, stop-smoking group work by a few health educators has grown into a huge mainstream NHS smoking cessation programme. A handful of health workers going into schools to give talks has developed into a European-wide health-promoting schools network with fully-fledged personal, social and health education school programmes.

We are gratified and humbled to think that our book has made a small contribution to these and other developments over the last 25 years. It has been widely used in the UK but also in over 50 countries around the world. It has been translated into seven European and Asian languages and has been useful in health development in Africa, parts of Asia and the Middle East. We are pleased to think that we must have got something right! We would also like to take this opportunity to thank all those people who, in so many different ways, have helped to make *Promoting Health* a success.

Of course, as Richard Parish points out in his Foreword, health promoters now face 21st-century challenges, such as obesity, alcohol consumption levels, climate change and new forms of communicable diseases. We hope that this edition continues to contribute to the spread of sound health promotion practice in tackling these and other issues which undermine health today. We also hope that it helps people to continue their efforts to reduce health inequalities in the UK and across the world.

Linda Ewles
Ina Simnett

Foreword

The need for effective health promotion has never been greater. We face immense challenges to health as we move through the 21st century. Regrettably, modern-day life is not always as conducive to health and wellbeing as we would wish. The current scourge of overweight and obesity is but one measure of our unhealthy lifestyles. To this we must add the growing impact of climate change and the emergence of new strains of communicable disease. Never before have we faced such an assault upon our health, with the disadvantaged suffering the greatest.

The forces waged against health are complex and comprehensive. We need a skilled and competent workforce if we are to improve health for all over the coming years. The earlier editions of *Promoting Health: A Practical Guide* have been heavily used by students, academic staff in universities and colleges, policy makers and planners, and by health promoters going about their everyday work. This new edition will continue the tradition of this seminal publication and will strongly influence the training of future practitioners. Building on its rich pedigree, this latest edition tackles the major health issues facing us today, focusing on practical interventions for better health.

Many strategies and techniques in health promotion are tried and tested. There is a sound and growing evidence base. We know what works in most situations, although we must be ever vigilant in pursuing new approaches and evaluating the outcomes. Effective health promotion draws on many disciplines, adapting to the emergence of new evidence. This book reflects contemporary thinking, referring to the application of new technologies and approaches such as social marketing.

The challenge of better health requires action at all levels of society. Government and the national agencies most certainly have a major role to play, not least in supporting those who work to improve health. The following pages provide an authoritative text for everyone involved in promoting health, both informing policy makers as to what is possible and acting as a toolkit for health promoters. From planning and management to monitoring and evaluation, this edition ranges across the full panoply of tools and techniques. It is genuinely a practical guide, helping to ensure effective practice in every area of health promotion work.

Promoting Health: A Practical Guide is not just for health promotion specialists responsible for delivering better health to the communities with which they work. It also describes the potential for health promotion. As such, it is an essential tool for commissioners and those who plan and procure health improvement services, helping to define how best to invest public resources.

Better health will only be achieved through actions at all levels of society. The state and the public sector, commercial organisations, voluntary agencies and individual citizens all have a role to play. This book will help ensure effective and efficient action. We must deploy our resources to maximum advantage, for the cost of not doing so will be measured in avoidable ill health, unnecessary expenditure and a loss of human potential. To this end *Promoting Health: A Practical Guide* is a valuable investment.

Richard Parish

Preface

The aim of this book is to provide an accessible practical guide for all those who practise health promotion in their everyday work. It was first published in 1985, and in response to demand a new updated edition has been produced approximately every five years. Earlier editions have also been published in German, Hungarian, Finnish, Greek, Indonesian, Italian and Swedish.

The book is addressed to all those who promote health, including health promotion and public health practitioners and specialists, hospital and community nurses, health visitors and midwives, hospital doctors and general practitioners, dentists and dental hygienists, pharmacists, health service managers and the professions allied to medicine. It is also for the wide range of health promoters in statutory and non-statutory agencies, for example local authority staff such as environmental health officers and social workers, voluntary organisations, youth and community workers, teachers in schools, colleges and universities, probation officers, prison officers and police officers.

Health promotion encompasses a wide variety of activities, with the common purpose of improving the health of individuals and communities. This book is concerned with the what, why, who and how of health promotion. It aims to help you explore important questions such as:

● What is health?
● What affects health?
● What is health promotion? How is it part of a wider public health movement?
● Who are the agents and agencies of health promotion?

● Who needs health promotion and what are these needs?
● How can priorities be set?
● How can health promotion be planned, managed and evaluated?
● How can health promoters best carry out health promotion? What are the competencies they require?
● What are the key issues for health promotion?

There is a focus on the theories, principles and competencies you need to consider, whatever your background and wherever you work. The range of health issues and settings for health promotion (such as communities, schools, workplaces, GP surgeries or hospitals) is clearly enormous, but it is beyond the scope of this book to cover all these in depth. Different professional groups will all have their own areas of expert knowledge and specialist skills to be employed alongside the specific expertise in promoting health addressed in this book.

As in previous editions, the book is organised into three parts. *Part 1 Thinking About Health and Health Promotion* deals with basic ideas of what health, health promotion and health education are about, and the different approaches and ethical issues that need to be considered, and identifies the agencies and people who have a part to play in health promotion and public health.

Part 2 Planning and Managing for Effective Practice looks at planning and evaluation at the level of a health promoter's daily work and starts by introducing a basic planning and evaluation framework. It continues with a discussion of how to identify and assess needs and priorities, and develop skills to manage yourself and your work effectively.

Part 3 Developing Competence in Health Promotion looks at how you can develop your competence in carrying out a range of activities, including enabling people to learn in one-to-one and group settings, enabling people towards healthier living, working with communities and changing policies and practices. The fundamentals of communication and of using communication tools are also addressed.

This sixth edition is fully revised and updated to take account of recent developments in public health, such as revised national strategies for health, reorganisations that have taken place in the National Health Service, and new policies that have a bearing on the promotion of health. It is important to note, however, that policies and strategies for health frequently change, particularly when governments change, and there will be a general election during the life of this sixth edition. It is likely, therefore, that some of the policies referred to in the text may have been replaced. New issues that are highlighted are:

- changes to the structure and organisation of the National Health Service in the UK
- national standards for work in health promotion and public health
- new research on the comparative effectiveness of different approaches to health promotion
- reference to new technology, especially the Internet
- new approaches, including social marketing.

The user-friendly style adopted in the previous editions has been retained. There are many more website addresses, to reflect the increased use of the internet to disseminate health information and evidence, with such networking sites as Twitter and YouTube being used in a health-promoting capacity by the Department of Health, non-governmental organisations and community health groups.

Non-sexist writing is used throughout the text, drawing on the ideas on non-sexist writing discussed in Chapter 11. Several terms have been used to describe the people that health promotion targets. These terms include 'patients' (referring mainly to those who receive their health promotion in a healthcare environment), 'clients' (for patients and non patients) or simply users, individuals or groups. The term 'health promoters' is used to cover the multidisciplinary workforces that have remits for promoting health, but whose job titles cover a wide spectrum, including public health practitioners (see Ch. 2 for a discussion on who promotes health).

The overall aim of the book is the same as in previous editions, to keep you involved, so that studying this book will be an active educational experience. Exercises are included to undertake as an individual or in a group, and examples and case studies are provided to help you to apply ideas to your own situation. Often the exercises are designed to stimulate thought and discussion and there may be no right answers. You will need to think it through, talk it over and reflect. In this way the answers will have personal meaning and application.

London, 2010   Angela Scriven

Acknowledgements

Linda Ewles and Ina Simnett, the authors of the first five editions of this book, produced a seminal text that I and many others have used in the training and education of health promoters over the last 25 years. Their book has shaped health promotion practice in the UK over this time. I am privileged to have been invited to take over the authorship and wish to thank Ewles and Simnett and Elsevier, the publishers, for giving me this opportunity. I also wish to thank all of those who had an involvement in the first five editions. Some of the exercises and elements of the book have been strongly influenced by the work of others. Many of these remain and have been further adjusted to suit the current needs of health promoters. Finally, I would like to thank Professor Richard Parish for his Foreword, and for their support and encouragement throughout the process of producing this new edition, Sally Davies and Mairi McCubbin from Elsevier, my colleague Sebastian Garman at Brunel University and my family and friends.

PART 1

Thinking about health and health promotion

PART CONTENTS

PART SUMMARY

Part 1 has three purposes:

- It sets the context for the whole book, by introducing key concepts, principles and ideas and by providing you with a common language in which to communicate about health promotion.

- It offers an introduction to the dimensions and scope of health and health promotion, which enables you to focus on the wide range of activities and approaches being utilised by health promoters.

- It highlights important philosophical and ethical issues, which are explored in a practical context later in the book.

Health is an extremely difficult word to define but it is clearly important that you know what it means. This is discussed in Chapter 1, along with a description of the major influences on health and inequalities in health.

There is also an historical overview of some of the international and national movements that have worked towards better health.

In Chapter 2 health promotion is defined and shown to encompass a wide range of activities. Frameworks are given for classifying the major areas of health promotion action. Occupational standards are outlined and an exercise is provided to help you to explore the scope of your health promotion work.

In Chapter 3 the aims and values associated with different approaches to health promotion are analysed, a number of ethical dilemmas are examined and guidance is provided on how to make ethical decisions.

In Chapter 4 the agents and agencies of health promotion are identified and there is an opportunity to clarify your own health promotion role.

Chapter 1

What is health?

SUMMARY

This chapter starts with an exercise which enables you to examine what being healthy means to you, and reviews the wide variation in people's concepts of health. Dimensions of health are considered (physical, mental, emotional, social, spiritual and societal) and health is explored as a holistic concept. Factors that affect health are identified, with a particular focus on medicine and inequalities in health. Case studies illustrate the factors that shape the health of people in differing circumstances. In the final section there is a historical overview of the contribution of international and national movements towards better health.

WHAT DOES BEING HEALTHY MEAN TO YOU?

Being healthy means different things to different people, and much has been researched and written about people's varying concepts of health (see, for example, Hughner & Kleine 2004 and Earle 2007). It is fundamental that you, as a health promoter, explore and define for yourself what being healthy means to you and what it may mean to your clients. This is the aim of Exercise 1.1.

Exercise 1.1 generally shows that different people identify different aspects of being healthy as important. What you choose is often a reflection of your particular circumstances at the time, your experiences and/or your professional background. For example, if you are feeling stressed at work you may consider enjoying work without too much

---

EXERCISE 1.1   What does being healthy mean to you?

In Column 1, tick any of the statements that seem to you to be important aspects of your health. Tick as many as you like.

For me, being healthy involves:	Column 1	Column 2	Column 3
1. Enjoying being with my family and friends	☐	☐	☐
2. Living to a ripe old age	☐	☐	☐
3. Feeling happy most of the time	☐	☐	☐
4. Having a job	☐	☐	☐
5. Hardly ever taking tablets or medicines	☐	☐	☐
6. Being the ideal weight for my height	☐	☐	☐
7. Taking regular exercise	☐	☐	☐
8. Feeling at peace with myself	☐	☐	☐
9. Never smoking	☐	☐	☐
10. Never suffering from anything more serious than a mild cold, flu or stomach upset	☐	☐	☐
11. Not getting things confused or out of proportion – assessing situations realistically	☐	☐	☐
12. Being able to adapt easily to big changes in my life such as moving house or a new job	☐	☐	☐
13. Drinking only moderate amounts of alcohol or none at all	☐	☐	☐
14. Enjoying my work without too much stress	☐	☐	☐
15. Having all the parts of my body in good working condition	☐	☐	☐
16. Getting on well with other people most of the time	☐	☐	☐
17. Eating the 'right' foods	☐	☐	☐
18. Enjoying some form of relaxation or recreation	☐	☐	☐

In Column 2, tick the six statements which are the most important aspects of 'being healthy' to you.

Then in Column 3, rank these six in the order of importance – put 1 by the most important, 2 by the next most important and so on down to 6.

If you are working in a group, compare your list with other people's. Look at the similarities and differences, and discuss the reasons for your choices.

(Adapted with kind permission from Open University 1980.)

---

stress as important, or if you work in a smoking cessation service you may prioritise not smoking as a crucial aspect of being healthy. As your circumstances change, your idea of what being healthy means to you is also likely to change.

CONCEPTS OF HEALTH

As Exercise 1.1 will have indicated, health is a difficult concept to define in absolute terms. The meaning can be culturally and professionally determined and has changed over time (Thomas 2003). A variety of definitions and explanations of what it means to be healthy exists (Duncan 2007) and none can be deemed to be right or wrong.

LAY PERCEPTIONS

It is important to understand the way lay people think about health and wellness, as this influences their health and wellness-related behaviours (Hughner & Kleine 2004). Researchers have found a wealth of complex lay notions about health. Some lay perceptions are based on pragmatism, where health is regarded as a relative phenomenon, experienced and evaluated according to what an individual finds reasonable to expect, given their age, medical condition and social situation. For them being healthy may just mean not having a health problem which interferes with their everyday lives (Bury 2005). Thomas (2003) has classified some personal constructs of health into models. The *functional model*, for example, is based on social role performance and social normality, rather than physical normality; the *psychological model* emphasises the ability to deal with stress and having resilience. Whatever the lay understandings of health are based on, however, they illustrate that lay accounts are unique, and health and strategies for health must be individualised. For example:

- Homeless, single young people in Scotland viewed their health in terms of functional concepts such as taking regular exercise and getting a good night's sleep. In this respect, health was seen as a tool for everyday living (Watts et al 2006).
- Lay men's understanding of health and wellbeing has been shown in a study to relate to notions of control, and the associated issues of risk and responsibility. Specifically, men saw health in more psychological terms (Robertson 2006).
- Exploration of children's concepts of health has shown that their ideas of being healthy and what makes them healthy are strongly tied up with notions of infection; health for them is the lack of symptoms like a cough or running nose. Children in the study also linked environmental pollution with health, with smoking seen as an environmental pollutant, but did not mention violence, being homeless or similar social factors among health determinants (Piko & Bak 2006).

Concepts of health, illness and disease have generally been linked with people's social and cultural situations. Knowledge of illness, prevention and treatment can also be powerful in shaping people's concept of health. Such knowledge may be part of a cultural heritage, passed on through generations (Kue Young 2005).

Standards of what may be considered healthy also vary. An elderly woman may say she is in good health on a day when her chronic arthritis has eased up enough to enable her to get to the shops. A man who smokes may not regard his early morning cough as a symptom of ill health, because to him it is normal. People assess their own health subjectively, according to their own norms and expectations.

People may also trade-off different aspects of health. A common example is that people may accept the physical health damage from smoking as the price they pay for the emotional benefit.

Because of this variety and complexity of the ways in which people conceptualise health, it is difficult to measure health.

For more about measuring health, see Chapter 6, section on finding and using information.

PROFESSIONAL CONCEPTS OF HEALTH

Professional concepts of health have changed over time. In the late 19th and 20th century, as medical discoveries were made and medical practice developed, there was a preoccupation with a mechanistic view of the body and consequently with physical health. Earlier still, there have been centuries of many philosophies of health in different civilisations, such as Greek and Chinese, where a more holistic view of health has been held. See Lloyd & Sivin (2002) for a comparison of these two cultures and their view on health, science and medicine.

One way of understanding the various meanings that the different professional groups hold is to put health into broad categories or models. Three models are identified below and include the *medical model*, the *holistic model*, and the *wellness model*.

The medical model
- The medical model dominated thinking about health for most of the 20th century.
- Health is defined and measured as the absence of disease and the presence of high levels of function.
- In its most extreme form, the medical model views the body as a machine, to be fixed when broken.
- It emphasises treating specific physical diseases, does not accommodate mental or social problems well and de-emphasises prevention.

The holistic model
- The holistic model was exemplified by the World Health Organization (WHO) constitution which referred to health as a state of complete physical, mental and social wellbeing and not merely the absence of disease or infirmity (WHO 1948).
- This broadened the medical model perspective, and highlighted the idea of positive health, although the WHO did not originally use that term, and linked health to wellbeing.

- The WHO definition is in many ways difficult to measure. This is less because of the complexity of measuring wellbeing, as psychologists have done (for example White 2007), but more because doing so required subjective assessments that contrast sharply with the objective indicators favoured by the medical model.

The wellness model

- In 1984, a WHO discussion document proposed moving away from viewing health as a state, toward a dynamic model that presented it as a process or a force (WHO 1984). This was amplified in the *Ottawa Charter for Health Promotion* which proposed that health is the extent to which an individual or group is able to realise aspirations and satisfy needs, and to change or cope with the environment. Health is seen as a resource for everyday life, not the objective of living; it is a positive concept, emphasising social and personal resources, as well as physical capacities (WHO 1986).
- Related to this is the notion of resiliency, such as the success with which individuals and communities adapt to changing circumstances (see Antonovsky 1979 and 1987, and his Sense of Coherence theory).

There are advantages and disadvantages to each of these models. The advantage of the medical model is that disease represents a major public health issue facing society, and disease states need to be treated and can be readily diagnosed and counted. But this approach is narrow, negative and reductionist, and in an extreme form implies that people with disabilities are unhealthy, and that health is only about the absence of morbidity. A further potential limitation to the medical model is its omission of a time dimension. Should we consider as equally healthy two people in equal functional status, one of whom is carrying a fatal gene that may lead to early death?

The holistic and wellness models have the advantage of allowing for mental as well as physical health, and on broader issues of active participation in life. They also allow for more subtle discrimination of people who succeed in living productive lives despite a physical impairment. The visually impaired or amputees, for example, may still be able to satisfy aspirations, be productive, happy and so be viewed as healthy. The disadvantage is

that these conceptions run the risk of excessive breadth, of incorporating all of life. Thus, they do not distinguish clearly between the *state* of being healthy and the *consequences* of being healthy; nor do they distinguish between health and the determinants of health (some of the above is adjusted from http://courseweb.edteched.uottawa.ca).

It is important to note that the WHO (1948) constitution definition of health mentioned above has been heavily criticised, mainly on two grounds: it is unrealistic and idealistic and it implies a static position. A study by Jadad & O'Grady (2008) found that some criticisms of the WHO definition focused on its lack of operational value and the problem created by use of the word 'complete'. An extreme critique, such as Smith (2008), call it a ludicrous definition that would leave most of us unhealthy most of the time. In support of the definition, Jadad & O'Grady (2008) argue that the WHO invited nations to expand the conceptual framework of their health systems beyond the traditional boundaries set by the physical condition of individuals and their diseases, and it challenged political, community and professional organisations devoted to improving or preserving health to pay more attention to the social determinants of health.

Even just using these three broad categories of health, it follows that there will be differences between health practitioners' concepts of health. To take one example, practitioners of complementary medicine hold to a range of beliefs about what health is and how health can be restored or improved which is based on holism and empowerment (Barrett et al 2004).

In exploring the concept of health further it is useful to consider the identification of different dimensions of health which began with the WHO definition but have been subsequently expanded. The dimensions now include:

Physical health. This is perhaps the most obvious dimension of health, and is concerned with the mechanistic functioning of the body.

Mental health. Mental health refers to the ability to think clearly and coherently. It can be distinguished from emotional and social health, although there is a close association between the three.

Emotional health. This means the ability to recognise emotions such as fear, joy, grief and anger and to express such emotions appropriately. Emotional (or affective) health also means coping with stress, tension, depression and anxiety.

Social health. Social health means the ability to make and maintain relationships with other people.

Spiritual health. For some people, spiritual health might be connected with religious beliefs and practices; for other people it might be associated with personal creeds, principles of behaviour and ways of achieving peace of mind and being at peace with oneself.

Societal health. So far, health has been considered at the level of the individual, but a person's health is inextricably related to everything surrounding that person. It is impossible to be healthy in a sick society that does not provide the resources for basic physical and emotional needs. For example, people obviously cannot be healthy if they cannot afford necessities like food, clothing and shelter, but neither can they be healthy in countries of extreme political oppression where basic human rights are denied. Women cannot be healthy when their contribution to society is undervalued, and neither black nor white can be healthy in a racist society where racism undermines human worth, self-esteem and social relationships. Unemployed people cannot be healthy in a society that values only people in paid employment, and it is very unlikely that anyone can be healthy if they live in an area that lacks basic services and facilities such as health care, transport and recreation.

The identification of these different aspects of health is a useful exercise in raising awareness of the complexity and the holistic nature of health. But in practice it is obvious that dividing people's health into categories such as physical and mental can impose artificial divisions and unhelpful distortions. Sexual health, for example, can cross all these boundaries proving that the dimensions of health are interrelated.

Some writers have provided useful analyses of what health means from different disciplinary perspectives. Seedhouse (2001), for example, proposes the idea of health as the foundation for achieving a person's realistic potential.

Similarly, when the WHO broadened their definition, as noted in the wellness model outlined earlier in the chapter, they also identified key aspects of health. The conception of health is the extent to which an individual or group is able to realise aspirations and satisfy needs, to change or cope with the environment, where health is seen as a resource for everyday life, not the objective of living; it is a positive concept emphasising social and personal resources, as well as physical capacities, not simply the absence of disease (WHO 1984).

This is a rich view of health. It encompasses ideas of:

- Personal growth and development ('realise aspirations').
- Meeting personal basic needs ('satisfy needs').
- The ability to adapt to environmental changes (resilience to change and cope with the environment').
- A means to an end, not an end in itself (a resource for everyday life, not the objective of living).
- Not just absence of disease (a positive concept).
- A holistic concept (social and personal resources … physical capacities).

This notion of health has much to offer the health promoter. It recognises that health is a dynamic state, that a person's potential is different, and that each person's health needs vary. Working for health is both an individual and a societal responsibility, and involves empowering people to improve their quality of life.

This discussion of health as a concept is an important prerequisite to thinking about what determines people's health. Before moving on to a consideration of what affects health, it might be useful to undertake Exercise 1.2 and to read Case studies 1.1 and 1.2 and answer the associated questions.

WHAT AFFECTS HEALTH?

Being healthy is rarely, if ever, the result of chance or luck. A state of health or ill health, however defined, is the result of a combination of factors having a particular effect on a particular individual at any one time. In order to work towards better health, we need to identify these influential factors. You can begin by identifying factors that influence your own health, using Exercise 1.3.

Exercise 1.3 will have identified a huge range of factors which affect health. They are likely to include genetic make-up, gender, family, religion, culture, friends, income, advertising, social life, social class, race, age, employment status, working conditions, health services, self-esteem, self-confidence, access to leisure facilities and shops, housing, education, national food policy, environmental pollution and many more.

EXERCISE 1.2   Dimensions of health

1. Go back to your answers in Exercise 1.1 'What does being healthy mean to you?' Tick if any of the following dimensions of health are reflected in the statements you ticked in Column 1:

Physical   ☐   Emotional   ☐
Mental   ☐   Spiritual   ☐
Social   ☐   Societal   ☐

Is any one of these dimensions more important to you than the others? How do they relate to each other?

2. Has your idea of health changed since childhood? If so, how and why? How do you think your idea of health may change as you grow older?
3. If you have had professional training in health or a related area of work, what difference has this made to your idea of health?
4. What do you think being healthy may mean to someone who:
   - has learning difficulties?
   - has a permanent physical disability such as deafness or paralysis?
   - has an illness or infection for which there is currently no known cure such as diabetes, arthritis, HIV, schizophrenia?
   - lives in poverty?
5. Identify three or four key points you have learnt from this exercise about your own ideas of being healthy.

HEALTH AND MEDICINE

There has been much debate since the 1970s about the relative importance of the many and varied determinants of health. There have also been concerns that medicine might have less effect on the population's overall health improvement than promoting lifestyle changes or social reforms, although some have argued that these concerns are not founded (see, for example, Bunker 2001). The National Health Service (NHS) has undoubtedly evolved in the main as a treatment and care service for people who are ill, not as the major means of improving public health (Baggott 2004, Klein 2006 and Ham 2009 offer further discussion of the NHS and healthcare policies).

Some people have claimed that the practice of scientific medicine has, in fact, done considerable harm. Examples are the side-effects of treatment, complications that set in after surgery and depend-

---

EXERCISE 1.3   What affects your health?

The aim of this radiating circle exercise is to identify factors that affect your health. The exercise can be done:
- individually
- individually, followed by comparing results with other people
- as a group, pooling your ideas about what influences your health.

You are at the centre of the rings:

In the inner ring, write in factors that influence your health and that are to do with yourself as an individual.

In the second ring, write in factors that influence your health and that are to do with your immediate social and physical environment.

In the outer ring, write in factors that influence your health and that are to do with your wider social, physical or political environment.

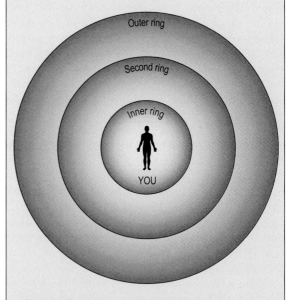

How do these factors influence your health – positively or negatively?

Which factors do you think are the most important?

Are there factors that you have not identified for yourself, but which may be important for other people?

(Burkitt 1982, reproduced with kind permission of Medical Education (International) Ltd.)

CASE STUDIES 1.1 AND 1.2 WHAT SHAPES PEOPLE'S HEALTH AND HEALTH BELIEFS?

Case 1.1 Salma

Salma had been widowed twice, and now believes that people are plotting against her. At the same time, she is in a desperate situation, living with her four children in a small, crumbling, two-bedroomed terraced house. She has no money for repairs, and no husband to support her or help put things right. The rooms are poorly decorated and the emersion heater is broken so there is only cold water in the bathroom. To have a bath, Salma has to heat water on the cooker downstairs and carry it up. The plumbing needs repair, and there is no water in the cold water tap of the washbasin. Salma sleeps with her daughter in one of the bedrooms and her three sons sleep in the other. One of the downstairs rooms cannot be used because it needs replastering, and the floor boards are dangerous in another. Salma applied for a repair grant about a year and a half ago. They came and took pictures and didn't do anything about it. She has also applied for a council house, but she has been told it will take a long time. She feels there is nothing wrong with her health; just nerves. She feels like her life is being squeezed out of her. She worries about her children. They cannot play outside or go to the park because the English children fight with them, and the house is too small and dangerous to play in.

- What affects the health of Salma and her children?
- What is Salma's own view about her health? Why do you think she holds this view?
- What should be done to improve and promote the health of Salma and her children? (Adjusted from Commission for Racial Equality 1993.)

Case 1.2 Anne and Charlie

Anne is 57 years old and has cancer. She had it for the first time 7 years ago, when a lump was discovered when she went along to her first mammography, and she had a mastectomy. Six months ago another lump was discovered and she had to have a second mastectomy and more chemotherapy. She is a primary school teacher and has just returned to work part time. She loves her work and has very supportive colleagues. She was divorced 2 years after the first mastectomy and now lives alone with her daughter, Charlie. Anne has lots of friends, a large extended family and a good social network. She feels healthy and is determined to overcome the cancer and has established a new diet and exercise programme to help her stay healthy. Like her parents, she wants to live to a very old age, and looks forward to Charlie being settled in life and to having grandchildren. She belongs to a cancer support group and is planning to undertake a half marathon to raise money for a cancer charity. While Charlie admires her mother and the way she is dealing with her illness, she is worried that she may die of cancer soon. Charlie is in her final year of university and while she considers herself to be fit and healthy, since she became a student she smokes heavily, frequently binge drinks, and when she is very stressed will occasionally use drugs. She often has casual and sometimes unprotected sex when drunk. Her diet is not good; she either skips meals or just eats take-away foods. She knows that her chances of getting breast cancer are higher because her mother has had it, so feels she should enjoy life to the full while she is young. She found her parents' divorce very difficult and hasn't seen her father in 5 years. She has been very depressed over the past 6 months but has continued with her university degree because she knows her mother would be very upset if she withdraws.

- What affects the health of Anne and Charlie?
- What are Anne's and Charlie's own views about their health? Why do you think they hold these views?
- What could be done to improve and promote the health of Anne and Charlie?

ence on prescribed drugs. But more important, perhaps, is that control over health and illness has been taken away from people themselves, who become dependent on doctors and medical drugs. Aspects of life that are natural, such as pregnancy and childbirth, the menopause and ageing, have become medicalised and the responsibility for health has shifted from the lay public to the medical profession. These arguments that medicine is, at best, a treatment and care service for the ill and, at worst, a means of undermining people's competence and confidence to improve their health reached a peak around 1980, led in part by the work of Illich (1977), but they are still relevant today (see, for example, Jackson 2001 and Meyer 2001). There are moves to change this perception of the health services and government policy is currently in place to attempt to make the healthcare services fairer, more personalised, effective and safe (Department of Health (DoH) 2007a).

THE WIDER DETERMINANTS OF HEALTH

The Black Report (Townsend & Davidson 1982) showed that, for almost every kind of illness and disability in the UK, people in the upper socio-economic groups had a greater chance of avoiding illness and staying healthy than those in the lower socioeconomic groups. It also established the differences in the risks to men and women, and variations in the apparent health consequences of living in different parts of the country.

All this pointed to the fact that the major determinants of health were socioeconomic conditions, geographical location and gender. Evidence from the late 1990s (Acheson 1998) demonstrated that the health gap was widening, so that while overall population health may be improving, the rate of improvement is not equal across all sections of society. The gap in the health status between the lower socioeconomic groups and the higher socio-economic groups continues to increase.

Work comparing data across different countries has shown another slant on the issue of inequalities. It is not the richest societies that have the best health, but those that have the smallest income differences between rich and poor. It is the *relative* difference in income levels which is crucial. The reason seems to be that small income differences across society mean an egalitarian society that has a strong community life and better quality of life in terms of strong social networks, less social stress, higher self-esteem, less depression and anxiety and more sense of control (Marmot 2005). All of this adds up to better health.

In recent years the UK government has implemented a programme of action to tackle health inequalities (see DoH 2007b for a status report on the strategies in place). At the time of writing the government has also commissioned a post-2010 strategic review of health inequalities (the Marmot Review; see References). It will be interesting to monitor whether the Marmot Review will repeat the findings of earlier reports, or whether the review will show that the *Programme for Action* set in place (DoH 2003) has been effective.

One way of addressing health inequalities and inequities is by building *social capital*. Social capital is the term used to describe investment in the social fabric of society, so that communities develop high levels of trust and many networks for the exchange of information, ideas and practical help. Social capital is produced when, for example, there are neighbourhood schemes of child care and crime prevention, community groups and social activities that engage a wide range of interests and people (Li 2007).

Differences in health experience may not be due entirely to socioeconomic determinants. There are important differences in rates of illness and death between ethnic groups, which may be related to differences in income, education and living conditions, cultural factors or genetic make-up. There are also differences associated with age, sex, occupation and where people live (Wilkinson & Marmot 2003). Addressing the distribution of wealth in society, reducing the gap between rich and poor and tackling socioeconomic disadvantage are clearly political issues (DoH 2003), and the post-2010 strategic review of health inequalities (the Marmot Review) demonstrates the government's continued commitment to reducing health inequalites.

IMPROVING HEALTH – HISTORICAL OVERVIEW

A number of conclusions can be drawn from the discussion above. First, health is a complex concept, meaning different things to different people. Second, health status is linked with people's ability to reach their full potential. Finally, health is affected by a wide range of factors, which may be broadly classified as:

- Lifestyle factors to do with individual health behaviour.
- Broader social, economic and environmental factors such as whether people live in an egalitarian society, what social support networks are available, and how they live in terms of employment, income and housing.

Early public health work in the first half of the 20th century concentrated on structural reforms such as slum clearance, improved sanitation and clean air. Then in the 1950s and 1960s the focus shifted towards the need for changes in individual health behaviour, for example, family planning, venereal disease (the original term to describe sexually transmitted infections), accident prevention, immunisation, cervical smear checks, weight control, alcohol consumption and smoking. This emphasis on the lifestyle approach meant a concentration of effort on health education, which was reflected in government statements at the time (see, for example, Department of Health and Social Security 1976). Over time, this emphasis has been heavily criticised because it distracts attention from the social and economic determinants of health, and tended to blame individuals for their own ill health. For example, people with heart disease could be blamed for it because they were overweight and smoked, but the reasons for being overweight and smoking, what Marmot (2005) refers to as the causes of the causes, were ignored. Reasons may have included lack of education, no help available to stop smoking, eating and smoking used as a way of coping with stresses such as poor housing or unemployment, lack of availability of cheap nutritious foods, and so on. This blaming people for their health behaviour became known as *victim-blaming* (see Dougherty (1993) and Caraher (1995) for early discussions of victim-blaming). In the 1980s a broader approach was used in conjunction with what was called the new public health movement (WHO 1986). It encompassed health education but also political and social action to address issues such as poverty, employment, discrimination and the environment in which people live. It also, importantly, focused on the grass-roots involvement of people in shaping their own health destiny.

See Chapter 4 for information on people and organisations working to improve public health.

INTERNATIONAL INITIATIVES FOR IMPROVING HEALTH

More is said about the role of the WHO and other international organisations in Chapter 4.

The WHO took a leading role in the evolution of health promotion in the 1980s and 1990s. It stated in 1978 that the main target of governments in the coming decades should be the attainment of all citizens of the world by the year 2000 of a level of health that will permit them to lead a socially and economically productive life (WHO 1978). This was the beginning of what came to be known as the *Health for All* (HFA) movement. It led to the development of a strategy for the WHO European Region in 1980 (WHO 1985).

This regional strategy called for fundamental changes in the health policy of member countries, including a much higher priority for health promotion and disease prevention. It called for not only health services but all public sectors with a potential impact on health to take positive steps to maintain and improve health. Specific regional targets were published; these have been subsequently updated and the movement is now called *Health 21* (WHO 1999a, b). The targets emphasised the following HFA principles:

- Reducing inequalities in health.
- Positive health through health promotion and disease prevention.
- Community participation.
- Cooperation between health authorities, local authorities and others with an impact on health.
- A focus on primary health care as the main basis of the healthcare system.

The *Health for All* targets for Europe, which European governments and the WHO aimed to reach by 2000, were reviewed and evaluated at the end of the century (http://www.euro.who.int). Progress had been made on many fronts, but targets had not been reached, mainly because of political, social and economic difficulties.

Health 21 sets out 21 targets for the European region. The targets cover a wide range, including reducing health inequalities. Target 2 states: 'By the year 2020, the health gap between socioeconomic groups within countries should be reduced by at least one fourth in all Member States, by substantially improving the level of health of disadvantaged groups' (WHO 1999b). Other *Health 21* targets cover better health for children and older people; reducing communicable and chronic diseases, injuries and harm from alcohol, drugs and tobacco; developing better health care, policies and strategies for health; and partnership working.

A major milestone for health promotion was the publication in 1986 of the *Ottawa Charter*, launched at the first WHO international conference on health promotion held in Ottawa, Canada (WHO 1986). This identified five key themes for health promotion:

1. Building a healthy public policy.
2. Creating supportive environments.
3. Developing personal skills through information and education in health and life skills.

4. Strengthening community action.
5. Reorienting health services towards prevention and health promotion.

(See Scriven & Speller (2007) for an overview of the global influence of Ottawa.)

The Jakarta declaration in 1997 (WHO 1997) reiterated the importance of the *Ottawa Charter* principles and added priorities for health promotion in the 21st century:

- Promote social responsibility for health.
- Increase investment for health development.
- Expand partnerships for health promotion.
- Increase community capacity and empower the individual.
- Secure an infrastructure for health promotion.

The Bangkok Charter for Health in a Globalized World is the most recent WHO declaration (WHO 2005). The Charter builds on Ottawa by asserting that progress towards a healthier world requires strong political action, broad participation and sustained advocacy.

The call is to ensure that health promotion's established repertoire of proven effective strategies will need to be fully utilised, with all sectors and settings acting to:

- **advocate** for health based on human rights and solidarity
- **invest** in sustainable policies, actions and infrastructure to address the determinants of health
- **build capacity** for policy development, leadership, health promotion practice, knowledge transfer and research, and health literacy
- **regulate and legislate** to ensure a high level of protection from harm and enable equal opportunity for health and wellbeing for all people
- **partner and build alliances** with public, private, nongovernmental and international organizations and civil society to create sustainable actions.

NATIONAL INITIATIVES

See Chapter 7, section on national health strategies, for more about national strategies for health and how they are implemented.

An important development for the UK in the early 1990s was the advent of national strategies for health improvement. The first was *The Health of the Nation* in England (DoH 1992), and comparable strategies for Wales, Scotland and Northern Ireland. These were the first national strategies to focus on health and health gain rather than illness and health services.

The most recent of these strategies are:

- 2001: the National Assembly for Wales (NAW) published Improving Health in Wales: a Summary Plan for the NHS with its Partners (NAW 2001a) and an action plan Promoting Health and Wellbeing: Implementing the National Health Promotion Strategy (NAW 2001b).
- 2002: in Northern Ireland the Department of Health and Social Services and Public Safety (DHSSPS) published Investing for Health: a Public Health Strategy for Northern Ireland (DHSSPS 2002).
- 2003: the Scottish Office (SO) published Improving Health in Scotland: the Challenge (SO 2003).
- 2004: in England the Department of Health published Choosing Health: Making Healthy Choices Easier (DoH 2004).

A further significant development was that in 2001 the Department of Health published national targets to reduce inequalities in England, and re-affirmed these in 2007 as part of the spending review. This welcome emphasis on reducing inequalities ensures that work to improve the health of the public will have inequalities in health at its core, at both local and national levels. The targets are as follows:

- Starting with children under 1 year, by 2010 to reduce by at least 10% the gap in mortality between routine and manual groups and the population as a whole.
- Starting with local authorities, by 2010 to reduce by at least 10% the gap in life expectancy between the fifth of areas with the worst health and deprivation indicators (the Spearhead Group) and the population as a whole (http://www.dh.gov.uk).

Also in 2001, a long-awaited report was produced by the Chief Medical Officer, setting out the role for a stronger public health function and building on targets set in national health strategies (DoH 2001). The report identified major themes relevant to achieving a stronger public health function, including:

- a wider understanding of health
- a better and more coordinated public health function
- partnership working
- community development and public involvement
- an increased and more capable public health workforce
- increased health protection.

WHERE ARE WE NOW?

It is clear from the above that there is a broad understanding of the wider determinants of people's health, and there are international and national health strategies which are reviewed and revised on an ongoing basis. There is a stronger national and local emphasis on prevention, health improvement and reducing inequalities, with health promotion playing a bigger part in the role of all the health and social welfare professions. Health issues feature more in public policy debate at both central and local government and in the health service.

But as yet these positive developments have failed to narrow the health gap between socio-economic groups in the UK (DoH 2007b, 2009). Health promoters in the UK are still faced with entrenched inequality in health status, and huge problems of poverty, unemployment and homelessness (Marmot 2005). This raises questions about the distribution of wealth in society and emphasises that health is a political issue.

PRACTICE POINTS

- Health and being healthy mean different things to different people, and you need to explore and understand what they mean to you and to your clients.
- A wide range of factors at many levels influence and determine people's health.
- There are wide inequalities in the health status of people from different social classes, ethnic groups, age groups, sexes and people who live in different geographical locations.
- Improving people's health means addressing the social, environmental and economic factors that affect their health, as well as individual health behaviour and lifestyle.
- International and national strategies and movements have emerged to tackle the lifestyle, socioeconomic and environmental determinants of health, and to reduce inequalities in health.

References

Acheson D 1998 Independent inquiry into inequalities in health. The Stationery Office, London.

Antonovsky A 1979 Health, stress and coping. Jossey-Bass, San Francisco.

Antonovsky A 1987 Unraveling the mystery of health – how people manage stress and stay well. Jossey-Bass, San Francisco.

Baggott R 2004 Health and health care in Britain, 3rd edn. Macmillan, Basingstoke.

Barrett B, Marchand L, Scheder J et al 2004 What complementary and alternative medicine practitioners say about health and health care. Annals of Family Medicine 2: 253–259.

Bunker JP 2001 The role of medical care in contributing to health improvements within societies. International Journal of Epidemiology 30: 1260–1263.

Burkitt A 1982 Providing education about health. Nursing, June 29–30.

Bury M 2005 Health and illness. Wiley/Polity, Chichester.

Caraher M 1995 Nursing and health education: victim blaming. British Journal of Nursing 4(20):1190–1192, 1209–1213.

Commission for Racial Equality 1993 The sorrow in my heart. Sixteen Asian women speak about depression. CRE, London.

Department of Health 1992 The health of the nation: a strategy for health in England. The Stationery Office, London.

Department of Health 2001 Report of the Chief Medical Officer's project to strengthen the public health function. The Stationery Office, London.

Department of Health 2003 Tackling health inequalities: a programme for action. The Stationery Office, London.

Department of Health 2004 Choosing health: making healthy choices easier. The Stationery Office, London.

Department of Health 2007a Our NHS, our future: NHS next stage review – interim report. The Stationery Office, London.

Department of Health 2007b Tackling health inequalities: status report on the Programme for Action. The Stationery Office, London.

Department of Health 2009 Tackling health inequalities: 10 years on. The Stationery Office, London.

Department of Health and Social Security 1976 Prevention and health – everybody's business. The Stationery Office, London.

Department of Health and Social Services and Public Safety Northern Ireland 2002 Investing for health: a public health strategy for Northern Ireland. The Stationery Office, Belfast.

Dougherty CJ 1993 Bad faith and victim-blaming: the limits of health promotion. Health Care Analysis 1993 1(2): 111–119.

Duncan P 2007 Critical perspectives on health. Palgrave Macmillan, Basingstoke.

Earle S 2007 Exploring health. In: Earle S, Lloyd CE, Sidell M, Spurr M (eds) Theory and research in promoting public health. Sage, in Association with the Open University, London.

Ham C 2009 Health policy in Britain. Palgrave/Macmillan, Basingstoke.

Hughner RS, Kleine SS 2004 Views of health in the lay sector: a compilation and review of how individuals think about health. Health 8(4): 395–422.

Illich I 1977 Limits to medicine – medical nemisis: the expropriation of health. Pelican, Harmondsworth.

Jackson E 2001 Regulating reproduction: law, technology and autonomy. Hart, Oxford.

Jadad AR, O'Grady L 2008 Editorial: How should health be defined? British Medical Journal 337: a2900.

Klein R 2006 The new politics of the NHS: from creation to reinvention. Radcliffe Medical Press, Oxford.

Kue Young T 2005 Population health: concepts and methods, 2nd edn.

Oxford University Press, Oxford.

Li Y 2007 Social capital, social exclusion and wellbeing. In: Scriven A, Garman S (eds) Public health: social context and action. McGraw Hill/Open University Press, London.

Lloyd G, Sivin N 2002 The way and the word: science and medicine in early China and Greece. Yale University Press, New Haven and London.

Marmot M 2005 Social determinants of health inequalities. Lancet 365: 1099–1104.

Marmot Review: http://www.ucl. ac.uk/gheg/marmotreview and http://www.dh.gov.uk/en/ Publichealth/Healthinequalities/ DH_094770

Meyer VF 2001 The medicalization of menopause: critique and consequences. International Journal of Health Services 31(4): 769–792.

National Assembly for Wales 2001a Improving health in Wales: a summary plan for the NHS with its partners. NAW, Cardiff.

National Assembly for Wales 2001b Promoting health and wellbeing: implementing the national health promotion strategy. NAW, Cardiff.

Open University 1980 The good health guide. Pan Books, Harmondsworth, p. 16.

Piko BF, Bak J 2006 Children's perceptions of health and illness: images and lay concepts in preadolescence. Health Education Research 21(5): 643–653.

Robertson S 2006 Not living life in too much of an excess: lay men understanding health and wellbeing. Health 10(2): 175–189.

Scottish Office 2003 Improving health in Scotland: the challenge. The Stationery Office, Edinburgh.

Scriven A, Speller V 2007 Global issues and challenges beyond Ottawa: the way forward. Promotion & Education 14(4): 194–198.

Seedhouse D 2001 Health: the foundations for achievement, 2nd

edn. John Wiley & Sons, Chichester.

Smith R 2008 The end of disease and the beginning of health. BMJ group blogs. http://blogs.bmj.com/ bmj/2008/07/08/richard-smith-the- end-of-disease-and-the-beginning- of-health/.

Thomas RK 2003 Society and health: sociology for health professionals. Springer, New York.

Townsend P, Davidson N 1982 Inequalities in health: Black Report. Penguin, Harmondsworth.

Watts G, Dorrans S, White D 2006 Young single homeless people: their perceptions of health and use of health promotion activities. NHS Scotland, Edinburgh.

White A 2007 A global projection of subjective wellbeing: a challenge to positive psychology? Psychtalk 56: 17–20.

Wilkinson R, Marmot M (eds) 2003 Social determinants of health: the solid facts, 2nd edn. WHO, Copenhagen.

World Health Organization 1948 Constitution of the World Health Organization. www.who.int/ governance/eb/who_constitution_ en.pdf.

World Health Organization 1978 Alma Ata Declaration. WHO, Geneva.

World Health Organization 1984 Health promotion: a discussion document on the concepts and principles. WHO, Copenhagen.

World Health Organization 1985 Regional targets for health for all. WHO, Geneva.

World Health Organization 1986 The Ottawa charter for health promotion. WHO, Geneva. http:// www.who.int/hpr/hpr/ documents/ottawa.html.

World Health Organization 1997 The Jakarta declaration on leading health promotion into the 21st century. WHO, Geneva. http:// www.who.int/hpr/hpr/ documents/jakarta/ english.html.

World Health Organization 1999a
Health 21: health for all in the 21st
century. WHO, Copenhagen.

World Health Organization 1999b
Health 21: the health for all
policy framework for the WHO
European Region. WHO,
Copenhagen.

World Health Organization 2005 The
Bangkok charter for health

promotion in a globalized world.
WHO, Geneva. http://www.who.
int/healthpromotion/
conferences/6gchp/bangkok_
charter/en/index.html.

Websites

http://courseweb.edteched.uottawa.
ca/epi5251/Index_notes/
Definitions%20of%20health.htm

http://www.dh.gov.uk/en/
Publichealth/Healthinequalities/
Healthinequalitiesguidance
publications/DH_064183

http://www.euro.who.int/
InformationSources

Chapter 2

What is health promotion?

CHAPTER CONTENTS

SUMMARY

This chapter starts with a discussion of the definitions of health promotion, and the related terms health gain, health improvement, health development, health education and social marketing. This is followed by an examination of the position of health promotion within the multidisciplinary public health movement. An outline of the scope of health promotion work is offered, with frameworks for activities for promoting health. Broad areas of practice covered by professional health promoters and the core competencies needed are set out with an outline of the framework for national occupational standards. Exercises are included to help you explore the range of health promotion activities and the extent of your own health promotion work.

DEFINING HEALTH PROMOTION

Health promotion is about raising the health status of individuals and communities. *Promotion* in the health context means improving, advancing, supporting, encouraging and placing health higher on personal and public agendas.

Given that major socioeconomic determinants of health are often outside individual or even collective control, a fundamental aspect of health promotion is that it aims to empower people to have more control over aspects of their lives that affect their health.

These twin elements of improving health and having more control over it are fundamental to the aims and processes of health promotion. The World

Health Organization (WHO) definition of health promotion as it appears in the *Ottawa Charter* has been widely adopted and neatly encompasses this: 'Health promotion is the process of enabling people to increase control over, and to improve, their health' (WHO 1986).

HEALTH GAIN, HEALTH IMPROVEMENT AND HEALTH DEVELOPMENT

Health development, **health improvement** and **health gain** are terms that are also employed when discussing the process of working to improve people's health. **Health development** is defined as the process of continuous, progressive improvement of health status of individuals and groups in a population (Nutbeam 1998). The *Jakarta Declaration* (WHO 1997) describes health promotion as an essential element of health development. **Health improvement** is frequently used by national health agencies. For example, there is a health improvement section on the Department of Health (DoH) website (http://www.dh.gov.uk) and NHS Scotland calls itself Scotland's health improvement agency (http://www.healthscotland.com). A research study undertaken by Abbott (2002), however, found that people's understanding of health improvement varied and ranged from explaining the term primarily as a government strategy – as a set of activities for the NHS – or in terms of the overarching purpose of health improvement. One definition sees health improvement as covering a wide range of activity, principally focused on improving the health and wellbeing of individuals and communities (so much like health promotion) (http://www.suffolkcoastal.gov.uk).

The term **health gain** emerged in policy documents in the late 1980s (for example, Welsh Health Planning Forum 1989). One useful early definition said health gain was a measurable improvement in health status, in an individual or population, attributable to earlier intervention (Nutbeam 1998).

Measurable means that it should be possible to put a value, usually a numerical value, onto health status, in order to demonstrate that a change has occurred.

Attributable means proving that the change in health status is the result of the intervention. This can be difficult. How will you be certain, for example, that a specific programme to reduce

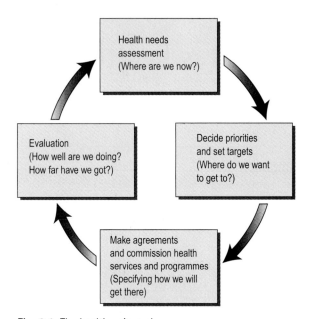

Fig. 2.1 The health gain cycle.

smoking has been effective when so many influences can affect smoking habits?

An **intervention** means a planned activity designed to improve health. It could be treatment, a care service or a health promotion activity.

The role of health promoters in assessing health needs, deciding on priorities, setting objectives and targets, allocating resources, and monitoring and reviewing outcomes can be seen as a **health gain cycle** (Fig. 2.1). Health gain is a useful concept. It focuses attention on health outcomes and on how different choices or priorities can be compared by considering the extent to which they contribute to health gains for individuals or groups.

HEALTH EDUCATION, HEALTH PROMOTION AND SOCIAL MARKETING

The WHO (1998) defined **health education** as the consciously constructed opportunities for learning involving some form of communication designed to improve health literacy, including improving knowledge, and developing life skills which are conducive to individual and community health (see Smith et al 2006 for updates on the WHO glossary of health promotion terms). In the 1970s the range of activities undertaken in the pursuit of better health began to diverge from health education (Scriven 2005). There was also criticism that the health education approach was too narrow, focused too much on individual lifestyle and could become victim-blaming (see Ch. 1, Improving Health – Historical Overview) and increasingly work was being undertaken on wider issues such as political action to change public policies. Such activities went beyond the scope of traditional health education.

Health promotion as a term was used for the first time in the mid 1970s (Lalonde 1974) and quickly became an umbrella term for a wide range of strategies designed to tackle the wider determinants of health. There is no clear, widely adopted consensus of what is meant by health promotion (see Scriven 2005 for a detailed discussion of the development and use of the term). Some definitions focus on activities, others on values and principles. The WHO (1986) definition defines health promotion as a *process* but implies an *aim* (enabling people to increase control over, and improve, their health) with a clear philosophical basis of self-empowerment.

Recently in the UK, health-related **social marketing** has emerged as a prominent health promoting strategy to achieve and sustain behaviour goals on a range of social issues. There are a number of definitions of social marketing, but the description most generally in use is the systematic application of marketing, alongside other concepts and techniques, to achieve specific behavioural goals, for a social good and to improve health and reduce inequalities (French & Blair-Stevens 2005). The exact relationship between social marketing and health promotion is currently being debated, so there is no consensus on whether social marketing comes under the health promotion umbrella of approaches to health gain.

MULTIDISCIPLINARY PUBLIC HEALTH

In the last decade, national and local policy has focused on the development of multidisciplinary public health (see Berridge 2007 for a critique and overview of these developments). Public health work has been defined by Acheson (DoH 1998) as the science and art of preventing disease, prolonging life and promoting health through the organised efforts of society. The Faculty of Public Health (FPH) also uses this definition but offers guidelines specifying that public health:

- Is population based.
- Emphasises collective responsibility for health, its protection and disease prevention.
- Recognises the key role of the state, linked to a concern for the underlying socioeconomic and wider determinants of health, as well as disease.
- Emphasises partnerships with all those who contribute to the health of the population (http://www.fphm.org.uk).

Three spheres of public health have been outlined by Griffiths et al (2005):

Health improvement
- Inequalities
- Education
- Housing
- Employment
- Family/community
- Lifestyles
- Surveillance and monitoring of specific diseases and risk factors.

Improving services
- Clinical effectiveness
- Efficiency
- Service planning
- Audit and evaluation
- Clinical governance
- Equity.

Health protection
- Infectious diseases
- Chemicals and poisons
- Radiation
- Emergency response
- Environmental health hazards.

It is clear from these definitions and explanations that public health requires a wide range of competencies (Evans & Dowling 2002), that it is a multidisciplinary activity involving people from many professions and backgrounds (DoH 2001, Coen & Wills 2007) and that health promotion activities overlap with and are an integral part of the UK public health function (DoH 2005).

INVOLVEMENT IN PUBLIC HEALTH

See also Chapter 1, section on national initiatives, for more about this report.

There are three levels of involvement in public health (DoH 2001):

1. Teachers, social workers, voluntary sector staff and health workers all have a role in health improvement. They need to adopt a public health mind set and appreciate how their work can make a difference to health and wellbeing, and where more specialist support can be obtained locally.
2. A smaller number of hands-on public health professionals, such as health visitors and environmental health officers, who spend a major part, or all, of their time in public health practice working with communities and groups.
3. A still smaller group of public health specialists from medical and other professional backgrounds, who work at a senior level with responsibility to manage strategic change and lead public health initiatives. This group includes health promotion specialists and medically qualified public health doctors.

The roles of professionals who contribute to health promotion work are discussed in Chapter 4.

THE SCOPE OF HEALTH PROMOTION

The questions in Exercise 2.1 give examples of the wide range of activities that may be classified as health promotion. Answering 'yes' to each one indicates a broad view of what may be included: mass media advertising, campaigning on health issues, patient education, self-help, environmental safety measures, public policy issues, health education, preventive and curative medical procedures, codes of practice on health issues, health-enhancing facilities in local communities, workplace health policies and social education for young people. Answering 'no' indicates that you identify criteria that you believe exclude these activities from the realms of health promotion. For example, you may have said 'no' to Item 2 because increasing tobacco taxation would place a heavier burden on smokers in poor financial circumstances, thus putting their health even more at risk.

Attempts to provide frameworks and models for classifying activities have helped to clarify the scope of health promotion (see Naidoo & Wills 2000 for an overview). Drawing on these, Fig. 2.2 identifies the activities that contribute to health gain and maps out all those activities which aim to improve people's health. There are two sets of activities, those about providing services for people who are ill or who have disabilities, and positive health

---

EXERCISE 2.1   Exploring the scope of health promotion

Consider each of the following activities and decide whether you think each is, or is not, health promotion:

	Yes	No
1. Using TV advertisements to encourage people to be more physically active.	☐	☐
2. Campaigning for increased tax on tobacco.	☐	☐
3. Explaining to patients how to carry out their doctor's advice.	☐	☐
4. Setting up a self-help group for people who have been sexually abused as children.	☐	☐
5. Providing schools with a crossing patrol to help children across the road outside schools.	☐	☐
6. Raising awareness of how poverty affects health.	☐	☐
7. Giving people information about the way their bodies work.	☐	☐
8. Immunising children against infectious diseases such as measles.	☐	☐
9. Protesting about a breach in the voluntary code of practice for alcohol advertising.	☐	☐
10. Running low-cost gentle exercise classes for older people at local leisure centres.	☐	☐
11. Providing healthier menu choices at workplace canteens.	☐	☐
12. Teaching a programme of personal and social education in a secondary school.	☐	☐
13. Providing support to people with learning disabilities living in the community.	☐	☐
14. Using social marketing tools to ensure behavioural change in a group of smokers.	☐	☐

What were your reasons for saying 'yes' or 'no'? Can you identify the criteria you are using for deciding whether an activity is 'health promotion'?

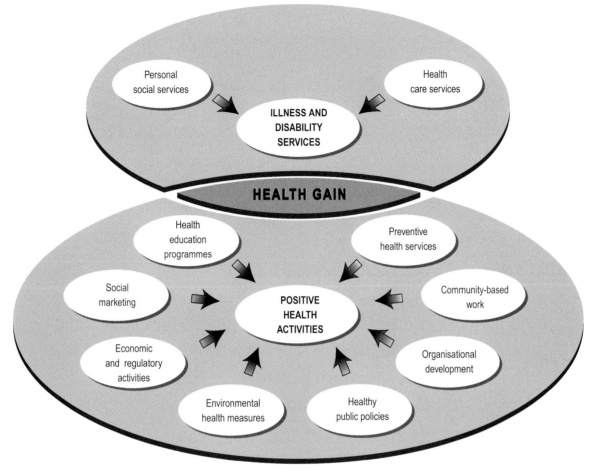

Fig. 2.2 Activities for health gain.

activities, which are about personal, social and environmental changes aiming to prevent ill health and develop healthier living conditions and lifestyles. These two sets of activities overlap, because they both contribute to health gain, and they are often closely related in practice. Ten categories of activities are identified, comprising two illness and disability services and eight types of positive health activities.

ILLNESS AND DISABILITY SERVICES

Personal social services. This includes all those social services aimed at addressing the needs of sick people and people with disabilities or disadvantages whose health (in its widest sense) is improved by those services. This includes, for example, community care of mentally ill people and home help services for the elderly.

Healthcare services. This includes the major work of the health services: treatment, cure and care in primary care and hospital settings.

An important question when considering the boundaries of service provision by health promoters is: 'If all illness and disability services improve health and produce varying amounts of health gain, are they all called health promotion?' For example, is taking out someone's appendix or placing a child in a foster home health promotion?

It is helpful to go back to the WHO (1986) definition of health promotion, about enabling people to increase control over and improve their health. Things that need to be done to people (like taking out their appendix or placing them in foster homes) are excluded from this definition, so are generally not considered to be health promotion activities (although they are health gain activities). But those aspects of care and treatment that are about enabling people to take control over their health and improve it (such as educating patients in the skills of self-care, or educating foster parents in the skills of parenting) are legitimate areas of health promotion. So is creating a health promoting environment by, for example, modifying a home to make it suitable for a person with disabilities or providing affordable housing for homeless people with health problems.

POSITIVE HEALTH ACTIVITIES

Health education programmes

These are planned opportunities for people to learn about health, and to undertake voluntary changes in their behaviour. Such programmes may include providing information, exploring values and attitudes, making health decisions and acquiring skills to enable behaviour change to take place. They involve developing self-esteem and self-empowerment so that people are enabled to take action about their health. This can happen on a personal one-to-one level such as health visitor/client, teacher/pupil, or in a group such as a smoking cessation group or exercise class, or reach large population groups through the mass media, health fairs or exhibitions.

> See Chapters 10–14 for detailed information on carrying out these health promotion activities.

Health education programmes may also be a part of healthcare and personal social services, and because of this it is useful to understand the concepts of primary, secondary and tertiary health education.

Primary health education. This would reflect McKinley's (1979) vision of upstream, preventative activity. It is directed at healthy people, and aims to prevent ill health arising. Most health education for children and young people falls into this category, dealing with such topics as sexual health, nutrition and social skills and personal relationships, and aiming to build up a positive sense of self-worth in children. Primary health education is concerned not merely with helping to prevent illness but with positive wellbeing.

Secondary health education. There is also often a major role for health education when people are ill. It may be possible to prevent ill health moving to a chronic or irreversible stage, and to restore people to their former state of health. This is known as secondary health education, educating patients about their condition and what to do about it. Restoring good health may involve the patient in changing behaviour (such as stopping smoking) or in complying with a therapeutic regime and, possibly, learning about self-care and self-help. Clearly, health education of the patient is of great importance if treatment and therapy are to be effective and illness is not to recur.

Tertiary health education. There are, of course, many patients whose ill health has not been, or could not be, prevented and who cannot be completely cured. There are also people with permanent disabilities. Tertiary health education is concerned with educating patients and their carers about how to make the most of the remaining potential for healthy living, and how to avoid unnecessary hardships, restrictions and complications. Rehabilitation programmes contain a considerable amount of tertiary health education with a focus on improving quality of life.

Quantenary health education. This concentrates on facilitating optimal states of empowerment and emotional, social and physical wellbeing during a terminal stage (see Hancock 2001, Scriven 2005).

It is not always easy to see where people fit into this primary, secondary or tertiary framework because a person's state of health is open to interpretation. For example, is educating an overweight person who appears to be perfectly well, despite being overweight, primary or secondary health education?

Social marketing

The National Social Marketing Centre (NSMC) identifies the primary aim of health-related social marketing as the achievement of a social good (rather than commercial benefit) in terms of specific, achievable and manageable behaviour goals, relevant to improving health and reducing health inequalities. Social marketing is a systematic process using a range of marketing techniques and approaches (a marketing mix) phased to address short-, medium- and long-term issues. The following six features and concepts are pertinent to understanding social marketing:

Customer or consumer orientation. A strong customer orientation with importance attached to understanding where the customer is starting from, their knowledge, attitudes and beliefs, along with the social context in which they live and work.

Behaviour and behavioural goals. Clear focus on understanding existing behaviour and key influences upon it, alongside developing clear behavioural goals. These can be divided into actionable and measurable steps or stages, phased over time.

Intervention mix and marketing mix. Using a mix of different interventions or methods to achieve a particular behavioural goal. When used at the strategic level this is commonly referred to as the intervention mix, and when used operationally it is described as the marketing mix.

Audience segmentation. Clarity of audience focus using audience segmentation to target effectively.

Exchange. Use of the exchange concept, understanding what is being expected of people, and the real cost to them.

Competition. This means understanding factors that impact on people and that compete for their attention and time (adjusted from http://www.nsmcentre.org.uk).

Social marketing uses the total process planning model summarised in Fig. 2.3. The front end scoping stage drives the whole process. The primary concern is establishing clear actionable and measurable behaviour goals to ensure focused development across the rest of the process. The ultimate effectiveness and success of social marketing rests on whether it is possible to demonstrate direct impact on behaviour. It is this feature that sets it apart from other communication or awareness raising approaches, such as health education, where the main focus is on imparting information and enabling people to understand and use it. The information on social marketing above has been adjusted from the NSMC website (http://www.nsmcentre.org.uk). For more details on how to engage in health-related social marketing, see Macdowall et al (2006) and NSMC (2007). To explore the effectiveness of social marketing as an approach, see McDermott et al (2005) and Stead et al (2007), and to examine in more detail the links between social marketing and health promotion, see NSMC (2008).

Preventive health services

These include medical services that aim to prevent ill health, such as immunisation, family planning and personal health checks, as well as wider preventive health services such as child protection services for children at risk of abuse.

Community-based work

This is a bottom-up approach to health promotion, working with and for people, involving communities in health work such as local campaigns for better facilities. It includes community development, which is essentially about communities identifying their own health needs and taking action to address them. The sort of activities that may result could include forming self-help and pressure groups, and developing local health-enhancing facilities and services.

See Chapter 15, Working with communities.

Organisational development

This is about developing and implementing policies within organisations to promote the health of staff and customers. Examples include implementing policies on equal opportunities, providing healthy food choices at places of work and working with commercial organisations to develop and promote healthier products.

See Chapter 16, Influencing and implementing policy.

Healthy public policies

Developing and implementing healthy public policies involves statutory and voluntary agencies, professionals and the public working together to develop changes in the conditions of living. It is about seeing the implications for health in policies about, for example, equal opportunities, housing, employment, transport and leisure. Good public transport, for example, would improve health by reducing the number of cars on the road, decreasing pollution, using less fuel and reducing the stress of the daily grind of travelling for commuters. It could also reduce isolation for those who do not own cars and enable people to have access to shopping and

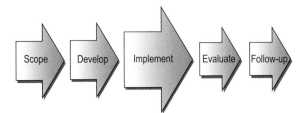

Fig. 2.3 Social marketing uses a total process planning model. *(NSMC and Consumer Focus 2007. Reproduced with permission).*

leisure facilities, all measures that improve well-being (See Scriven 2007 for a detailed overview of healthy public policies).

See Chapter 16, Influencing and implementing policy.

Environmental health measures

Environmental health is about making the physical environment conducive to health, whether at home, at work or in public places. It includes public health measures such as ensuring clean food and water and controlling traffic and other pollution.

Economic and regulatory activities

These are political and educational activities directed at politicians, policy makers and planners, involving lobbying for and implementing legislative changes such as food labelling regulations, pressing for voluntary codes of practice such as those relating to alcohol advertising or advocating financial measures such as increases in tobacco taxation.

A FRAMEWORK FOR HEALTH PROMOTION ACTIVITIES

There are two important points to make about the use of the framework of health promotion activities

in Fig. 2.4. The first is that activities do not always fall neatly into categories. For example, would a health visitor who was supporting a local women's health group be engaged in a health education programme because they provided health information to the group and set up stress management sessions, or in community-based work because some members of the group had got together to lobby their local health services for better sexual health advice clinics for young people?

Obviously areas of activity overlap, but this is not important. What *is* important is to appreciate the range of activities encompassed by health promotion, and the many ways in which you can contribute to health improvements.

The second point about using this framework is to note that it reflects planned, deliberate activities, and it is important to recognise that a great deal of health promotion happens informally and incidentally. For example, portrayal of damage caused by excessive drinking on television soaps and an advertising campaign to promote wholewheat breakfast cereals are all health promotion activities which are not likely to be planned with specific health promotion aims in mind. They may, however, be significant influences for change.

See Chapter 11, section on mass media.

Exercise 2.2 is designed to help you to identify your own contribution to health promotion.

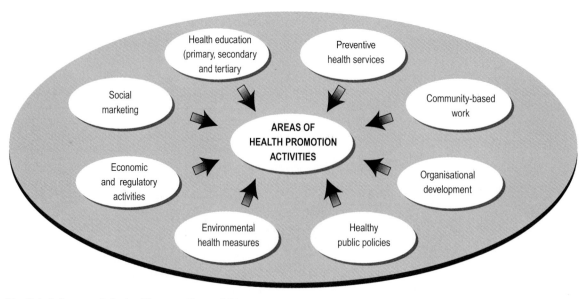

Fig. 2.4 A framework for health promotion activities.

EXERCISE 2.2 Identifying your health promotion work

> **EXERCISE 2.2   Identifying your health promotion work**
>
> Look at Fig. 2.4 again, which identifies eight major areas of health promotion activity. By each of the eight headings, note down any parts of your work you think come into that category. If you are not sure what each category includes, look back at the explanations. Then think about each category again, and consider whether there is scope for developing your work within each category.

BROAD AREAS OF COMPETENCIES IMPORTANT TO HEALTH PROMOTION PRACTICE

In order to engage in the activities outlined in the framework in Fig. 2.4, health promoters require a range of competencies. There are two aspects of work to consider. One is the technical/specialist aspect such as immunising a child, taking a cervical smear test, recording blood pressure or undertaking microbiological tests for food hygiene purposes. All of these are the subject of specialist training, and outside the scope of this book.

The other aspect of your work is about working with people to promote health in many different situations with a variety of different aims. To do this, health promoters need to have knowledge of particular methods and acquire specialist competencies in the following areas:

Managing, planning and evaluating

All these are addressed in Part 2: Planning and managing for effective practice, Chapters 5–9.

Managing resources for health promotion, including money, materials, oneself and other people, is crucial. Systematic planning is needed for effective and efficient health promotion. All health promotion work also requires evaluation, and different methods are appropriate for different approaches.

Communicating and educating

Communication and educating are addressed in Chapters 8–14.

Health promotion is about people, so competence in communication is essential and fundamental. A high level of competence is needed in one-to-one communication and in working with groups in various ways, both formal and informal.

Effective communication is an educational competence, but health promoters also need to understand how people receive information and learn. For example, patient education requires communication and educational competencies.

Marketing and publicising

Marketing and publicising are addressed in Chapter 11.

This requires competence in, for example, marketing and advertising, using local radio and getting local press coverage of health issues. It may be used when undertaking any health promotion activities that would benefit from wider publicity.

Facilitating, networking, partnership working

This means enabling others to promote their own and other people's health, using various means such as sharing skills and information and building up confidence and trust. These competencies are particularly important when working with communities. They are also vital for working with other agencies and forming partnerships for health that cross barriers of organisations and disciplines.

Facilitating, networking and partnership working are addressed in Chapters 9, 13 and 15.

Influencing policy and practice

Health promoters are in the business of influencing policies and practices that affect health. These can be at any level, from national (such as policies set by government or political parties about, for example, housing, transport and future directions for the NHS) to the level of day-to-day work of a health promoter (such as what sort of health promotion programmes will be run in a GP practice, or what resources will be devoted to specific health promotion activities in an environmental health department).

Influencing policy and practice is addressed in Chapter 16.

In order to influence policy and practice, you need to understand how power is distributed and exercised between people at any level, from a group of colleagues to those in positions of great authority or influence. You need to be able to use that knowledge to affect decisions. This includes working with statutory, voluntary and commercial organisations to influence them to develop health promoting policies for their staff and to produce health enhancing products and services. It also includes working for healthy public policies and economic and regulatory changes requiring lobbying and taking political action.

It is unrealistic to expect all health promoters to be highly competent in all aspects of health promotion. Practice nurses, for example, will work predominantly in health education and preventive health services, needing a high level of competence in communication and education. However, they also needs other competencies in order to plan and evaluate their work, market health promotion programmes to their patients, facilitate change in their patients and be able to refer them to a network of helpful contacts. They will also need to be able to influence the development of health promotion policy in their practice.

OCCUPATIONAL STANDARDS IN HEALTH PROMOTION

At the time of writing there are a number of different initiatives taking place in the UK and in Europe that will result in a much clearer set of core competencies for health promotion. Currently in the UK competencies set out in the form of occupational standards are available for specialists and practitioners in public health (Skills for Health 2007). There is currently no agreed route through these standards for health promotion specialists or practitioners.

At an international level, the Galway Consensus Statement (http://www.sophe.org; see also Morales et al 2009) sets out eight domains of core competency in health promotion. They are: catalysing change, leadership, assessment, planning, implementation, evaluation, advocacy and partnerships. At the time of writing there is broad consultation on the consensus statement, so it will be interesting to monitor the development of both UK and international health promotion competency statements over the coming years.

The standards developed for specialist practice in public health set out in Box 2.1 are applicable (at least in part) to health promotion. It is useful to examine these standards and to think about the areas of health promotion work you are involved in and which standards are important for your work. It is also important to recognise the areas you do *not* use in your work and to think about the implications for working collaboratively with other professionals. Exercise 2.3 is designed to encourage you to think about your health promotion work and how it contributes to the wider public health

---

BOX 2.1   Overview of the national standards for public health (Skills for Health 2007)

Area 1: Surveillance and assessment of the population's health and wellbeing – see Chapter 6

1. Collect and form data and information about health and wellbeing and/or stressors to health and wellbeing.
2. Obtain and link data and information about health and wellbeing and/or stressors to health and wellbeing.
3. Analyse and interpret data and information about health and wellbeing and/or stressors to health and wellbeing.
4. Communicate and disseminate data and information about health and wellbeing and/or stressors to health and wellbeing.
5. Facilitate others' collection, analysis, interpretation, communication and use of data and information about health and wellbeing and/or stressors to health and wellbeing.

6. Collect, structure and analyse data on the health and wellbeing and related needs for a defined population.
7. Undertake surveillance and assessment of the population's health and wellbeing.

Area 2: Promoting and protecting the population's health and wellbeing – see Chapters 5–7 and 16

1. Communicate with individuals, groups and communities about promoting their health and wellbeing.
2. Encourage behavioural change in people and agencies to promote health and wellbeing.
3. Work in partnership with others to promote health and wellbeing and reduce risks within settings.
4. Work in partnership with others to prevent the onset of adverse effects on health and wellbeing in populations.

Continued

BOX 2.1	Overview of the national standards for public health (Skills for Health 2007) – cont'd

5. Work in partnership with others to contact, assess and support individuals in populations who are at risk from identified hazards to health and wellbeing.
6. Work in partnership with others to protect the public's health and wellbeing from specific risks.
7. Promote and protect the population's health and wellbeing.

Area 3: Developing quality and risk management within an evaluative culture – see Chapter 7

1. Develop one's own knowledge and practice.
2. Contribute to the development of the knowledge and practice of others.
3. Support and challenge workers on specific aspects of their practice.
4. Manage the performance of teams and individuals.
5. Contribute to improvements at work.
6. Develop quality and risk management within an evaluative culture.

Area 4: Collaborative working for health and wellbeing – see Chapters 4 and 9–14

1. Build relationships within and with communities and organisations.
2. Develop, sustain and evaluate collaborative work with others.
3. Represent one's own agency at other agencies' meetings.
4. Work in partnership with communities to improve their health and wellbeing.
5. Enable the views of groups and communities to be heard through advocating on their behalf.
6. Provide information and advice to the media about health and wellbeing and related issues.
7. Improve health and wellbeing through working collaboratively.

Area 5: Developing health programmes and services and reducing inequalities – see Chapters 5–8

1. Work in partnership with others to plan, implement and review programmes and projects to improve health and wellbeing.
2. Manage change in organisational activities.
3. Develop people's skills and roles within community groups/networks.
4. Assess, negotiate and secure sources of funding.
5. Develop health programmes and services and reduce inequalities.

Area 6: Policy and strategy development and implementation to improve health and wellbeing – see Chapter 16

1. Work in partnership with others to plan, implement, monitor and review strategies to improve health and wellbeing.
2. Work in partnership with others to assess the impact of policies and strategies on health and wellbeing.
3. Work in partnership with others to develop policies to improve health and wellbeing.
4. Appraise policies and recommend changes to improve health and wellbeing.
5. Improve health and wellbeing through policy and strategy development and implementation.

Area 7: Working with and for communities to improve health and wellbeing – see Chapter 15

1. Facilitate the development of people and learning in communities.
2. Create opportunities for learning from practice and experience.
3. Support communities to plan and take collective action.
4. Facilitate the development of community groups/networks.
5. Enable people to address issues related to health and wellbeing.
6. Enable people to improve others' health and wellbeing.
7. Work with individuals and others to minimise the effects of specific health conditions.
8. Improve health and wellbeing through working with and for communities.

Area 8: Strategic leadership for health and wellbeing – see Chapters 8 and 13

1. Use leadership skills to improve health and wellbeing.
2. Promote the value of, and need for, health and wellbeing.
3. Lead the work of teams and individuals to achieve objectives.
4. Design learning programmes.
5. Enable learning through presentations.
6. Evaluate and improve learning and development programmes.

Continued

BOX 2.1   Overview of the national standards for public health (Skills for Health 2007) – cont'd

7. Strategically lead the improvement of health and wellbeing and the reduction of inequalities.

Area 9: Research and development to improve health and wellbeing – see Chapter 7

1. Plan, undertake, evaluate and disseminate research and development about improving health and wellbeing.
2. Develop and maintain a strategic overview of developments in knowledge and practice.
3. Develop, implement and evaluate strategies to advance knowledge and practice.
4. Commission, monitor and evaluate projects to advance knowledge and practice.
5. Contribute to the evaluation and implementation of research and development outcomes.

6. Improve health and wellbeing through research and development.

Area 10: Ethically managing self, people and resources to improve health and wellbeing – see Chapters 3 and 5–9

1. Promote people's equality, diversity and rights.
2. Prioritise and manage own work and the focus of activities.
3. Manage the use of financial resources.
4. Monitor and review progress with learners.
5. Facilitate individual learning and development through mentoring.
6. Enable individual learning through coaching.
7. Ethically manage self, people and resources to improve health and wellbeing.

EXERCISE 2.3   Mapping your health promotion work against the standards for specialist practice in public health

Study the areas identified as specialist public health practice and tick the level of activity you are involved in. Look at Box 2.1 for details of the work covered by each area of activity.

Note the areas you work in and the areas that are outside your current job responsibilities or which you are not trained to do.

Compare this mapping with that of colleagues or other health workers.

Area of public health practice	Very high level of activity	High level of activity	Fair level of activity	Some level of activity	No activity in this area
Area 1: Surveillance and assessment of the population's health and wellbeing.	☐	☐	☐	☐	☐
Area 2: Promoting and protecting the population's health and wellbeing.	☐	☐	☐	☐	☐
Area 3: Developing quality and risk management within an evaluative culture.	☐	☐	☐	☐	☐
Area 4: Collaborative working for health and wellbeing.	☐	☐	☐	☐	☐
Area 5: Developing health programmes and services and reducing inequalities.	☐	☐	☐	☐	☐
Area 6: Policy and strategy development and implementation to improve health and wellbeing.	☐	☐	☐	☐	☐
Area 7: Working with and for communities to improve heath and wellbeing.	☐	☐	☐	☐	☐
Area 8: Strategic leadership for health.	☐	☐	☐	☐	☐
Area 9: Research and development.	☐	☐	☐	☐	☐
Area 10: Ethically managing self, people and resources.	☐	☐	☐	☐	☐

Standards taken from Skills for Health (2007)

function. It will also help you to think about the differences between health promotion and public health.

USING THE NATIONAL OCCUPATIONAL STANDARDS

Broadly speaking there are three uses for the national occupational standards:

1. Employers and managers can use the standards to improve the quality of the performance of their staff. An organisation can map what it is trying to achieve against the areas and sub-areas of practice. It can then look at its service specifications and its management of human resources through job specifications, staff appraisal and performance review. The standards could also be used as the basis for auditing a service and checking whether it meets quality standards.

Audit is discussed in more detail in Chapter 7.

2. Individuals can use the standards to improve their competence through identifying their key areas of work, assessing their own performance, identifying their learning needs and defining the learning outcomes needed to meet the national standards.

3. Education and training providers can use the standards to modify their programmes to enable practitioners to develop appropriate competencies, or use the standards as the basis of their programme design.

PRACTICE POINTS

- Health promotion practice encompasses a wide range of approaches that are united by the same goal, to enable people to increase control over and improve their health.
- It is important for you to identify the full scope of your health promotion work and to see how this fits with the work of your organisation or employer and the wider remit of public health.
- The national standards for specialist practice in public health provide a map which can be used by organisations, managers, education and training providers, and individuals to improve the quality of public health and health promotion work.

References

Abbott S 2002 The meaning of health improvement. Health Education Journal 61(4): 299–308.

Berridge V 2007 Multidisciplinary public health: what sort of victory? Public Health 121(6): 404–408.

Coen C, Wills J 2007 Specialist health promotion as a career choice in public health. The Journal of the Royal Society for the Promotion of Health 127(5): 231–238.

Department of Health 1998 Independent inquiry into inequalities in health. London, The The Stationery Office.

Department of Health 2001 Chief Medical Officer's report to strengthen the public health function of England. London, The The Stationery Office.

Department of Health 2005 Shaping the future of public health: Promoting health in the NHS. London: The Stationery Office.

Evans D, Dowling S 2002 Developing a multi-disciplinary public health specialist workforce: training implications of current UK policy. Journal of Epidemiology and Community Health 56: 744–747.

French J, Blair Stevens C 2005 Social marketing pocket guide. London, National Social Marketing Centre for Excellence (http://www.nsms.org.uk).

Griffiths S, Jewell T, Donnelly P 2005 Public health in practice: the three domains of public health. Public Health 119: 907–913.

Hancock T 2001 Healthy people in healthy communities in a healthy world: the science, art and politics of public health in the 21st century. Paper presented at the launch of the OU School of Health and Social Welfare Health Promotion and Public Health Research Group, 12 September. Milton Keynes, The Open University.

Lalonde M 1974 A new perspective on the health of Canadians. Ottawa, Information Canada.

Macdowall W, Bonell C, Davies M 2006 Social marketing. In: Macdowall W, Bonell C, Davies M (eds) Health promotion practice. Maidenhead, Open University Press.

McDermott L, Stead M, Hastings GB et al 2005 A systematic review of the effectiveness of social marketing nutrition and food safety interventions – final report prepared for Safefood. Stirling, University of Stirling, Institute for Social Marketing.

McKinley JB 1979 A case for refocusing upstream: the political economy of health. In: Javco, EG (ed.) Patients, physicians and illness. Basingstoke, Macmillan.

Morales AS-M, Battel-Kirk B, Barry MM et al 2009 Perspectives on health promotion competencies and accreditation in Europe. Global Health Promotion 16(2): 21–30.

Naidoo J, Wills J 2000 Models and approaches to health promotion. In: Naidoo J, Wills J (eds) Public health and health promotion practice: foundations for health promotion, 3rd edn. London, Elsevier.

National Social Marketing Centre 2007 Big pocket guide: social marketing. London, NSMC.

National Social Marketing Centre 2008 Social marketing for health and specialised health promotion: stronger together – weaker apart. London, NSMC.

Nutbeam D 1998 Health promotion glossary. Health Promotion International 13(4): 349–364.

Scriven A 2005 Promoting health: policies, principles and perspectives. In: Scriven A (ed.) Health promoting practice: the contribution of nurses and allied health professions. Basingstoke, Palgrave.

Scriven A 2007 Healthy public policies: rhetoric or reality. In: Scriven A, Garman G (eds) 2007 Public health: social context and action. Maidenhead, Open University Press.

Skills for Health 2007 Public health national occupational standards – practice and specialist. http://www.skillsforhealth.org.uk/competences/~/media/Resource-Library/Word/PHstdstracking6.ashx.

Smith BJ, Cho Tang K, Nutbeam D 2006 WHO health promotion glossary: new terms. Health Promotion International 21(4): 340–345.

Stead M, Hastings G, McDermott L 2007 The meaning, effectiveness and future of social marketing. Obesity Reviews 8(1): 189–193.

Welsh Health Planning Forum 1989 Strategic intent and direction for the NHS in Wales. Cardiff, Welsh Office.

World Health Organization 1986 The Ottawa charter for health promotion. Geneva, WHO (http://www.who.int/hpr/NPH/docs/ottawa_charter_hp.pdf).

World Health Organization 1997 The Jakarta declaration on health promotion in the 21st century. Geneva, WHO.

World Health Organization 1998 List of basic terms. Health promotion glossary. Geneva, WHO.

Websites

http://www.dh.gov.uk/en/Publichealth/Healthimprovement/index.htm

http://www.fphm.org.uk/about_faculty/what_public_health/default.asp

http://www.healthscotland.com

http://www.nsmcentre.org.uk

http://www.sophe.org

http://www.suffolkcoastal.gov.uk

Chapter 3

Aims, values and ethical considerations

SUMMARY

In this chapter some key philosophical issues about aims and values in health promotion practice will be identified and explored. Two fundamental dilemmas about the aims of health promotion will be addressed. First, whether health promoters should aim to change the individual or to change society, and second, whether they should set out to ensure compliance with a health promotion programme or to enable clients to make an informed choice. A framework of five approaches to health promotion is provided as a tool for analysing key aims and values, along with exercises and case studies. Ethical issues are discussed, four ethical principles are described and there is a series of questions designed to help health promoters to make ethical choices. Exercises on making ethical decisions are included.

This chapter establishes some of the key philosophical issues in health promotion. You are encouraged to think deeply about why you are engaging in specific activities, what values are reflected in your work and what ethical dilemmas are presented. Guidelines on how to approach ethical decision making are considered and some key principles of practice are explored.

Philosophical issues are fundamental to practice, but as Seedhouse (2004) argues, the values of health promotion are sometimes muddled. Health promotion work, if successful, will influence the lives of individuals and communities and it would be irresponsible to develop and apply health promotion practical skills without understanding the values and ethics that should underpin health promotion interventions.

CLARIFYING HEALTH PROMOTION AIMS

Should health promoters aim to change individual behaviour and lifestyles or aim to influence the socioeconomic determinants that directly influence people's health, or both? Health promoters have been criticised in the past for focusing on changing the attitudes and behaviour of individuals and communities towards healthier lifestyles and neglecting the importance of the social, political and physical environments on people's lives (Jones 2003). This focus on behaviour can result in victim-blaming, which is a significant ethical dilemma that health promoters need to address (see, for example, Richards et al 2003). It is important to note that individuals often *can* change behaviour and may *want* to take responsibility to improve their health. Health promotion is an essential tool in enabling that process, by promoting people's self-esteem, confidence and empowering them to take more control over their own health. Proponents of the lifestyle behavioural change approach also maintain that medical and health experts have knowledge that enables them to know what is in the best interests of their patients and the public at large, and that it is their responsibility to persuade people to make healthier choices. Furthermore, society has vested that responsibility in health professionals, and people often seek advice and help in health matters; it is not necessarily a matter of persuading them against their will. Sometimes, too, individuals may not be in a position to take responsibility because they may, for example, be too young, too ill or have severe learning difficulties. See Godin (2007) and Taylor (2007) for a fuller debate on the advantages and disadvantages of a lifestyle approach.

There are several points to be taken into account if the aim to change lifestyle is pursued:

- You cannot assume that lay people believe that health professionals know best. Sometimes health experts are proved wrong and new evidence can contradict existing health messages. For example, over the years there has been much contradictory advice on what constitutes a good diet (Taubes 2009), with some people finding the barrage of information confusing (Health and Social Care Information Centre 2008).

- There is a danger of imposing alien or opposing values. For example, a doctor may perceive that the most important thing for a patient's physical health is to lose weight and cut down on alcohol consumption, but drinking beer in the pub with friends may be far more important in terms of overall wellbeing to the overweight, middle-aged, unemployed patient. Who is right?

- Linked to this, a health promoter advocating lifestyle changes can be seen as making a moral judgment on clients' failure to change, that it is their own fault if, for example, they develop an obesity-related or smoking-related illness.

- Promoting a lifestyle change approach may produce negative and counterproductive feelings in the targeted individual or community, such as guilt for failing to comply, or of rebelliousness and anger at being told what to do, as some parents and children felt when Jamie Oliver attempted to change school dinners. The fall in numbers taking school dinners was regarded as a clear indication of this resistance to comply (Butler 2008).

- It cannot be assumed that individual behaviour is the primary cause of ill health. This is a limited view and there is a danger that focusing on the individual's behaviour distracts attention from the significant and politically sensitive determinants of health such as the social and economic factors of racism, relative deprivation, poverty, housing and unemployment as outlined in Chapter 1 in the section What Affects Health?

- Finally, it also cannot be assumed that individuals have genuine freedom to choose healthy lifestyles. Freedom of choice is often limited by socioeconomic influences (Contoyannis & Jones 2004). Economic factors may affect the choice of food; for example, fresh fruit and wholemeal bread are relatively more expensive than biscuits and white bread (Oldfield 2008, and for information on food poverty see http://www.combatpoverty.ie).

Social factors are also important. Freedom of choice about smoking for adolescents where both parents smoke, for example, is a complex issue (Action on Smoking and Health 2007). Also, how much freedom do people really have to change other health-demoting factors such as stressful living or working conditions and unemployment? It is easy to blame an individual for their own ill health, become victim-blaming, when in reality they might be the victims of their socioeconomic circumstances. In some disadvantaged situations and where resources of time, energy and income are limited, health choices may become health compromises. What a health promoter may see as irresponsibility may actually be what the client sees as the most responsible action in the circumstances. For example, mothers confronted with the day-to-day pressures of parenting may smoke as a way of relieving their stress. Research by Robinson & Kirkclady (2007) indicates that while mothers who smoked in their sample acknowledged the health promotion messages and were aware of the health dangers to their children of environmental tobacco smoke, they resisted these messages and found alternative explanations for their children's illnesses which discounted their smoking.

Part 3 of this book is about how to promote health in a way that is sensitive to these issues. Chapter 16 looks at what you can do to challenge and change health-related policies.

It is crucially important that everyone engaged in health promotion should be aware of these ethical concerns and have an opportunity to consider them in relation to their own work, particularly if they are engaged in interventions that aim to change individual lifestyles. Exercise 3.1 is designed to help you to think through your views on the aims of health promotion.

AIMING FOR COMPLIANCE OR INFORMED CHOICE?

Another key question about the aims of health promotion centres on what you aim to do with or for the client (whether the client is a single individual, a community or an organisation). Is your aim to ensure that your client complies with your programme and changes behaviour, as is the case with a social marketing approach? Or is it to enable your client to make an informed choice, and have the skills and confidence to carry that choice through into action, whatever that choice may be?

For example, a health promoter is working with a client whose sexual behaviour is such that there is a serious risk of catching sexually transmitted infections, including HIV. If the aim is compliance,

---

EXERCISE 3.1	Analysing your philosophy of health promotion

Consider the following statements A and B:

A: The key aim of health promotion is to inform people about the ways in which their behaviour and lifestyle can affect their health, to ensure that they understand the information, to help them explore their values and attitudes, and (where appropriate) to help them to change their behaviour.

B: The key aim of health promotion is to raise awareness of the many socioeconomic policies at national and local level (e.g. employment, housing, food, transport and health) that are not conducive to good health, and to work actively towards a change in those policies.

1. Taking statement A:
   - List arguments in support of this view.
   - List any points about the limitations of this view, and any arguments against it.
2. Do the same with statement B.
3. Do you think that the views in A and B are *complementary* or *incompatible*? Why?
4. Imagine these two views at either end of a spectrum:

A|. . . . .|. . . . .|. . . . .|. . . . .|. . . . .|B
    1   2   3   4   5

Indicate the two positions on the scale of 1 to 5 which most closely reflect (a) *what you actually do* in practice and (b) *what you would like to do* if you were free to work exactly as you would choose.

(The exercise is based on an idea in the *Schools Health Education Project 5–13*, published by the Health Education Council and reproduced here by kind permission of the Council)

---

it is more likely that the health promoter will be persuasive, will stress the risks to the client and will consider the session a failure if the client does not choose to behave differently. If, on the other hand, the health promoter's aim is to enable the client to make an informed choice, the health promoter will ensure that the client understands the facts and the risks, will encourage and support the client and accept that if the client chooses not to change their behaviour then this choice will be respected. It would not be interpreted as a failure, because the client made an informed choice.

The same issues arise with health promotion work on a larger scale. For example, is the aim of a campaign to change diets and to promote the consumption of five pieces of fruit or vegetables a day (Department of Health (DoH) 2007a), to persuade people to a particular point of view or to give them the information on which to make up their own minds? This is a difficult question. Most health promoters are doing their jobs because they believe that the action they are advocating is in the best interests of individuals, and of society as a whole. It raises questions about how far to go in imposing your own values and ideas of what are appropriate lifestyle choices on other people.

While considering this question it is also worth noting that it raises the issue of defining success in health promotion. In the first example (about sexual health behaviour), if the aim is to change behaviour then success is likely to be measured in terms of a drop in rates of sexually transmitted infections and unplanned pregnancies. But if the aim is solely to educate in order that people can make empowered, informed choices, success will be measured in terms of changes in people's knowledge of health risks.

ANALYSING YOUR AIMS AND VALUES: FIVE APPROACHES

There is no consensus on what is the right aim for health promotion or the right approach or set of activities. Health promoters need to work out for themselves which aim and which activities they use, in accordance with professional codes of conduct (if they exist), professional values and an assessment of the clients' needs.

Different models of health promotion are useful tools of analysis, which can help you to clarify your own aims and values. A framework of five approaches to health promotion is suggested with the values implicit in any particular approach identified.

1. The medical approach

The aim is freedom from medically defined disease and disability, such as infectious diseases, cancers and heart disease. The approach involves medical intervention to prevent or ameliorate ill health, possibly using a persuasive or paternalistic method: persuading, for example, parents to bring their children for immunisation (DoH 2006) and men over 50 screened for cholesterol and high blood pressure

to comply with prescribed medication (DoH 2007b). This approach values preventive medical procedures and the medical profession's responsibility to ensure that patients comply with recommended procedures.

2. The behaviour change approach

The aim is to change people's individual attitudes and behaviours, so that they adopt what is deemed a healthy lifestyle (DoH 2004). Examples include supporting people in stopping smoking through smoking cessation programmes (see National Institute for Health and Clinical Excellence (NICE) 2006), encouraging people to be more physically active through exercise prescription or referral schemes (Morgan 2005), changing people's diet through the School Fruit and Vegetable Scheme, part of the five-a-day programme to increase fruit and vegetable consumption (Blenkinsop et al 2007). See also NICE (2007) for evidence on the behavioural change approach.

Health promoters using this approach will be convinced that a lifestyle change is in the best interests of their clients, and will see it as their responsibility to encourage as many people as possible to adopt the healthy lifestyle they advocate. Health-related social marketing fits in to this approach when the aim is to change behaviour.

3. The educational approach

The aim is to give information, ensure knowledge and understanding of health issues, and to enable the skills required to make well-informed decisions. Information about health is presented, and people are helped to explore their values and attitudes, develop appropriate skills and to make their own decisions. Help in carrying out those decisions and adopting new health practices may also be offered. School personal social and health education (PSHE) programmes, for example, emphasise helping pupils to learn the skills of healthy living, not merely to acquire knowledge (OFSTED 2005; and up-to-date guidance on the PSHE curriculum at http://www.pshe-association.org.uk).

Those favouring this approach will value the educational process, will respect individuals' right to choose, and will see it as their responsibility to raise with clients the health issues which they think will be in the clients' best interests.

4. The client-centred approach

The aim is to work in partnership with clients to help them identify what they want to know about and take action on, and make their own decisions and choices according to their own interests and values. The health promoter's role is to act as a facilitator, helping people to identify their concerns and gain the knowledge and skills they require to make changes happen. Self-empowerment (or community empowerment) (Laverack 2004 and 2007) of the client is seen as central. Clients are valued as equals, who have knowledge, skills and abilities to contribute, and who have an absolute right to control their own health destinies.

5. The societal change approach

The aim is to effect changes on the physical, social and economic environment, to make it more conducive to good health. The focus is on changing society, not on changing the behaviour of individuals.

Those using this approach will value their democratic right to change society, and will be committed to putting health on the political agenda at all levels and to the importance of shaping the health environment rather than shaping the individual lives of the people who live in it (Bambra et al 2005).

Table 3.1 summarises and illustrates these five approaches to health promotion. This framework

Table 3.1	Five approaches to health promotion – summary and example			
	AIM	HEALTH PROMOTION ACTIVITY	IMPORTANT VALUES	EXAMPLE – SMOKING
Medical	Freedom from medically defined disease and disability	Promotion of medical intervention to prevent or ameliorate ill health	Patient compliance with preventive medical procedures	*Aim* – freedom from lung disease, heart disease and other smoking-related disorders *Activity* – encourage people to seek early detection and treatment of smoking-related disorders
Behaviour change	Individual behaviour conducive to freedom from disease	Attitude and behaviour change to encourage adoption of 'healthier' lifestyle	Healthy lifestyle as defined by health promoter	*Aim* – behaviour changes from smoking to not smoking *Activity* – persuasive education to prevent nonsmokers from starting and to persuade smokers to stop
Educational	Individuals with knowledge and understanding enabling well-informed decisions to be made and acted upon	Information about cause and effects of health-demoting factors. Exploration of values and attitudes. Development of skills required for healthy living	Individual right of free choice. Health promoter's responsibility to identify educational content	*Aim* – clients will have understanding of the effects of smoking on health. They will make a decision whether or not to smoke and act on the decision *Activity* – giving information to clients about the effects of smoking. Helping them to explore their own values and attitudes and come to a decision. Helping them to learn how to stop smoking if they want to
Client-centred	Working with clients on their own terms	Working with health issues, choices and actions that clients identify. Empowering the client	Clients as equals. Clients' right to set agenda. Self-empowerment of client	Anti-smoking issue is considered only if clients identify it as a concern. Clients identify what, if anything, they want to know and do about it
Societal change	Physical and social environment that enables choice of healthier lifestyle	Political/social action to change physical/social environment	Right and need to make environment health enhancing	*Aim* – make smoking socially unacceptable so it is easier not to smoke than to smoke *Activity* – no-smoking policy in all public places. Cigarette sales less accessible, especially to children, promotion of nonsmoking as social norm. Banning tobacco advertising and sports' sponsorship

has been used because it is a simple one that helps health promoters to appreciate that there are many approaches to health promotion, and that these different approaches reflect differing viewpoints and values. The framework has been questioned and challenged, and this is part of a healthy debate as the theory and practice of health promotion continue to develop. There are well-known models, such as the Tannahill model (Tannahill 2008) which have helped frame approaches to health promotion. See also Scriven (2005, p. 10) for an alternative framework. An important point to note is that some of these approaches can be used together. For example, a client-centred approach may also use educational processes and a comprehensive health promotion strategy to deal with a public health problem. (See Box 3.1 for examples of using approaches in practice). Exercise 3.2 is designed to enable you to think through the aims and values of your health promotion practice.

ETHICAL DILEMMAS

The following are some of the more common ethical dilemmas that health promoters may encounter.

BOTTOM UP OR TOP DOWN?

There is a key issue of control and power at the heart of health promotion: who decides what health issue to target and how; who sets the agenda? Is it bottom up, set by people themselves identifying issues they perceive as relevant, or is it top down, set by health promoters who often have the power (supported by government policy) and the resources to impose strategies? There is a spectrum of possible modes of interventions, from those that eliminate choice and remove freedom to those that just involve information giving (see Fig. 3.1). The interplay and interaction between individuals, communities and the wider population is important and central to deciding on whether a top down or bottom up approach is used. One of the difficulties in applying ethical principles in health promotion is the tension between the individual and population. Decisions have to be taken about when an individual's rights should be overridden in the interests of the greater good. Is it ever an ethical choice to initiate health promotion action that ultimately leads to an infringement of individual

---

BOX 3.1   Approaches A and B

Approach A

Jill is a hospital nurse running a programme of rehabilitation for patients who have had heart attacks. She decides that she is working with an educational approach, aiming for her patients to make informed decisions and have knowledge and skills about taking exercise and modifying their diet and other risk factors like smoking. She accepts that some patients will choose not to do so. She thinks that sometimes she may be working in a behaviour change model, because she sincerely believes that her patients would be better off if they changed their behaviour, and she finds that she sometimes really wants to persuade them. In the end, she decides that it is their choice and their life, and that she will not pressure them into doing what they do not want to do. Jill is aware, though, that some of her colleagues (who favour the behaviour change approach) think she should be tougher and shock patients into complying by horror stories of what may happen to them if they do not adjust their lifestyles.

Approach B

Terry is a community worker, based in a deprived housing estate. Facilities for recreation, exercise and buying good food, among other things, are poor. He decides that he is working with a mixture of client-centred and societal change approaches, because people in the community have identified that they want a better diet, and he is helping them to set up a food cooperative and help each other to learn new cooking skills. He is also helping them to lobby their local councillor for better green spaces on the estate where the children can play.

---

liberty in order to achieve overall health gain within the population?

There is also a danger that, when the public is involved in health promotion at a local level, local people can be manipulated into changing their agenda to match that of the health promoters. Community development approaches to health promotion should be about empowering the public to work on their own agendas of health issues, even if these are radically different from the agendas of those working for health in a professional capacity (Mittelmark 2007). But health promoters also raise awareness of health issues; they provide information about them and in doing so create demand for

---

EXERCISE 3.2   Identifying your health promotion aims and values

Select two or three specific health promotion activities you are engaged in or have been engaged in, such as a group health education programme, a media campaign, a patient education scheme, an immunisation programme, a one-to-one meeting with a client, a community activity or working on a health policy. Select different kinds of activities if you can or use Case studies 3.1 and 3.2.

With reference to Table 3.1, identify which approach you are using for each activity (you may find that you will identify more than one approach).

For each activity, define the aim and the important values implicit in your work. You may find it helpful to look at Case studies 3.1 and 3.2

Discuss your findings with a partner or in a small group.

CASE STUDY 3.1

A group of local people, led by a woman whose son died of a heroin overdose, has got together because they are concerned about drug misuse in the neighbourhood. They are afraid for the safety of their teenagers and younger children: drugs seem to be an established part of the teenage social scene, are easily available in the neighbourhood, and needles and syringes are found in local alleyways.

The group has decided that the best way to combat drugs is to go into local schools and scare the children off drugs with horror stories of bad 'trips' and addiction. They have recruited a former drug addict who is prepared to tell his story. They have asked the school nurse to help by providing supplies of leaflets and supporting them in their approach to the schools.

The school nurse believes that the shock-horror approach the group proposes has been shown by research into drug education to be ineffective. At best it will do no good, and at worst it could glamorise the drug scene and a make a hero out of the ex-addict. She believes that the local schools' approach is best: education on the facts of drug taking and how to minimise harm from taking drugs, coupled with building up self-esteem, social skills and confidence for young people to deal with drug situations. The parents think this is inadequate, and believe that their idea for a hard-hitting approach will work for their children.

■ Identify the ethical issues in this situation.
■ What do you think the school nurse should do, and why?

CASE STUDY 3.2

An environmental health officer (EHO) wants to undertake some research into the impact of air pollution on asthma rates in a neighbourhood that straddles a main road. Town planning colleagues have told the EHO that they expect this road to become even busier soon because it will become the feeder road to a new bypass leading to a massive new out-of-town office development. The EHO has a well worked out research proposal and has the cooperation of local GPs, which will enable him to see if there is any correlation between traffic flow, air pollution levels and asthma rates. If he can show a correlation, it will help to put health issues on the agenda of the council's planning committee, so that the health impact of planning decisions will be taken into account in future.

He needs to secure a research grant to pay for the additional pollution measurements and traffic flow counts, and to collect and process the data from the GPs. If he does not start within the next month, he will miss the chance to collect vital baseline measurements before the expected increase in traffic when the bypass opens.

Despite applications to many sources, the only offer of research money he has received has come from a research trust which specialises in the impact of environmental pollution on respiratory disease. It is funded primarily by the tobacco industry. The trust assures the EHO that that they will not interfere with the research in any way, and the grant will be given with 'no strings attached'. The EHO is unhappy about accepting money from the tobacco industry, but this is now his only chance to get the research under way.

■ Identify the ethical issues in this situation.
■ What do you think the EHO should do, and why?

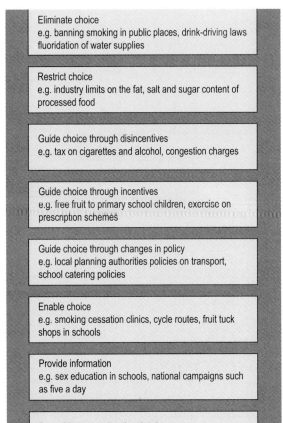

Fig. 3.1 **Health promotion intervention ladder.** *(Adjusted from Nuffield Council on Bioethics (2007, p. 42). Reproduced with permission).*

change. So where does this process differ from manipulating the community into wanting what the health promoters wanted in the first place?

See Chapter 15.

JUST WIDENING THE INEQUALITIES?

As discussed in Chapter 1, there are wide differences in the health status of different groups of people; generally those in poorer social and economic circumstances are the least healthy, with a widening gap between the health status of rich and poor.

There is a danger that health promotion activities only reach the people who have the resources and education to make use of health information and take health action. Those who are trapped in poor financial circumstances are often less likely to be in a position to change their lifestyle, to have the health literacy to fully understand the health messages, to effectively access health services or to have the other competencies necessary to lobby for social or political changes. There is clearly a need to be sensitive to this (Wanless 2004).

Some ways of working with those most in need, and often hardest to reach, are discussed in Chapter 15.

Efforts to change people's physical environments in order to improve health may have negative outcomes. Evaluation of studies on community regeneration has revealed a mixed impact, with one study showing an overall deterioration in health (Thomson et al 2006).

THE HEALTH PROMOTER: A SHINING EXAMPLE?

Consider the cases of an overweight dietitian, a nurse who smokes and an environmental health officer whose own kitchen is unhygienic. All three are in a position where they need to address these issues as part of their work and may be asked for advice which they clearly do not follow themselves.

Few health promoters would claim that they are perfect examples of healthy living, but we suggest that they have a responsibility to consider their own health, and think of ways in which it could be improved and in which they could contribute to a healthier environment. Health promoters are teaching by example, and the examples discussed above convey silent messages that it is okay to be overweight, to smoke, or to risk health by cooking unhygienically. It is probably best to be open and honest in situations where health promoters' own lifestyles are at odds with the health promoting ways they are advocating. Personal experience can also be turned to good advantage: for example, if the dietitian has a constant struggle to control her own weight, she can use that experience to develop a greater understanding of her clients' difficulties.

FACTS, FADS OR FASHIONS?

A concern for the public is that health advice changes. A difficulty is that research continuously turns up new evidence. At what point do you decide that the evidence is sufficiently convincing to begin publicising a new message, or to campaign to change an aspect of health policy or legislation?

If you have insufficient knowledge or experience to judge questions that may be medically or technically complex, on what basis do you make your decision? Is it more ethical to discuss the conflicting views openly and just air the debate more widely?

See Chapter 11 for an overview of the mass media in health promotion.

Another problem is that health issues are regularly covered in the media (see *The Guardian* at http://www.guardian.co.uk for an article on change in exercise advice) and media attention often focuses on the novel and controversial and often distorts the facts (Goldacre 2008).

HEALTH AT ANY COST?

What being healthy means to different people is discussed in Chapter 1.

In their enthusiasm for improving health, there is a danger that health promoters might lose sight that health means different things to different people and is shaped by their various values and experiences. Health may become a stereotyped image of the health promoter's own idea of perfection, leading to a prescription of what people should and should not do. This is clearly contrary to the concept that health promotion is about enabling people to increase control over their health and improve it in ways they see as appropriate.

HEALTH INFORMATION: AN INSENSITIVE BLUNDERBUSS?

Health promoters should be sensitive to the social, ethnic, economic and cultural background of the individuals and communities with which they work. Health information and large-scale health promotion programmes which portray only white Caucasians, are available only in the English language, or assume a common set of values are unethical.

EMPOWER THE PEOPLE?

Health promotion requires special competencies, some of which are the subject of this book. It is a whole or part of the work of very many professions, including health, education and community work.

Health promoters from this wide range of disciplinary backgrounds, if they are to empower people to take more control over their own health, need to seek to share their knowledge and experience with lay people, to learn from them, and to see them and other workers as valued partners in health promotion (Scriven 2007).

HEALTH FOR SALE?

With a scarcity of resources available for health promotion and in a climate of market economy and income generation, some health promotion activities are sponsored by commercial companies. One pitfall is the issue of perceived endorsement of products. For example, an NHS organisation could be seen as promoting the use of vitamins if it accepted sponsorship of appointment cards printed with the name of the sponsoring vitamin manufacturer.

There is also a move to involve commercial companies in promoting products in a way that also promotes health. For example, food manufacturers may be involved in special promotions for lower fat products. There are dangers here, the most obvious one being that the interests of the company may not be in harmony with those of the health promoter, who will be perceived as endorsing the product. There is also a possibility that the independent credibility of the health promoter is compromised.

Another pitfall is that health promotion, which should be a fundamental part of the free NHS, is seen as a potential money maker. Basic services, such as health information materials, health teaching, and giving advice to commercial companies on health promotion for employees, become subject to charges.

INDIVIDUAL FREEDOM OR COMMUNITY HEALTH?

Health promotion can be seen as paternalistic, interfering with personal liberty and freedom. Some might hold the view that doing nothing is the most morally acceptable option as it gives individuals the greatest freedom. However, this does not redress the distribution of power in society which may limit the ability of individuals (particularly vulnerable groups) to act autonomously. Health promotion addresses this by empowering individuals and communities to increase control over factors that affect their health and wellbeing. However, the interplay and interaction between individuals, communities and the wider populations is important. One of the difficulties in applying ethical principles in health promotion is the tension between the individual and population. In what instances should an individual's rights be over-ridden in the interests of the greater good? See Shaping the Future of Health Promotion and Society of Health Education and Promotion Specialists (SFHP/SHEPS) Cymru (2009) for a further over-view of ethical issues, and Taylor & Harvey (2006) for a discussion on health promotion and the freedom of the individual.

MAKING ETHICAL DECISIONS

Areas of ethical concern have been raised that do not present easy resolutions or answers. Beau-champ & Childress (2001) offer four ethical princi-ples which can act as a guide to ethical practice:

Respect for autonomy. Respecting the decision-making capacities of autonomous persons; enabling individuals to make reasoned informed choices. Are there groups in society who might be seen as incapable of autonomy, such as people with learn-ing disabilities, young children, prisoners, and if so will this affect your health promotion approach? If an individual makes a choice that you consider harmful, the dilemma may be how to respect that person's autonomy while doing good and avoiding harm. The key question is: by what right am I intervening and how do I justify the action I am taking?

Beneficence. This considers the balancing of ben-efits of an intervention against the risks and costs; the health promoter should act in a way that benefits the client.

Non-maleficence. Avoiding the causation of harm; the health promoter should not harm the client. The harm should not be disproportionate to the benefits of intervention. Victim-blaming would be consid-ered a harm. It may not always be possible to simul-taneously do good and avoid harm. For example, a mass media campaign showing the dangers of drink driving may have the effect of reducing the rates of drink driving but may also impact nega-tively on those who have been convicted of drink driving by labelling them and/or increasing their feelings of guilt. You will be able to think of other examples.

Justice. This involves distributing benefits, risks and costs fairly; the notion that clients in similar positions should be treated in a similar manner.

Health promotion involves difficult decisions in the dividing of time and resources between individuals and communities, between high-risk groups and whole populations. How do you balance general campaigns on healthy eating for the whole popula-tion with targeted interventions, such as setting up a food cooperative in a deprived area?

The principles provide a framework for consist-ent moral decision making, but health promotion action can encapsulate complex and sometimes conflicting choices between these principles (some of the examples above are taken from SFHP/SHEPS Cymru 2009). The following sets of questions (taken from Seedhouse 1988) draw on the four ethical prin-ciples and are designed for you to think about inter-vention ethics (see also Seedhouse 2009).

1. Questions fundamental to decisions about health

● Will I be creating autonomy in my clients, enabling them to choose freely for themselves and direct their own lives?
● Will I be respecting the autonomy of my clients, whether or not I approve of what they are doing?
● Will I be respecting persons equally, without discrimination?
● Will I be serving basic needs before any other wants?

2. Questions about duties and principles

● Will I be doing good and preventing harm?
● Will I be telling the truth, based on current evidence?
● Will I be minimising harm in the long term?
● Will I be honouring promises and agreements?

3. Questions about consequences

● Will I be increasing individual good?
● Will I be increasing the good of a particular group?
● Will I be increasing the social good?

4. Questions about external considerations

● Am I putting resources to best use: what is the most effective and efficient thing to do?
● What is the degree of risk involved?

- Is there a professional code of practice that has a bearing on this?
- How certain am I of the evidence?
- Is there any disputed evidence and will I make this clear?
- Are there legal implications? If so, do I understand them?
- What are the views and wishes of other relevant people?
- Can I justify my actions in terms of the evidence I have before me?

These questions are tools to help decision making and moral reasoning. They are not substitutes for personal judgements, but they help you to think through your proposed actions and come to an ethical decision. Not all the questions will be relevant, but they act as a useful checklist which will enable careful consideration to be given to health promotion interventions.

Exercise 3.3 and Exercise 3.4 (which uses Fig. 3.1) are designed to help you to think about intervention ethics. Please also refer to Fig. 3.2 which provides an overview of ethical ways of working that highlight goals and principles.

TOWARDS A CODE OF PRACTICE

Many professions have codes of practice, which are broad principles and guidelines on how professionals should and should not act. They reflect the

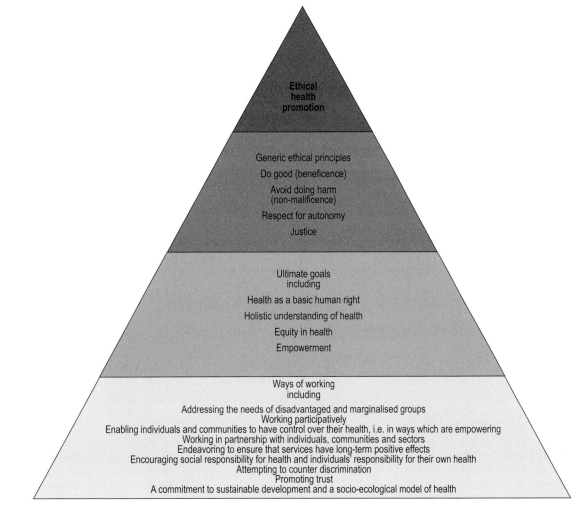

Fig. 3.2 A framework for ethical health promotion. *(Taken from Shaping the Future of Health Promotion (SFHP) and Society of Health Education and Promotion Specialists (SHEPS) Cymru 2009. Reproduced with permission).*

EXERCISE 3.3   Ethical decisions in health promotion

Look again at Case studies 3.1 and 3.2. You may find it helpful to use the questions in the section above on making ethical decisions to identify the issues relevant to each situation, and to decide what you would do.

EXERCISE 3.4   Ladder of health promotion action

Work in small groups of three or four.
  Consider the health promotion intervention ladder in Fig 3.1 and discuss the following.
- The ethical issues that might be relevant to each rung of the ladder.
- Would you encounter any difficulties with any of the modes of interventions in practice?
- Are there modes of intervention that you would reject on ethical grounds?

---

values accepted as underpinning sound professional practice. Health promoters should ensure they are familiar with the codes of practice of their own professional bodies See SHEPS Cymru, (2007) for a specific code of practice relating to health promotion.

PRACTICE POINTS

- In choosing approaches to health promotion, take account of the different aims and values they reflect.
- Remember that ethical issues and dilemmas are inherent in health promotion practice and you need to think through the process of how you will make ethical decisions.
- Be familiar with the code of professional practice of any profession to which you belong.
- Good practice in health promotion involves working to the specific values and principles of practice.

References

Action on Smoking and Heath 2007 Young people and smoking fact sheet number 3. London, ASH.

Bambra C, Fox D, Scott-Samuel A 2005 Towards a politics of health. Health Promotion International 20(2): 187–193.

Beauchamp TL, Childress JF 2001 Principles of biomedical ethics, 5th edn. Oxford, Oxford University Press.

Blenkinsop S, Bradshaw S, Cade J et al 2007 Further evaluation of the school fruit and vegetable scheme. London, Department of Health.

Butler P 2008 Social change isn't won by lone heroes. The Guardian, Joe Public Blog. http://www.guardian.co.uk/society/joepublic/2008/sep/03/jamieoliver.schoolmeals.

Contoyannis P, Jones AM 2004 Socio-economic status, health and lifestyle. Journal of Health Economics 23(5): 965–995.

Department of Health 2004 Choosing health: making healthy choices easier. London, The Stationery Office.

Department of Health 2006 Immunisation against infectious disease – the Green Book. London, The Stationery Office.

Department of Health 2007a The health benefits of fruit and vegetables. http://www.dh.gov.uk/en/Publichealth/Healthimprovement/FiveADay/FiveADaygeneralinformation/DH_4002343.

Department of Health 2007b The coronary heart disease national service framework– shaping the future. Progress report for 2006. London, The Stationery Office.

Godin G 2007 Has the individual vanished from Canadian health promotion? In: O'Neil M, Pederson A, Dupere S, Rootman I (eds) Health promotion in Canada: critical perspectives, 2nd edn. Toronto, Canadian Scholars Press.

Goldacre B 2008 Bad Science. London, Fourth Estate.

Health and Social Care Information Centre 2008 Health survey for England 2007: healthy lifestyles: knowledge, attitudes and behaviour. Leeds, NHS Health and Social Care Information Centre.

Jones IR 2003 Health promotion and the new public health. In: Scambler G 2003 Sociology as applied to medicine, 5th edn. Burlington MA, Saunders.

Laverack G 2004 Health promotion practice: power and empowerment. London, Sage.

Laverack G 2007 Health promotion practice: building empowered communities. Maidenhead, Open University Press.

Mittelmark M 2007 Editorial: community empowerment and participation. Promotion & Education XIV(2) (plus other articles and case studies in this edition of the journal on current health promotion practices in communities).

Morgan O 2005 Approaches to increase physical activity: reviewing the evidence for exercise-referral schemes. Public Health 119(5): 361–370.

National Institute for Health and Clinical Excellence 2006 Public health programme guidance draft scope: national provision of smoking cessation services. London, NICE.

National Institute for Health and Clinical Excellence 2007 The most appropriate means of generic and specific interventions to support attitude and behaviour change at population and community levels. London, NICE.

Nuffield Council on Bioethics 2007 Public health: ethical issues. London, Nuffield Council on Bioethics. http://www. nuffieldbioethics.org.

OFSTED 2005 OFSTED subject conference report: PSHE developments in personal, social and health education. London, 23–24 November 2005. Document reference number HMI2515. http://www.ofsted.gov.uk.

Oldfield L 2008 The cost of a socially acceptable healthy diet for low-income families. The Food Magazine 83 (December).

Richards H, Reid M, Watt G 2003 Victim-blaming revisited: a qualitative study of beliefs about illness causation, and responses to chest pain. Family Practice 20(6): 711–716.

Robinson J, Kirkclady AJ 2007 'You think that I'm smoking and they're not': why mothers still smoke in the home. Social Science and Medicine 65(4): 641–652.

Scriven A 2005 Promoting health: policies, principles and perspectives. In: Scriven A (ed.) Health promoting practice: the contribution of nurses and allied health professions. Basingstoke, Palgrave.

Scriven A 2007 Developing local alliance partnerships through community collaboration and participation. In: Handsley S, Lloyd CE, Douglas J et al (eds) Policy and practice in promoting public health. London, Sage.

Seedhouse D 1988 Ethics – the heart of health care. Chichester, Wiley.

Seedhouse D 2004 Health promotion: philosophy, prejudice, and practice, 2nd edn. Chichester, Wiley.

Seedhouse D 2009 Ethics – the heart of health care, 3rd edn. Chichester, Wiley Blackwell.

Shaping the Future of Health Promotion and Society of Health Education and Promotion Specialists Cymru 2009 A framework for ethical health promotion (draft). London, Royal Society for Public Health and SHEPS Wales.

Society of Health Education and Promotion Specialists Cymru 2007 The principles and practice and code of professional conduct for health education and promotion specialists in Wales. Cardiff, National Assembly for Wales.

Tannahill A 2008 Health promotion: the Tannahill model revisited. Public Health 122(12): 1387–1391.

Taubes G 2009 The diet delusion: challenging the conventional wisdom on diet, weight loss and disease. London, Vermillion.

Taylor G, Harvey H 2006 Health promotion and the freedom of the individual. Health Care Analysis 14(1): 15–24.

Taylor S 2007 Approaches to health and illness. In: Taylor S, Field D (eds) Sociology of health and health care, 4th edn. Oxford, Blackwell.

Thomson H, Atkinson R, Petticrew M, Kearns A 2006 Do urban regeneration programmes improve public health and reduce health inequalities? A synthesis of the evidence from UK policy and practice (1980–2004). Journal of Epidemiology and Community Health 60(2): 108–115.

Wanless D 2004 Securing good health for the whole population: final report. London, Royal College of General Practitioners summary paper 2004/2/, HMS Treasury.

Websites
http://www.combatpoverty.ie/research/foodpoverty.html
http://www.guardian.co.uk/uk/2007/aug/17/health.topstories3
http://www.pshe-association.org.uk

Chapter 4

Who promotes health?

SUMMARY

In this chapter the major agents and agencies of health promotion are identified, and their roles discussed. Included are international and national organisations, the government, the NHS, local authorities and voluntary organisations. There is an exercise on identifying key local health promoters and the chapter ends with suggestions for practice and an exercise about how you can improve your own health promotion role.

This chapter provides an overview of the people and organisations that support and enable better health. To some extent many lay people are health promoters, because they discuss health matters and offer support, advice and guidance to others. This can happen informally. The unofficial networks of family, friends and neighbours are of great significance in shaping people's health beliefs and behaviour, in providing healthy living conditions and creating social capital. Health promotion may also occur incidentally. The availability of a wide variety of cheap fruit and vegetables in the summer, for example, means that it is easier for people to choose a healthy diet, so the greengrocer is inadvertently promoting health. These informal and unplanned sources of health promotion are very significant. The aim here, however, is to identify the agents and agencies through which planned, deliberate programmes and policies are delivered.

England, Wales, Scotland and Northern Ireland have public health systems which differ slightly but all countries support the following health policy themes:

- Modernisation: using up-to-date streamlined methods of management and communication in health (Department of Health (DoH)/NHS Modernisation Board 2003 and http://www.dh.gov.uk).
- Equity and inequalities: equal opportunities for everyone and reducing health inequalities between different social groups (DoH 2007).
- Social and economic regeneration: addressing poverty, unemployment, poor living conditions and social exclusion (a sense of not being a part of a community, of not belonging) (http://www.publicservice.co.uk).
- Democratic renewal: ensuring that the process of democracy is applied through all levels of public service (http://www.communities.gov.uk).
- Public involvement: getting people involved with decisions and actions that affect them, such as consulting people about proposed changes to local health services (http://www.publicinvolvement.org.uk).

AGENTS AND AGENCIES OF HEALTH PROMOTION

Fig. 4.1 identifies a wide range of the most important agents and agencies of health promotion. Most have a variety of health promotion roles.

See Chapter 9, section on working in partnership with other organisations.

An increasing number of agencies work together in collaborative partnerships, in an effort to make their work more effective. Partnership working has been a dominant theme in national and international health promotion and public health directives since the *Ottawa Charter* (World Health Organization (WHO) 1986). In the UK it has been part of all the national strategies for health (see, for example, DoH 1992, 1999, 2004) and these have been accompanied by guidance on how agencies could work together for better health (see for example, the Welsh Partnership Forum constitution at http://www.cymru.gov.uk). Government strategies and guidelines continue to focus on the importance of partnerships for health between agencies and across government departments.

INTERNATIONAL AGENCIES

THE EUROPEAN COMMUNITY

In 2007 the EU developed a new public health strategy, *Together for Health: a strategic approach for the EU 2008–2013* (Commission of the European Communities 2007). The strategy brings together and extends the public health programme and the programme in support of EU consumer policy. As public health and consumer protection policies share many objectives, such as promoting health protection safety information and education, the commission aimed, in combining the two programmes, to exploit synergies and to generate greater health policy coherence.

The WHO's role in promoting health is also discussed in Chapter 1.

THE WHO

The WHO (http://www.who.int) has a role in guiding both European and global health policy. It has issued many statements in the form of declarations and charters addressing important and broad areas of health promotion and public health-related policy. It coordinates European networks such as Health Promoting Schools and Hospitals, and Healthy Cities. These initiatives are discussed more fully in Chapter 16.

OTHER INTERNATIONAL AGENCIES

The International Union for Health Promotion and Education (IUHPE)

The IUHPE (http://www.iuhpe.org) is half a century old, and is the only global organisation entirely devoted to advancing health promotion and health education. It is a leading global network working to promote health worldwide and contribute to the achievement of equity in health between and within countries. It has an established track record in advancing the knowledge base and improving the quality and effectiveness of health promotion and health education practice, with members ranging from government bodies, to universities and institutes, to nongovernmental organisations (NGOs) and individuals across all continents.

The IUHPE decentralises its activity through regional offices and works in close cooperation with

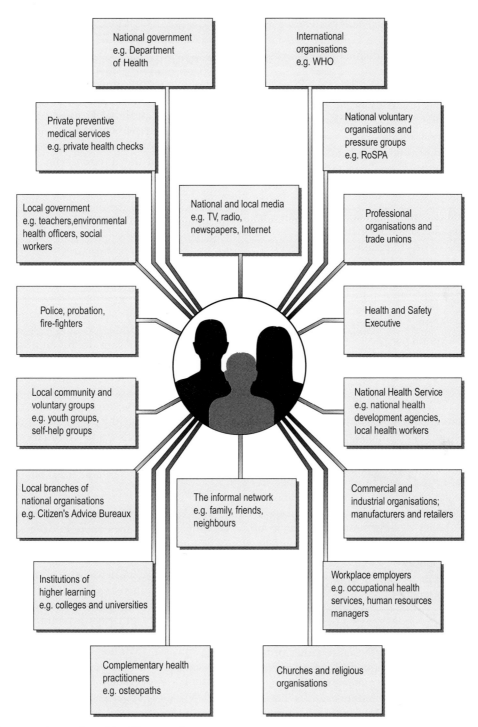

Fig. 4.1 Agents and agencies of health promotion.

the major intergovernmental and NGOs such as WHO, UNESCO, UNICEF, to influence and facilitate the development of health promotion strategies and projects.

The IUHPE has four goals:

1. Advocate for health: to advocate for actions that promote the health of populations throughout the world.

2. Build knowledge of effective health promotion and health education: to develop the knowledge base for health promotion and health education.

3. Improve effectiveness of policy and practice: to improve and advance the quality and effectiveness of health promotion and health education practice and knowledge.

4. Build capacity for health promotion and health education: to contribute to the development of capacity in countries to undertake health promotion and health education activities (http://www.iuhpe.org).

European Public Health Alliance (EPHA)

The EPHA (http://www.epha.org) is a network of NGOs (NGOs are organisations that are independent of government control) and other agencies actively involved in protecting and promoting public health. EPHA's mission is to promote and protect the health of all people living in Europe and to advocate for greater participation of citizens in health-related policy making at the European level.

World Federation of Public Health Associations (WFPHA)

The WFPHA (http://www.wfpha.org) is an international, nongovernmental, multiprofessional and civil society organisation bringing together public health professionals interested and active in safeguarding and promoting the public's health through professional exchange, collaboration and action. It is the only worldwide professional society representing and serving the broad area of public health, as distinct from single disciplines or occupations (such as the IUHPE). The Federation's members are national and regional public health associations, as well as regional associations of schools of public health.

NATIONAL AGENCIES

THE GOVERNMENT

Government departments in the UK (and their devolved counterparts in Wales, Scotland and Northern Ireland), such as the Department of Health, the Department of Work and Pensions, the Department for Education and Skills (DfES), the Department of the Environment, Food and Rural Affairs and the Department of Transport, Local Government and the Regions, have an interest in and responsibility for the promotion of health and therefore have to take account of the impact of legislation and economic and fiscal policies on health.

The national public health strategies for health in England, Wales, Scotland and Northern Ireland demonstrate a commitment towards the pursuit of improved health and a reduction in health inequalities, rather than focusing just on treatment services and health care. To this end, key units have been established, for example, neighbourhood renewal (http://www.neighbourhood.gov.uk) and the social exclusion taskforce (http://www.cabinet office.gov.uk) to produce national directives to be implemented locally by partnerships of health services, local authorities, and voluntary and community organisations.

See Chapters 1 and 7 for more on national strategies for health.

The UK government has also taken a lead in tackling health issues such as drug misuse (DoH 2008a) and teenage pregnancy (Department for Children, Schools and Families (DCSF) 2007, DoH/ DfES 2008). In relation to drug misuse, for example, its aims are to increase the safety of communities from drug-related harm, to reduce the acceptability and availability of drugs to young people and to reduce the health risks and other damage related to drug misuse. Multiagency drug action teams produce local plans, coordinate work and bring together a wide range of people and agencies to work at a local level.

OTHER NATIONAL AND LOCAL AGENCIES

Non-governmental organisations

There are a number of NGOs concerned specifically with public health in the UK, such as The Royal

Society for Public Health, the UK Public Health Association and The Institute of Health Education and Health Promotion.

The Royal Society for Public Health (RSPH)

The RSPH (http://www.rsph.org.uk) is an independent organisation dedicated to the promotion and protection of population health and wellbeing. It advises on policy development, provides education and training services, encourages scientific research, disseminates information and certifies products, training centres and processes. The RSPH is the largest multidisciplinary public health organisation in the UK and is an independent charity formed in 2008 by the merger of the Royal Society of Health (RSH) and the Royal Institute of Public Health (RIPH). *Shaping the Future of Health Promotion* is hosted and led by the Royal Society for Public Health (in collaboration with the Faculty of Public Health, UK Public Health Register and Institute of Health Promotion and Education). This important project derived from the main recommendations of the 2005 report *Shaping the Future of Public Health: Promoting Health in the NHS* (DoH/Welsh Assembly Government 2005). Through this project the RSPH advocates for the importance of specialised health promotion within public health and supports the specialised health promotion workforce.

The UK Public Health Association (UKPHA)

The UKPHA (http://www.ukpha.org.uk) is an independent voluntary organisation which aims to be a unifying and powerful voice for the public's health and wellbeing in the UK, focusing on the development of healthy public policy at all levels of government and across all sectors. Their mission includes three aims:

1. To combat health inequalities and work for a fairer, more equitable and healthier society.
2. To promote sustainable development, ensuring healthy environments for future generations.
3. To challenge anti-health forces, collaborating with business to promote health-sustaining production, consumption, employment and socially responsible products and services.

The Institute of Health Promotion and Education (IHPE)

The IHPE (http://www.ihpe.org.uk) was established to bring together professionals on the basis of their common interest in health education and health promotion with a view to sharing experiences, ideas and information. It is a professional association with a recognised role in the field of prevention and management of illness and promotion of health. Its activities have been mainly concerned with health education, and following the *Declaration of Alma Ata* (WHO 1978) they also include health promotion. The IHPE has been in the forefront of health promotion developments with special contributions to the advancement of a settings approach.

Voluntary organisations and pressure groups

There are many voluntary organisations concerned with health promotion, some of which have regional and/or local branches. Examples of these are The Advisory Council on Alcohol and Drug Education (TACADE) (http://www.tacade.com) and the National Association for Mental Health (MIND) (http://www.mind.org.uk). Most of these organisations produce educational material, and some run training courses for professionals and/or the public. Some organisations act mainly as pressure groups, such as Friends of the Earth (http://www.foe. co.uk).

Professional associations

Professional associations, such as the British Medical Association (BMA) (http://www.bma.org. uk), the Royal College of Nursing (RCN) (http://www.rcn.org.uk), the Chartered Institute for Environmental Health (CIEH) (http://www.cieh.org) and the Faculty of Public Health (FPH) (http://www.fphm.org.uk) have been highly influential in policy and legislative changes and in the practice and training of their members in health promotion.

Trade unions

Trade unions are active in promoting health and safety at work, both through negotiating workplace conditions and through their health and safety representatives (Barbeau et al 2005). In the UK, The Health and Safety Executive (HSE) (http://www. hse.gov.uk) also oversees the implementation of health and safety at work legislation.

Commercial and industrial organisations

These have a role in safeguarding public health. Examples include companies providing water and refuse removal companies. In recent years in the UK, some facilities with a public health protection function have been privatised, which has raised public health dilemmas. For example, should water companies have the right to cut off supplies to consumers who do not pay their bills, when a possible consequence of this is the occurrence and spread of infectious diseases such as dysentery?

Manufacturers and retailers

Manufacturers have increasingly taken the health and safety aspects of their products into account. These include manufacturers of children's toys, food manufacturers and producers of green eco household products. Large supermarket chains have made a wide range of healthy options available to the public, such as fat-reduced and low-sugar foods. These trends are often as a result of increased consumer demands, reflecting heightened awareness of health issues (House of Commons 2002).

The mass media

Health promotion is undertaken by national and local mass media organisations, including television, radio, newspapers and magazines (Hubley & Copeman 2008), and through the Internet many people have easy access to a huge range of health information (Korp 2006).

See Chapter 11 for more about mass media in health promotion.

Churches and religious organisations

Churches and religious organisations play an important part in developing values, attitudes and beliefs that affect health. Kramish Campbell et al (2007) show how church-based health promotion can influence members' lifestyle at multiple levels of change and produce significant impacts on a variety of behaviours.

THE NATIONAL HEALTH SERVICE (NHS)

The structure of the NHS

The NHS, established in 1948, has been reorganised on a regular basis, usually as a new government is voted into power. The most significant and fundamental reorganisation happened in the 1990s, starting with the *National Health Service and Community Care Act* reforms (DoH 1990). During the 1990s, a key feature of the NHS was the internal market and the division into *purchasers* and *providers*. Local health authorities were the purchasers, who decided what health care was required and purchased it, setting and monitoring contracts with provider local hospitals and community services. These providers became NHS trusts, in competition with one another to win contracts from the purchasers. The election of a new government in 1997 brought an approach which emphasised integrated care, and working in a spirit of cooperation. *The New NHS: Modern, Dependable* (DoH 1997) set out the plan for the health service, with partnership, quality and performance at the heart of the NHS, a focus on improving health and wellbeing, and tackling the root causes of ill health and inequalities. A separate White Paper was published for Scotland (DoH/Scottish Office 1997). In a shift towards a primary care-led NHS, primary care groups (PCGs) were set up in the late 1990s. These were basically groups of GP practices that worked closely with local authorities, especially social services, to assess local health needs and develop local health services. *The NHS Plan* (DoH 2000) set out a further programme for reform, investment and expansion of the NHS, including a central role for the wider public health function, including health promotion.

See below for information on primary care trusts.

Shifting the Balance of Power Within the NHS – Securing Delivery (DoH 2001) set out further change with a power shift to frontline staff. Primary care groups were given additional responsibilities to run services; they developed into primary care trusts (PCTs) with a responsibility to work closely with social services.

Larger strategic health authorities replaced the existing smaller health authorities in England in 2002. Strategic health authorities support the PCTs and NHS trusts in delivering *The NHS Plan*, to build capacity and support performance improvement, ensuring that all NHS organisations work together to meet government targets. (See http://www.nhs.uk for an interactive timeline which details milestones in the history of the NHS from its very beginning in 1948 to the present day.)

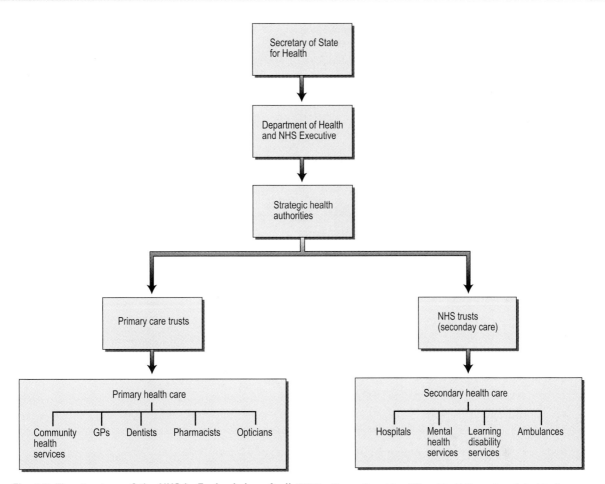

Fig. 4.2 The structure of the NHS in England since April 2002. *(Figure adjusted from Office of Health Economics website: http://www. ohe.org/page/knowledge/schools/hc_in_uk/nhs_structure.cfm. Reproduced with permission).*

In 2002, the Department of Health was refocused. Figs 4.2 and 4.3 show the overall structure of the NHS in England. At the top in Fig. 4.2 is the Secretary of State for Health, the government minister in charge of the Department of Health, responsible for the NHS in England and answerable to Parliament. The Department of Health and the NHS Executive are responsible for the strategic planning of the health service as a whole. Under the Department of Health are strategic health authorities which plan health care for the population of the region they cover.

Health services are divided between primary and secondary. Primary care services include general medical practitioners (GPs), dentists, pharmacists, opticians, district nursing and numerous other services. Secondary care includes not only hospitals but also ambulances and specialised health services for the mentally ill and the learning disabled, as shown in Fig. 4.2.

Services are provided by NHS organisations called trusts. NHS trusts supply secondary care. PCTs provide primary care services and are responsible for buying almost all of the health care, both primary and secondary, required by the local populations they serve (see more on PCTs and NHS trusts under Agents of Health Promotion, below).

The structures in Scotland, Wales and Northern Ireland differ. In the interests of keeping the text in this book short, the terms used are applicable to England but readers in all countries will need to familiarise themselves with the structure in the country where they work by undertaking Exercise 4.1.

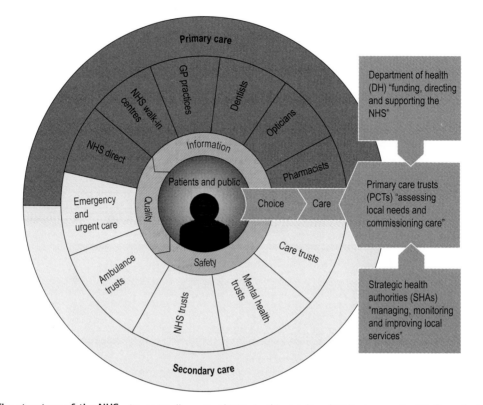

Fig. 4.3 The structure of the NHS. *(Source http://www.nhs.uk/NHSEngland/aboutnhs/Pages/NHSstructure.aspx. See http://www.nhs.uk for further details on the diagram and the structure, core principles and history of the NHS. Reproduced with the permission of NHS Choices).*

EXERCISE 4.1   What's on your patch? Finding out about your local NHS and agents and agencies of health promotion

Exercise 4.1 is designed to help you to find out how your local NHS is organised and to identify the health promotion agents and agencies which are important for your work. There is much to gain by having good local knowledge of health promoters you can refer clients to or work with in partnerships.

1. Find out about the structure of the NHS in the area where you work:
   - What is the name and function of the local organisation with responsibility for public health? (This will be your local primary care trust/care trust or its equivalent in Scotland, Wales or Northern Ireland. Try http://www.nhs.uk for information.)
   - What regional and/or national organisations are responsible for public health where you work?
2. Find out about the agencies and people on your patch:
   - Think of the geographical patch where you work, and identify its boundaries as clearly as you can.

It could be the area served by a GP practice, the catchment area of a hospital, the population of a primary care trust/care trust or the geographical patch that is your responsibility as an environmental health officer or community worker.
   - Identify as many health promotion agents and agencies on your patch as you can, using Fig. 4.1 and the information about agents and agencies in health promotion in this chapter as checklists.

It is likely that you will know some very well and others not at all. Identify those you would find it helpful to know more about and plan to find out about them. If there are some you know nothing about, such as the voluntary and community groups on your patch, identify people who are likely to know about them (such as health promotion practitioners/specialists) and contact them to find out more.

National Institute for Health and Clinical Excellence (NICE)

NICE is currently the national agency responsible for providing national guidance on promoting good health and preventing and treating ill health (http://www.nice.org.uk). NICE took over the functions of its predecessor, the Health Development Agency (HDA) on 1 April 2005. The HDA was a special health authority established in 2000 to develop the evidence base to improve health and reduce health inequalities. If you would like to know more about the HDA, see the White Paper *Saving Lives: our Healthier Nation* (DoH 1999).

Health Scotland

The work of Health Scotland covers every aspect of health improvement, from gathering evidence, to planning, delivery and evaluation, and spans the range of health topics, settings and life stages (http://www.healthscotland.com).

Public Health Agency for Northern Ireland

The Agency began work in 2009 following a review, which saw a range of functions in the health and social care system brought together to focus on improving the health and wellbeing of everyone in Northern Ireland. The Agency works with a wide range of partners from the health, voluntary and community sectors, as well as local government (http://www.publichealth.hscni.net).

Health promotion division: the National Assembly for Wales

The National Assembly for Wales approach to health improvement is to promote positive health throughout life, from healthy children to healthy ageing. Lifestyle changes that will improve health are encouraged, and by supporting communities to change a range of factors affecting health in the environment, the workplace and local government. The focus is on preventing ill health and on addressing problems at an early stage (http://wales.gov.uk).

Primary care trusts

PCTs have control of local healthcare while strategic health authorities monitor performance and standards. Since 2008, PCTs can choose to adopt the NHS prefix before their place name. The *Next Stage Review* report (DoH 2008b) signalled that PCTs have the freedom to re-name to NHS Local. This will allow PCTs to position themselves as the local leader of the NHS and frontline commissioners of patient care. It is integral to the objectives of world class commissioning (http://www.dh.gov.uk) and, in particular, that PCTs have responsibility for all primary care services (pharmacy, dental, medical and optical).

Improving the health of the local community involves PCTs in programmes of community development, health promotion and education. One means of doing this is through local strategic partnerships (LSPs) involving all the local NHS organisations, local authorities, voluntary and community groups and local businesses. LSPs ensure that priority is given to shared plans and integrated multi-agency programmes (http://www.neighbourhood.gov.uk). An example of this is teenage pregnancies (DoH/DfES 2008) with those LSPs in receipt of neighbourhood renewal funding (NRF) asked to work towards reducing teenage conception rates. All NRF and their LSPs operate within the context of local area agreements (LAAs). LAAs set out the priorities for a local area agreed between central government and a local area (the local authority and LSP) and other key partners at the local level.

For more detail, see Chapter 7, section on local health strategies and initiatives.

NHS and foundation trusts

NHS trusts provide patient-centred hospital services based on local agreements and national standards; some trusts provide specialised services such as mental health services or ambulance services. NHS trusts are expected to take account of patients' views as they plan their services, and to ensure that local people are involved in decisions about service planning. NHS trusts have a part to play in health promotion, particularly health education and preventive health work with patients, their carers and families.

Foundation trusts are a new type of NHS hospital introduced in 2004 and run by local managers, staff and members of the public, which are tailored to the needs of the local population. Foundation trusts have been given much more financial and operational freedom than other NHS trusts and have come to represent the government's commitment to decentralising the control of public services. These trusts remain within the NHS and its performance inspection system (http://www.nhs.uk).

Patient advice and liaison services

Patient advice and liaison services (PALS) are designed to bring citizens more closely into decision making processes. They provide:

- Confidential advice and support to families and their carers, information on the NHS and health-related matters.
- Confidential assistance in resolving problems and concerns quickly.
- Explanations of complaints procedures and how to get in touch with someone who can help.
- Information on how people can get more involved in their own healthcare.

Each NHS hospital has its own PALS. In addition, each primary care trust, ambulance trust, acute trust, care trust and mental health trust has its own PALS (see DoH 2006 and http://www.nhs.uk).

NHS Direct

NHS Direct is a national telephone helpline in England which is staffed by specially trained nurses 24 hours a day, 365 days a year. They have the knowledge and experience to give help and reassurance but also offer commissioned services to other parts of the NHS to help them meet their patients' needs.

These services include out-of-hours support for GPs and dental services, telephone support for patients with long-term conditions and pre- and postoperative support for patients (http://www.nhsdirect.nhs.uk).

NHS walk-in centres

NHS walk-in centres (WiCs) offer access to a range of NHS services. WiCs are managed by PCTs and deal with minor illnesses and injuries. They are predominantly nurse-led first-contact services available to everyone without making an appointment or requiring patients to register. Most centres are open 365 days a year and are situated in convenient locations that give patients access to services beyond regular office hours (http://www.nhs.uk).

Public health observatories

The Association of Public Health Observatories (APHO) represents a network of public health observatories (PHOs) working across the five nations of England, Scotland, Wales, Northern Ireland and the Republic of Ireland. They produce Health Profiles which provide information, data and intelligence on people's health and health care. Health Profiles provide a snapshot of health for each local council using key health indicators, which enables comparison locally, regionally and over time (http://www.apho.org.uk).

AGENTS OF HEALTH PROMOTION

Primary healthcare teams

Primary healthcare teams are usually the first point of contact that the general public has with the NHS. The exact membership of each primary healthcare team varies but it usually includes the following:

Health promotion specialists

Health promotion specialists (sometimes known by other professional titles such as public health practitioners) are mostly located within the public health directorate in PCTs and are responsible for the provision of expert advice, leadership, partnership development, training, programme development (including strategy and policy) and resources to support local health promotion initiatives. They liaise with other health promotion agents and agencies, both within and outside the NHS, to ensure that activities, wherever initiated, are coordinated and supported.

General practitioners

GPs provide a comprehensive range of diagnosis and treatment medical services for patients registered with their practice, and for those outside the practice in an emergency. They refer patients to other healthcare workers as necessary, for example to counsellors, practice nurses, health visitors, physiotherapists or consultants specialising in a particular disease area. Encouraging healthier living is an important part of a GP's work. Health promotion via GPs can come in the form of guidance on lifestyle choices or it can be implemented through immunisation or screening programmes (Kula 2007). The Royal College of General Practitioners' GP curriculum statements say that GPs have 'a crucial role to play in promoting health' (http://www.rcgp-curriculum.org.uk).

GP practice managers

These are key people in enabling the smooth running of practices and for ensuring that patients are efficiently, confidentially and caringly received. They have an important role in health promotion because they can control access to health information for patients.

Community nurses

PCTs depend on the contribution of a range of community nurses to achieve their objectives; their work in health promotion and in assessing health needs of the local population is particularly important (Weeks et al 2005). There is a range of nursing roles and professions within community nursing, including:

- district nurses
- health visitors
- school nurses
- community mental health nurses
- community midwives
- practice nurses
- others, such as diabetes specialist nurses.

Other health professions

Many other health professionals, such as hospital nurses (Whitehead 2005a,b), dentists, hospital and retail pharmacists (Armstrong et al 2005) and the full range of professions allied to medicine (Scriven 2005) have a part to play in health promotion, especially in patient education.

Health trainers

Health trainers are a new workforce recruited from the community and working in the NHS, local organisations including local authorities, businesses, the voluntary and community sector. Health trainers motivate and help people to set goals by developing personal health plans, give practical support to carry out those plans and identify with the individuals their barriers to change (DoH

2008c). The initiative was first targeted at the most disadvantaged areas to make it easier for individuals in these communities to make healthier choices (http://www.dh.gov.uk).

HEALTH PROMOTION AGENTS AND AGENCIES OUTSIDE THE NHS

Complementary and alternative medicine (CAM) practitioners

Those practising CAM include homoeopaths, chiropractors, osteopaths, acupuncturists, reflexologists, practitioners of herbal medicine, yoga, massage and shiatsu, among others. These practitioners can play a part in promoting health and relieving health problems, often using a more holistic approach than conventional medicine. Therapies may be available on the NHS, either by a member of the primary care team or through referral to a complementary practitioner. There is potential for collaboration and closer integration between health promotion and complementary therapies, with Hill (2003) arguing that health promoters cannot afford to ignore developments in CAM.

Local authorities

Local authorities have responsibilities that impact on the social, economic and environmental factors that affect health, such as poverty, low wages, unemployment, poor education, substandard housing, crime and disorder, and pollution. Working with others, they will be able to develop strategies for tackling many of the fundamental causes of ill health; for example, either by targeting housing maintenance or coordinating different types of information services. In doing so, they are fundamental to health development in the communities they serve (http://www.direct.gov.uk).

See also Chapter 9 section on working in partnership with other organisations.

A host of initiatives has been developed over the last decade to promote and improve economic, social and environmental wellbeing, through regeneration and partnership working. These have been encouraged by the Beacon Scheme, a prestigious award scheme that recognises excellence in local government (http://www.beacons.idea.gov.uk). See the example in Case study 4.1.

CASE STUDY 4.1 CALDERDALE LOCAL HEALTH STRATEGY

Through its strong and committed partnerships, Calderdale has developed effective structures for the development of strategies and delivery of the health agenda. The partnership between the council and the Calderdale and Kirklees Health Authority, Calderdale NHS Trust, Calderdale Primary Care Group and the voluntary sector in the borough has embraced the issues of broader regeneration and quality of life agenda in both the health improvement programme and the council's community plan.

The council and its partners have been able to recognise complex causes of ill health, making clear links with national policies, and have set out a vision to promote social equality and economic and environmental wellbeing. The key outcome has been the effective joint planning and strategy development between chief executives and leaders from the council and the health service through the multiagency health policy group.

(http://www.beacons.idea.gov.uk)

For more detail see Chapter 7, section on local health strategies and initiatives.

Environmental health officers/practitioners

Environmental health officers (EHOs) work in environmental protection, food safety and nutrition, health and safety, housing and public health (see http://www.cieh.org for specific details on EHOs roles and functions).

The organisation of environmental health services is mainly the function of local authority environmental health departments, but may be combined with other departments such as housing, community development and leisure. National and local legislation gives these departments power to take advisory and legal action on behalf of people who visit, live or work in an area. The scope for health promotion is wide. Many departments appoint specialist officers to work on specific health issues, such as home safety. Some environmental health services have full-time environmental health promotion officers (EHPOs) who work in supporting the role and function of environmental health as well as delivering and developing a number of health promotion projects. For a specific example of an EHPO, see East Herts LA (http://www.eastherts.gov.uk).

The local education authority

Local education authorities (LEAs) have responsibility for personal, social and health education (PSHE) in schools. They may employ advisors to provide advice, support and training for teachers in PSHE. PSHE includes everything schools do to promote pupils' good health and wellbeing. It is backed by the National Healthy Schools Programme (http://www.teachernet.gov.uk) and is linked to Citizenship (http://www.standards.dfes.gov.uk).

Social services

Social services staff, including social workers and staff of care homes, are concerned with improving or maintaining the health of clients. With the policy of providing care in the community rather than hospital, the role of social services departments in promoting the health of vulnerable groups such as older people, people with mental health problems and people with learning difficulties has increased greatly (see http://www.direct.gov.uk for the range of social services available).

Many other local authority staff have a health promotion role, such as recreation and leisure officers, housing officers, regeneration, youth and community workers, trading standards and community safety officers.

OTHER LOCAL ORGANISATIONS AND GROUPS

There are numerous individuals and groups at local level who help to promote particular aspects of health. Some notable ones are described here.

HIGHER EDUCATION INSTITUTES

Universities are responsible for the basic training of health promotion professionals. They are also involved in post-basic and continuing education for health promoters, including running postgraduate diplomas and masters level courses (König 2008).

VOLUNTARY AND COMMUNITY GROUPS

A huge range of voluntary and community groups exists that undertake education and support activities on health matters. Patients' associations, self-help groups, environmental action groups and youth groups are just a few examples. The importance of the voluntary sector in health improvement is demonstrated by the government's commitment to funding these organisations (Jerrom 2007).

EMPLOYERS

Employers can be active in developing and implementing health promoting policies in the workplace. Human resource officers and occupational health staff, in particular, are vital to implementing the government's *The Health, Work and Well-being Strategy* (Department for Work and Pensions et al 2005).

POLICE AND PROBATION OFFICERS

The police protect the public from crime and violence, take action to prevent misuse of drugs and alcohol and help to ensure road safety. Prison officers and probation officers are involved in the health and wellbeing of prisoners and their families, and may be involved in initiatives such as health promoting prisons (DoH 2002), education about HIV/AIDS, and educational programmes on sensible drinking for drink/drive offenders.

FIRE FIGHTERS

The fire service has a key role to play in preventing injuries at home and on the roads; they may run innovative projects such as schemes inviting people to bring in electric blankets for a safety check (http://www.fireservice.co.uk).

IMPROVING YOUR HEALTH PROMOTION ROLE

A number of factors affect the development of the health promotion role of professionals. The need for building capacity and capability is recognised (WHO 2005, Scriven & Spellar 2007), but one of the difficulties is how to fit more into the already crowded curriculum of basic professional training courses.

Postgraduate diplomas and masters degrees in health education, health promotion and public health are available, often in a range of learning modes. More recently, training in health promotion is being adapted to meet the public health occupational standards of competence and to move towards a professional registration system for those who want to work in a specialist capacity in health promotion.

See Chapter 2 for details of the national occupational standards relevant to health promotion.

All these developments help to ensure the quality of health promotion work. Resource constraints caused by staff shortages or work overload may hinder the professions from achieving their potential in health promotion. On a positive note, some strategies, such as partnership working, will improve the capacity in health promotion. The continued building of multiprofessional understanding, partnerships and capabilities and pulling together of the different professional groups under the banner of health promotion is vital to future success (Scriven 2005).

Exercise 4.2 is designed to enable you identify factors that help and hinder you in carrying out health promotion work, and consider what you might do to improve the situation.

PRACTICE POINTS

- It is important to appreciate the whole range of agents and agencies with a health promotion role: informal and formal, local, national and international.
- Think about how you can best work with other people and agencies.
- Ensure that you are clear about your role and responsibilities in health promotion.
- Consider how you could improve your health promotion role, through education and training or through identifying what helps and hinders your health promotion work and how the situation could be improved.

EXERCISE 4.2   What helps and hinders your health promotion work?

This exercise is designed to help you identify helping and hindering forces in your own situation.

In a stable system, the forces for producing changes are balanced by forces opposed to change. It is essential to pinpoint all the possible helping and hindering forces, so that you can take steps to increase the power of helping forces and decrease the power of hindering forces. The disruption of the balance results in progress towards change.

For your own situation:

■ Make a list of forces that *help you* in your health promotion work.

■ Make a list of forces that *hinder you* in your health promotion work.

■ Identify ways of *increasing the helpful forces.*

■ Identify ways of *decreasing the hindering forces.*

helping forces

	→	health	←	
helping forces	→	promotion	←	hindering forces
	→	work	←	

→

Direction you want to go

References

Armstrong M, Anderson C, Blenkinsopp A, Lewis R 2005 Promoting health through community pharmacies. In: Scriven A (ed.) Health promoting practice: the contribution of nurses and allied health professions. Basingstoke, Palgrave.

Barbeau EM, Goldman R, Roelofs C et al 2005 A new channel for health promotion: building trade unions. American Journal of Health Promotion 19(4): 297–303.

Commission of the European Communities 2007 Together for health: a strategic approach for the EU 2008–2013. Brussels, Commission of the European Communities.

Department for Children, Schools and Families 2007 Teenage parents' next steps: guidance for local authorities and primary care trusts. London, The Stationery Office.

Department of Health 1990 National Health Service and Community Care Act. London, HMSO.

Department of Health 1992 The health of the nation. London, HMSO.

Department of Health 1997 The new NHS: modern, dependable. London, The Stationery Office.

Department of Health 1999 Saving lives: our healthier nation. London, The Stationery Office.

Department of Health 2000 The NHS plan: a plan for investment, a plan for reform. London, The Stationery Office.

Department of Health 2001 Shifting the balance of power within the NHS – securing delivery. London, The Stationery Office.

Department of Health 2002 Health promoting prisons: a shared approach. London, The Stationery Office.

Department of Health 2004 Choosing health: making healthier choices easier. London, The Stationery Office.

Department of Health 2006 Developing the patient advice & liaison service: key messages for NHS organisations from the national evaluation of PALS. London, The Stationery Office.

Department of Health 2007 Tackling health inequalities 2004–2006 data and policy update for the 2010 national target. London, The Stationery Office.

Department of Health 2008a Drugs: protecting families and communities. London, The Stationery Office.

Department of Health 2008b High quality care for all: NHS next stage review final report. London, The Stationery Office.

Department of Health 2008c Improving health: changing behaviour – NHS health trainer handbook. London, The Stationery Office.

Department of Health/Department for Education and Skills 2008 Common themes – local strategic partnerships and teenage pregnancies. London, The Stationery Office.

Department of Health/NHS Modernisation Board 2003 The NHS plan – a progress report. London, The Stationery Office.

Department of Health/Scottish Office 1997 Designed to care: renewing the National Health Service in Scotland. London, The Stationery Office.

Department of Health/Welsh Assembly Government 2005 Shaping the future of public health: promoting health in the NHS. London, The Stationery Office.

Department for Work and Pensions, Department of Health, Health and Safety Executive 2005 The health, work and wellbeing strategy – caring for our future: a strategy for the health and wellbeing of working age people. London, The Stationery Office.

Hill F 2003 Complementary and alternative medicine: the next generation of health promotion? Health Promotion International 18(3): 265–272.

House of Commons 2002 Select Committee on Environment, Food and Rural Affairs ninth report. http://www.parliament.the-stationery-office.com/pa/cm200102/cmselect/cmenvfru/550/55017.htm.

Hubley H, Copeman J 2008 Mass media. In: Hubley H, Copeman J (eds) Practical health promotion. Cambridge, Polity Press.

Jerrom C 2007 Ivan Lewis pledges £25m for voluntary sector health and social care projects. http://www.communitycare.co.uk/Articles/2007/01/30/103089/ivan-lewis-pledges-25m-for-voluntary-sector-health-and-social-care-projects.html.

König C 2008 Higher education in health promotion in Europe: a comparative analysis of master's level training programmes using HP-Source.net. Promotion & Education 15(1): 30–35.

Korp P 2006 Health on the Internet: implications for health promotion. Health Education Research 21(1): 78–86.

Kramish Campbell M, Allicock Hudson M, Resnicow K et al 2007 Church-based health promotion interventions: evidence and lessons learned. Annual Review of Public Health 28: 213–234.

Kula M 2007 GPs are crucial to health promotion. http://www.healthcarerepublic.com//news/index.cfm?fuseaction=HCR.RSS.Education.registrar.Article&nNewsID=764593#Add Comment.

Scriven A 2005 Health promoting practice: the contribution of nurses and allied health professions. Basingstoke, Palgrave.

Scriven A, Spellar V 2007 Global issues and challenges beyond Ottawa: the way forward. Promotion and Education 14(4): 194–198, 255–259, 269–273.

Weeks J, Scriven A, Sayer L 2005 The health promoting role of heath visitors: adjunct or synergy? In: Scriven A (ed.) Health promoting practice: the contribution of nurses and allied health professions. Basingstoke, Palgrave.

Whitehead D 2005a The culture, context and progress of health promotion in nursing. In: Scriven A (ed.) Health promoting practice: the contribution of nurses and allied health professions. Basingstoke, Palgrave.

Whitehead D 2005b Hospital nursing based osteoporosis prevention study: action research in action. In: Scriven A (ed.) Health promoting practice: the contribution of nurses and allied health professions. Basingstoke, Palgrave.

World Health Organization 1978 Declaration of Alma Ata. Geneva, WHO.

World Health Organization 1986 Ottawa charter for health promotion. Geneva, WHO.

World Health Organization 2005 Bangkok charter for health promotion. Geneva, WHO.

Websites

http://www.apho.org.uk
http://www.apho.org.uk/resource/view.aspx?QN=P_HEALTH_PROFILES
http://www.heacons.idea.gov.uk
http://www.beacons.idea.gov.uk/idx/core/page.do?pageId=72385
http://www.bma.org.uk
http://www.cabinetoffice.gov.uk
http://www.cabinetoffice.gov.uk/social_exclusion_task_force.aspx
http://www.cieh.org
http://www.cieh.org/policy.html
http://www.communities.gov.uk
http://www.cymru.gov.uk
http://www.dh.gov.uk/en/Managingyourorganisation
http://www.dh.gov.uk/en/Managingyourorganisation/Commissioning/Worldclasscommissioning/DH_083204

http://www.dh.gov.uk/en/Publicationsandstatistics
http://www.dh.gov.uk/en/Publichealth
http://www.dh.gov.uk/en/Publichealth/Healthinequalities/HealthTrainersusefullinks/DH_6590
http://www.direct.gov.uk
http://www.direct.gov.uk/en/Hl1/Help/Socialservices/index.htm
http://www.eastherts.gov.uk/index.jsp?articleid=9305
http://www.epha.org
http://www.fireservice.co.uk
http://www.fireservice.co.uk/safety/electricblankets.php
http://www.foe.co.uk
http://www.fphm.org.uk
http://www.healthscotland.com
http://www.hse.gov.uk
http://www.ihpe.org.uk
http://www.iuhpe.org
http://www.iuhpe.org/?page=7&lang=en
http://www.mind.org.uk
http://www.neighbourhood.gov.uk
http://www.neighbourhood.gov.uk/page.asp?id=531
http://www.nhs.uk
http://www.nhs.uk/chq/Pages/1082.aspx?CategoryID=68&SubCategoryID=153
http://www.nhs.uk/NHSEngland/aboutnhs
http://www.nhs.uk/NHSEngland/aboutnhs/Pages/authoritiesandtrusts.aspx
http://www.nhs.uk/NHSEngland/aboutnhs/Pages/NHSstructure.aspx
http://www.nhs.uk/NHSEngland/AboutNHSservices
http://www.nhs.uk/NHSEngland/AboutNHSservices/Emergencyandurgentcareservices/Pages/Walk-incentresSummary.aspx
http://www.nhs.uk/Tools
http://www.nhs.uk/Tools/Pages/NHSTimeline.aspx
http://www.nhsdirect.nhs.uk

http://www.nice.org.uk

http://www.ohe.org/page/
knowledge/schools/hc_in_uk/
nhs_structure.cfm

http://www.publichealth.hscni.net

http://www.publicinvolvement.
org.uk

http://www.publicservice.co.uk

http://www.rcgp-curriculum.org.uk

http://www.rcn.org.uk

http://www.rsph.org.uk

http://www.rsph.org.uk/en/
health-promotion

http://www.standards.dfes.gov.uk

http://www.standards.dfes.gov.uk/
schemes2/citizenship/sec_pshe

http://www.tacade.com

http://www.ukpha.org.uk

http://www.wales.gov.uk

http://www.wfpha.org

http://www.who.int

PART 2

Planning and managing for effective practice

PART CONTENTS

PART SUMMARY

Part 2 aims to provide guidance on how you can:

- Plan and evaluate your health promotion work using a basic framework.
- Identify the views and needs of the clients/users/ receivers of health promotion, and set priorities for your work.
- Link your work to the efforts of colleagues and to local and national strategies.
- Use an evidence-based approach, through using published research, doing your own research when necessary and auditing your work, thus ensuring that your efforts are effective and provide value for money.
- Organise yourself and manage your work in order to be effective and efficient.
- Develop skills to work more effectively with colleagues and people from other organisations.

Chapter 5 sets out a seven-stage planning and evaluation cycle, which will help you to clarify what you are trying to achieve, what you are going to do and how you will know whether you are succeeding. The meaning of terms such as aims, objectives and targets are discussed, and there is guidance on how to specify them.

Chapter 6 explains how to identify need, and describes the sources of information you require to establish the needs of a community, a group or an individual. Guidelines are provided on how to gather and apply information in order to assess needs and set priorities.

Chapter 7 provides an overview of the knowledge and skills required to plan health promotion activities effectively, including how to find and use published research. Guidance is included on how you can contribute to national and local public health strategic plans and complement what other people are doing. Evidence-based health promotion is discussed and advice offered on how you can carry out small-scale research, audit your activities and ensure value for money. The chapter ends with a description of the key steps required to undertake a health impact assessment.

Chapter 8 focuses on how you can develop the skills to manage yourself and your work effectively, including managing information, writing reports, using time effectively, planning project work, managing change and working for quality.

Chapter 9 is about how to work with other people, including communicating with colleagues, coordination and teamwork, participating in meetings and working in health partnerships with other organisations.

Chapter 5

Planning and evaluating health promotion

CHAPTER CONTENTS

SUMMARY

This chapter presents an outline of a planning and evaluation cycle for use in the everyday work of health promoters. It involves seven stages which include the measurement and specification of needs and priorities; the setting of aims and objectives; decisions on the best way of achieving aims; the identification of resources; the planning of evaluation methods and the establishment of an action plan followed by action. Examples are given of aims, objectives and action plans, and exercises are provided on setting aims and objectives and using the planning framework to turn ideas into action.

This chapter is about planning and evaluation at the level of your daily work in health promotion. It provides a basic framework for you to use to plan and evaluate your health promotion activities, whether you work with clients on a one-to-one or group basis, or undertake specific projects or programmes.

THE PLANNING PROCESS

Planning is a process that, at its very simplest, should give you the answers to three questions:

1. **What am I trying to achieve?** This question is concerned with identifying needs and priorities, then with being clear about your specific aims and objectives.
2. **What am I going to do?** This can be helpfully broken down into smaller steps:

- Select the best approach to achieving your aims.
- Identify the resources you are going to use.
- Set a clear action plan of who does what and when.

3. **How will I know whether I have been successful?** This question highlights the importance of evaluation and the integral part it plays in planning health promotion interventions. It should not be an afterthought or left too late to capture the information you need.

The planning process has been put together in the seven-stage flowchart in Fig. 5.1. The arrows on the flowchart lead you round in a circle. This is because, as you carry out your plan and evaluation, you will probably find things that make you re-think and change your original ideas. For example, things you might want to change could include: working on a need you found you had overlooked; scaling down your objectives because they were too ambitious; or changing the educational or publicity materials because you found that they were not as useful or effective as you had hoped. The direction of the arrows is anticlockwise, but in reality planning is not always an orderly process. You may actually

start at Stage 6, with a basic idea of a health promotion intervention. Thinking more about it may lead you to clarify exactly what your aims are (Stage 2). Next, you might think about what resources you are going to need (Stage 4) and realise that you do not have enough time or money to do what you had in mind, so you go back to Stage 2 and modify your aims. Then you think about the best way of achieving your aims (Stage 3) and work out an action plan (Stage 6). After that, you start to think seriously about how you will know whether you are successful (Stage 5) and you put your evaluation plans into your action plan (Stage 6 again). In effect, you are continually reviewing and improving your plan, using the framework appropriately to help you keep on course.

Planning takes place at many levels. If you are embarking on a major project, you will need to take time to plan it in depth and detail. If you are simply planning a short one-to-one session with a client you will still need to plan, and to go through all the stages, but the process might be quick and may not even be written down.

For example, a chiropodist seeing a patient with a foot care problem may identify that the patient needs knowledge and skills in cutting toenails correctly. They decide that their aim is to give the

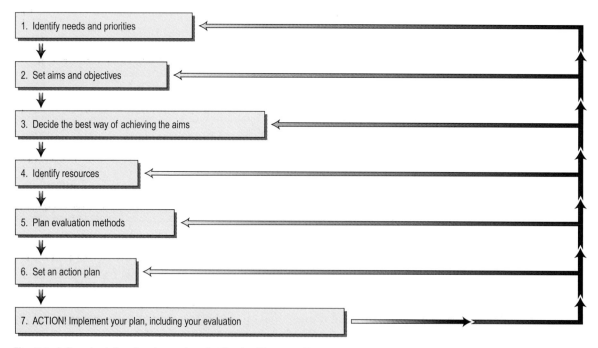

Fig. 5.1 A flowchart for planning and evaluating health promotion.

patient basic information and training on this. They will know if they have been successful by getting feedback from the patient about how they managed next time they see them. They identify an information leaflet that they can give the patient as reinforcement. They decide on an action plan of explanation, demonstration and then get the patient to practise. They review the patient's toenail cutting skills next time they see them, reinforcing or correcting as necessary. All this planning takes place inside the chiropodist's head, and is an integral part of their everyday professional practice.

THE PLANNING FRAMEWORK

STAGE 1: IDENTIFY NEEDS AND PRIORITIES

How do you find out what health promotion is needed? If you think you already know, what are you basing your judgement on? Who has identified the need: you, your clients or someone else? Identifying need is a complex process, which is looked at it in depth in the next chapter.

See Chapter 6.

You may have a long list of health promotion needs you would like to respond to, so another issue is how to establish your priorities. Again, this is discussed in detail in the next chapter, but an important point is that you must have a clear view about which needs you are responding to, and what your priorities are.

STAGE 2: SET AIMS AND OBJECTIVES

People use a range of words to describe statements about what they are trying to achieve, such as aims, objectives, targets, goals, mission, purpose, result, product, outcomes. It can be helpful to think of

them as forming a hierarchy as in Fig. 5.2. At the top of the hierarchy are words that tell you why your job exists, such as your job purpose or remit, or your overall mission. In the middle of the hierarchy are words that describe what you are trying to do in general terms, such as your goals or aims. At the bottom of the hierarchy are words that describe in specific detail what you are trying to do, such as targets or objectives.

It is worth noting that objectives can be of different kinds. *Health* objectives are usually expressed as the outcome or end state to be achieved in terms of health status, such as reduced rates of illness or death. However, in health promotion work objectives are often expressed in terms of a step along the way towards an ultimate improvement in the health of individuals or populations, such as increasing exercise levels.

In health education work, *educational* objectives are framed in terms of the knowledge, attitudes or behaviour to be exhibited by the learner. Objectives can also be in terms of other kinds of changes, for example a change in health policy (introducing a healthy eating policy in the workplace) or health promotion practice (providing health information in minority ethnic languages).

See the section below on setting educational objectives.

The term target is increasingly used in health promotion. Targets usually specify how the achievement of an objective will be *measured*, in terms of quantity, quality and time (the date by which the objective will be achieved). So a *health target* can be defined as a measurable improvement in health status, by a given date, which achieves a health objective. This is the approach used in national strategies for health, such as *Choosing Health: Making Healthier Choices Easier* (Department of Health (DoH) 2004) and in the *National service frameworks* (http://www.dh.gov.uk). An example of targets

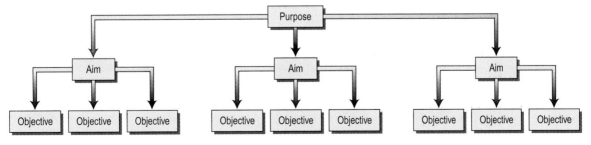

Fig. 5.2 A hierarchy of aims.

and ways of measuring progress can be found in the *Delivering Choosing Health: Making Healthier Choices Easier* (DoH 2005).

There is more about national strategies and targets in Chapter 7, section on national public health strategies.

The objectives are framed as *health objectives,* and the targets are framed as *health targets* (changes in rates of death or illness by a specific date), *behaviour targets* (such as changes in population rates of smoking or drinking by a specific date) or *progress measures* (such as the number of people attending a smoking cessation service and the number setting a date when they plan to stop smoking).

When you plan health promotion initiatives, you need to set aims, objectives and targets or goals and outcomes.

Your aims (or aim, as there does not have to be more than one) are broad statements of what you are trying to achieve. Your objectives are much more specific, and setting these is a critical stage in the planning process.

Objectives are the desired end state (or result, or outcome) to be achieved within a specified time period. They are not tasks or activities. Objectives should be as follows:

- **Challenging.** The objective should provide you with a health promotion challenge in relation to what needs to be achieved.
- **Attainable.** On the other hand, it should be both realistic and achievable within the constraints of your situation.
- **Relevant.** It should be consistent with the aims of the organisation and with the overall aims of your job.
- **Measurable.** You should try to identify objectives that are measurable, for example specifying quantity, quality and a time when they will be achieved. For instance (using the example in Exercise 5.1), an objective of 'to improve access to health information through the use of videos…' has been improved by working out the appropriate number of videos and languages, and then specifying the target as 'to have ten videos in six languages…'

It is sometimes difficult to distinguish between aims, objectives and action plans. For example, a dietician who wants to improve the information they give to patients may describe their aim as 'to produce an information leaflet' but this is also their objective and their action plan. The answer is to

---

EXERCISE 5.1   Clarifying your purpose, aims and objectives

Read this example of a health promoter's purpose, aims and objectives.

Mark is a health promoter working for a local authority. His *purpose* is to reduce inequalities in health in the population living and working in the borough. To do this, one of his *aims* is to improve levels of health knowledge of the black and ethnic minority groups. One of his *objectives* is to improve access to health information through the use of videos. He sets a target of having a selection of ten health videos in six languages available in 25 shops within 4 months.

Now:
1. Thinking of your own job, write down what you believe to be its mission or purpose.
2. Then give an example of one of the health promotion aims you are trying to achieve.
3. Finally, give an example of an objective you are trying to achieve, in fulfillment of the aim you selected.

If you can't find an example from your practice, make up an example of what you would like to do if you had the opportunity.

---

think it through further, and ask 'Why produce a leaflet? What am I aiming to achieve by producing the leaflet?' It then becomes clearer that the aim is to improve patient compliance with dietary treatment, and one of the objectives is to improve patients' understanding of their dietary instructions. The action is to produce the leaflet. The importance of actually thinking through your aims and objectives in this way is that it helps you to be absolutely clear about *why* you are doing something, not just *what* you are doing. Failure to think through this stage means that health promoters waste time and energy proceeding with what seems like a good idea only to realise, too late, that what they are doing is not actually achieving what they want.

Setting educational objectives

If your health promotion activity is based on a health education approach, it is useful to plan in terms of *educational* objectives.

Educationalists traditionally often think of objectives (sometimes called learning outcomes) in terms of what the clients will gain. Furthermore, the objectives are considered to be of three kinds: what the educator would like the clients to *know*, *feel* and *do* as a result of the education. In the language of the educationalist, these may be referred to as cognitive, affective and behavioural objectives.

Objectives about 'knowing'

These are concerned with giving information, explaining it, ensuring that the client understands it, and thus increasing the client's knowledge: for example, explaining the weight loss advantages of increasing exercise levels to someone who is obese. Here the objective would be to develop in the client an understanding of the value of exercise with regard to their weight loss programme to enable them to make informed choices in terms of their weight loss strategies.

Objectives about 'feeling'

These objectives are concerned with attitudes, beliefs, values and opinions. These are complex psychological concepts, but the important feature to note now is that they are all concerned with how people feel. Objectives about feelings are about clarifying, forming or changing attitudes, beliefs, values or opinions. In the example above, when the health promoter is educating a client about exercise and weight loss, in addition to the knowledge objective, there may be an objective about helping the client to explore their attitude towards exercise and any values, beliefs or opinions that might be forming a barrier to increasing exercise levels.

Objectives about 'doing'

These objectives are concerned with a client's skills and actions. For example, teaching a routine of aerobic or yoga exercises has the objective that clients acquire practical skills and are able to do exercise-related specific tasks.

In the health education approach to health promotion, a combination of the knowing, feeling or doing educational objectives is usually required. For example, when a health visitor is advising a parent about feeding their toddler, they may be planning to achieve the following objectives within three home visits:

- The objective of ensuring that the parent knows which foods constitute a healthy eating programme for their child and which are best given in restricted amounts.

- The objective of changing the parent's erroneous belief that sugar is essential to give their child energy, and relieving their anxiety that their healthy child's food fads may cause serious ill health.
- The objective that the parent learns what to do at meal times when her child has a tantrum about eating.

To summarise the key points about setting aims and objectives:

- The focus is on what you are trying to achieve.
- Be as specific as possible. Avoid vague or subjective notions of what you want to achieve.
- Express your objectives in ways that can be measured. How much? How many? When?
- Do not get bogged down in terminology. It does not matter whether you talk about goals, aims, objectives, targets or outcomes. The key principle is to be very clear about what you are trying to achieve.

In order to practise setting aims and objectives, undertake Exercise 5.1 and Exercise 5.2.

STAGE 3: DECIDE THE BEST WAY OF ACHIEVING THE AIMS

Occasionally, there might be only one possible way of accomplishing your aims and objectives. Usually, however, there will be a range of options. In Case study 5.1 Jim has a number of options about how to achieve his objective of increasing the sun safety measures being taken by the school and the children. He could write to the schools or to parents of school-age children, he could hand out leaflets at school gates, he could lobby parents to take up the cause, he could find out if there are any school governors' meetings and ask to speak at them, he could conduct a sun safety campaign in the local media, he could write an article on the issue of sun safety in school playgrounds for the education journals that teachers read, or he could try to meet each Head Teacher face-to-face. Or he could do two or more of these together.

Health promoters such as Jim in Case study 5.1 and Sue in Case study 5.2 are faced with the problem of how to identify the best strategy for achieving their objectives. Factors to consider include:

- Which methods are the most appropriate and effective in meeting your aims and objectives?

CASE STUDY 5.1

Jim is an environmental health officer. His project is to tackle sun safety in schools. This fits in with the overall purpose of his job, which is to ensure safer environments. Jim works out that his *aim* is to work with local schools to set up a scheme that will result in sun safety measures being taken by the school and the children. He researches the subject in detail, looking at the results achieved from similar projects and working out how much time and money it is likely to take. He then decides that it is reasonable to set his *objective* as follows:

■ Within 6 months to have raised awareness of the feasibility and advantages of developing shaded play areas with 10 primary schools, and worked with at least five to set up shaded areas.

EXERCISE 5.2   Setting aims and objectives

Yewtree scheme

The three practices at Yewtree Health Centre have agreed to establish physical activity assessment sessions, backed up by a display in the shared waiting area, with the aim of reducing the incidence of coronary heart disease in the practice populations.

The detailed objectives are:

1. To raise the users' awareness of the link between inadequate exercise and coronary heart disease, and the part which individuals can play in reducing their own vulnerability to the disease.
2. To assess, and advise about, individuals' physical fitness levels and help them to prepare an appropriate exercise action programme based on those results.
3. To monitor and evaluate, on a continuing basis, the effectiveness of the fitness testing, in respect of the resources involved and the reduction in vulnerability to heart disease.

Ask yourself the following questions:

1. Do the objectives match the characteristics of objectives described above? Are they challenging, attainable, as measurable as possible and relevant?
2. How would you suggest changing the objectives?

● Which methods will be most acceptable to the individual or population group?
● Which methods will be easiest?
● Which methods are cheapest?
● Which methods do you find comfortable to use?

There is more about evidence for success, cost-effectiveness and value for money in Chapter 7, and Part 3 of this book covers how to use these methods to develop the necessary competency.

Looking at the first of these questions about which methods are most appropriate and effective for

CASE STUDY 5.2

Sue is a nurse specialising in coronary care. Her project is to run patient education programmes so that discharged patients know how to look after themselves. This fits in with the overall purpose of her job, which is to care for patients while they are in hospital, and maximise their chances of a healthy life following discharge.

Sue decides that her *aim* is that patients will have participated in a cardiac rehabilitation programme for post-heart attack patients. Her *objectives* are:

■ That every patient, before leaving hospital, knows what they are advised to do about diet, exercise, smoking and stress control.
■ That every patient will be confident and competent to put this advice into practice.
■ That every patient, and their carers and relatives, will have had an opportunity to discuss questions and anxieties with a qualified member of the staff.

Sue's programme is a continuous course of group sessions each week, with each session focusing on a specific issue. So each individual session also has a set of objectives. Objectives for the session on 'Eating well when you go home', for example, include:

■ Patients will understand the basic principles of a healthy diet: low fat, low salt, low sugar and high fibre.
■ Patients will know which foods they can eat in unlimited amounts, which they should restrict and which they should avoid.
■ Patients will know what their ideal weight should be.
■ Patients who are overweight will have devised a personal weight loss plan.

your aims, there is an accumulated body of evidence that helps to identify effective methods for particular aims at the National Institute for Health and Clinical Evidence (NICE) (http://www.nice.org.uk) and at the Cochrane Database of Systematic Reviews (http://www.cochrane.org). (See also http://www.who.int.) Table 5.1 identifies the range of aims, grouped into categories, and the appropriate and effective methods for achieving them. This provides a general guideline, to which there may be exceptions.

Table 5.1	Aims and methods in health promotion	
AIM	APPROPRIATE METHOD
Health awareness goal	Talks
Raising awareness, or	Group work
consciousness, of	Mass media
health issues	Displays and exhibitions
	Campaigns
Improving knowledge	One-to-one teaching
Providing information	Displays and exhibitions
	Written materials
	Mass media (including the Internet)
	Campaigns
	Group teaching
Self-empowering	Group work
Improving self-	Practising decision making
awareness,	Values clarification
self-esteem,	Social skills training
decision making	Simulation, gaming and role play
	Assertiveness training
	Counselling
Changing attitudes	Group work
and behaviour	Skills training
Changing the lifestyles	Self-help groups
of individuals	One-to-one advice and instruction
	Group or individual therapy
	Written material
	Social marketing approach
Societal/environmental	Positive action for under-served
change	groups
Changing the physical	Lobbying for fiscal and legislative
or social	change
environment	Pressure groups
	Community development
	Community-based work
	Advocacy schemes
	Environmental measures
	Planning and policy making
	Organisational change
	Enforcement of laws and
	regulations

You may have decided on more than one of these categories of aims. For example, the inputs that contribute towards changing the behaviour of individuals can be complemented by societal changes, so that together they are more effective than either intervention alone by creating synergy. So, for example, to reduce the over-consumption of alcohol by young people, you could:

● Provide health education about alcohol as part of schools' personal and social education programmes.
● Provide educational rehabilitation programmes for young drink-drive offenders.
● Work with young people to promote the social acceptability of consuming nonalcoholic drinks.
● Lobby for an increase in alcohol taxation or for increasing the age at which young people can buy alcohol.

The example in Fig. 5.3 shows the range of aims and methods that might be used to promote healthy eating. These may not all be used by a health promoter at any one time, but they are given here to illustrate the range of possibilities.

STAGE 4: IDENTIFY RESOURCES

What resources are you going to use? You have to establish what resources you are going to need and what are already available, what additional resources you are going to have to acquire, and whether you will need extra funding. A number of different kinds of resources can be identified.

Professional input

Your experience, knowledge, skills, time, enthusiasm and energy are vital resources. It helps to identify all the other professional and lay people with something to offer. This may include colleagues and others in your professional networks with relevant expertise that can advise and help you make your plans, clerical and secretarial staff that can help with administration, technicians, graphic designers and artists who can help with exhibitions, displays and teaching/publicity materials.

Your client or client group

These are another key resource. Clients may have knowledge, skills, enthusiasm, energy and time,

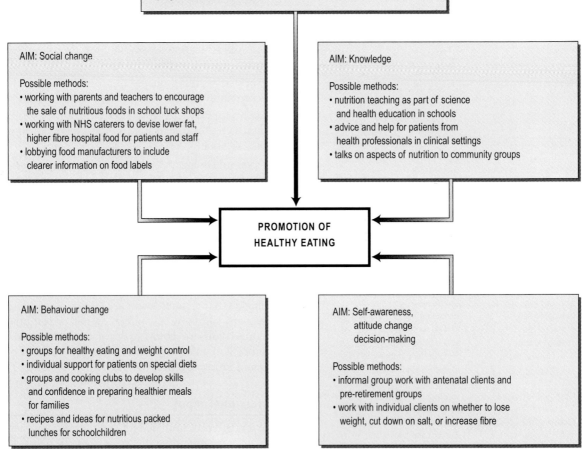

Fig. 5.3 Aims and methods for the promotion of healthy eating.

which can be used and built upon. In a group, clients can share their knowledge and previous experience and in this way help each other to learn and change. An ex-client can be a very valuable resource too. For example, someone who has successfully lost weight, an ex-smoker or a person who has undergone a particular health-related experience can be a great help to clients who are grappling with similar problems and experiences.

People who influence your client or client group

These may include clients' relatives, friends, volunteers, patients' associations and self-help groups. It may also be possible to harness the help of significant people in the community who are regarded as opinion leaders or trendsetters, such as political figures, religious leaders or media celebrities.

Existing policies and public health strategies

National and local policies and strategies for public health are useful to locate in terms of the work that you are planning. If, for example, you are planning to develop an intervention to help prevent the spread of sexually transmitted infections and HIV and reduce unwanted pregnancies, find out if there is already a policy on promoting sexual health in your area. Also find out whether your work fits into the *National Strategy for Sexual Health and HIV* (DoH 2001) and use the associated national guidance and evaluation reports to inform your work (such as Medical Foundation for AIDS and Sexual Health 2008).

> National and local plans, which your work could contribute to, are discussed in Chapter 7.

Existing facilities and services

Find out what relevant local facilities already exist and whether they are fully utilised; for example, sports centres offering facilities for exercise and local classes or groups on cooking for healthy eating.

Material resources

These might include leaflets, posters and display/publicity materials or, if you are planning health promotion involving group work, you need resources such as rooms, space, seats, audiovisual equipment and teaching/learning materials.

STAGE 5: PLAN EVALUATION METHODS

How will you measure success and know whether your health promotion is successful? Sophisticated methods are required to evaluate large-scale health promotion interventions. However, this should not deter health promoters; less complex methods of evaluating the everyday practice of health promotion can, and should, be used routinely.

What is meant by evaluation?

Evaluation is about making a judgement about the value of a health promotion intervention, whether it is a health education programme, for example, a community project or an awareness-raising campaign to change local policy. Evaluation is the process of assessing *what* has been achieved and *how* it has been achieved. It means looking critically at the activity or programme, working out what were its strengths and its weaknesses, and how it could be improved.

The judgement can be about the *outcome* (what has been achieved): whether you achieved the objectives which you set. So, for example, you should judge whether people understood the recommended limits for alcohol consumption as a result of your sensible drinking education, whether people in a particular community became more articulate about their health needs as a result of your community empowerment work, whether you achieved media coverage for your health campaign, etc.

Judgements can also be about the *process* (how it has been achieved): whether the most appropriate methods were used, whether they were used in the most effective way and whether they gave value for money. So, for example, you could consider whether the video-based discussion you used in your teaching programme was the best teaching method to use, whether the community development approach you chose was the most appropriate one in the circumstances, or whether you would have achieved more public awareness with less money if you had opted for a media stunt with possible free news coverage rather than an expensive advertising and leaflet campaign.

Key terms often used in discussions about evaluation are defined in the Glossary at the end of this book (see also Green & South 2007).

Why evaluate?

You need to be clear about why you are evaluating your work, because this will affect the way you do it and the amount of effort you put in. Some reasons could be:

● To improve your own practice: next time you deliver a similar intervention, you will build on your successes and learn from any mistakes.
● To help other people to improve their practice: if you disseminate your evaluation, it can help others improve their practice as well. It is vital to publicise failures as well as successes.
● To justify the use of the resources that went into the intervention, and to provide evidence to support the case for doing this type of health promotion in the future.

- To give you the satisfaction of knowing how useful or effective your work has been; in other words, for your own job satisfaction.
- To identify any unplanned or unexpected outcomes that could be important. For example, a publicity campaign to deter young people from taking drugs could have the opposite effect by unwittingly glamorising drug-taking and making it appear to be a more common activity than it really is.

Who is the evaluation for?

Who will be using your evaluation data? The answer to this affects what questions you ask, how much depth and detail you go into and how you present the information.

If you are solely assessing how well a health promotion intervention went, for your own benefit so you can change it appropriately next time you run a similar session, you will simply make a judgement on how you think it went based on your observation and the clients' reactions, and make a few notes. But if you are writing a report for your manager or for a body that you want to fund the work, you need to think through what questions those people will expect to be answered, and how much detail they will want.

For example, a group of health visitors evaluating a pilot scheme for a telephone advisory service at evenings and weekends need an evaluation report after 6 months for their manager, who is funding the service. What will the manager need to know? At the very least, they will probably need a clear indication of the use made of the service. This might include how many people used it, the characteristics of the users (for example, whether they were first-time parents), how much it was used, what sort of issues people rang about, what the clients gained from it and how much it cost. It would be helpful for the health visitors to ask their manager what evaluation data will be required at the planning stage of the project, so that the appropriate data can be collected from the start.

Assessing the outcome

Looking first at outcome measures, which are called summative evaluation, you need to go back to the objectives you set, and plan how you are going to determine whether you have achieved the objectives. Objectives are about the changes the

intervention was designed to achieve and might have included changes in people's knowledge or behaviour or changes in policies or ways of working. Long-term health promotion projects may also have objectives about changes in health status. The following list indicates the kinds of changes that may be reflected in your objectives, and what methods you might use to assess or measure those changes.

Changes in health awareness can be assessed by:
- Measuring the interest shown by consumers, for example how many people took up offers of leaflets, how many people enquired about preventive services, how many people visited a website.
- Monitoring changes in demand for health-related services.
- Analysis of media coverage.
- Questionnaires, interviews, focus group discussion, observation with individuals or groups.

Changes in knowledge or attitude can be assessed by:
- Observing changes in what clients say and do: does this show a change in understanding and attitude?
- Interviews and discussions involving question-and-answer between health promoter and clients.
- Discussion and observation on how clients apply knowledge to real-life situations and how they solve problems.
- Observing how clients demonstrate their knowledge of newly acquired skills.
- Written tests or questionnaires that require clients to answer questions about what they know. The results can be compared with those of tests taken before the health promotion activity or from a comparable group that has not received the health promotion.

Behaviour change can be assessed by:
- Observing clients' behaviour.
- Recording behaviour. This could be based on records, such as numbers attending a smoking cessation clinic or clients keeping a diary which is used at the end to assess behaviour change. It could be a periodical inventory, such as a follow-up questionnaire or interview to check on smoking habits 6 and 12 months after attending the smoking cessation clinic. Records

of client behaviour can be compared with those of comparable groups in other areas, or with national average figures.

Policy changes can be assessed by:
- Policy statements and implementation, such as increased introduction of healthy eating choices in workplaces and schools.
- Legislative changes, such as increased restriction on alcohol advertising.
- Changes in the availability of health promoting products, facilities and services such as exercise prescription schemes.
- Changes in procedures or organisation, such as more time being given to patient education.

Changes to the physical environment can be assessed by:
- Measuring changes in such things as air quality, traffic or pedestrian flows or the amount of open green space available to the public within a defined area.

Changes in health status can be assessed by:
- Keeping records of simple health indicators such as weight, blood pressure rates, pulse rates on standard exercise, or cholesterol levels.
- Health surveys to identify larger scale changes in health behaviour or self-reported health status.
- Analysis of trends in routine health statistics such as infant mortality rates or hospital admission rates.

It will be seen from this list that common evaluative methods are the generation of data from observation, holding discussions and distributing questionnaires and data analysis of health and other records.

Help with these is in Chapter 7, section on doing your own small-scale research, and Part 3 of this book.

Assessing the process

Assessing intervention processes, or formative evaluation, is an important aspect of a comprehensive evaluation of health promotion activities (see Parry-Langdon et al 2003 for an overview of process evaluations in health promotion). This requires examining what went on during the process of implementation, and making judgements about effectiveness and efficiency. Was it done as cheaply and quickly as possible? Was the quality as good as you wished? Were the appropriate methods and materials used? You may, for instance, achieve your objectives, but in a time-consuming, costly or inefficient way, so it is important to evaluate the process as well as identify whether you have achieved your desired outcome. Formative evaluation can be ongoing so that changes can be made to the intervention if it is found not to be working while it is in the process of delivery.

How are you going to assess the process? There are key aspects to process evaluation which involve measuring the input, self-evaluation by asking yourself questions and getting feedback from other people.

Measuring the input
This is essential if you are going to make judgements about whether the outcome was worthwhile. You need to record everything that went into your health promotion activity, in terms of time, money and materials. Then you can make an informed judgement about cost–benefit and whether the outcome justified the cost.

Self-evaluation
Ask yourself 'What did I do well?', 'What would I like to change?' and 'How could I improve that next time?' All kinds of health promotion approaches can be subjected to process evaluation, whether it is a one-to-one health education intervention with a client, facilitating a self-help group, undertaking community empowerment work, developing and implementing a health policy or lobbying for organisational and structural changes.

An important point to note about self-evaluation is the need for a balanced objective critique which highlights both the positive and the negative aspects. Identify the things that have worked and look for constructive ways forward about things that could be improved.

Feedback from other people
Giving and receiving feedback is an essential skill for every health promoter. Getting feedback from a trusted colleague on your health promotion initiatives is a valuable form of peer evaluation. Asking for, and getting, feedback from your manager should be part of the regular monitoring of your performance.

See section in Chapter 10 on asking questions and getting feedback.

Obtaining feedback from the clients or users themselves should also be part of assessing the process of every intervention. The important thing is to encourage a nonjudgemental atmosphere of openness and honesty. It can be done in many ways; simply observing clients and users accurately is an important tool. Do they look anxious or relaxed? Do they look interested and alert or bored and detached? You can also ask for feedback in such ways as a suggestions box, through noting any spontaneous verbal feedback you receive or through asking questions.

STAGE 6: SET AN ACTION PLAN

Now that you know:

- what you are trying to achieve and have identified the best way to go about it
- how to evaluate it
- what resources you need

you can get down to planning in detail exactly what you are going to do. This means writing a detailed statement of who will do what, with what resources and by when.

It is helpful, especially if you are tackling a large project, to break down your plan into smaller, manageable elements. One way of doing this is by thinking in terms of *key events*. Draw up a schedule showing the key events that are planned to happen at particular points in time. The schedule should specify deadlines that must be met by the people involved. Another way of breaking down a large project is by *milestone* planning. This is different from key events planning: instead of listing events, it lists a series of significant dates at fixed intervals (the milestones) and shows what must have happened by each of them. Box 5.1 illustrates both types of action plans.

For more discussion about the skills of project management, see Chapter 8, section on managing project work.

STAGE 7: ACTION!

This is the stage in which you actually *do* your health promotion, remembering to evaluate the process as you go along.

Exercise 5.3 gives you the opportunity to apply this planning framework.

To summarise, the planning process consists of a series of stages which enable you to more systematically organise your health promotion work by focusing on key questions around What? Why? When? Who? Where? and How? Useful additional reading to support planning and evaluation are Rootman et al (2001), Tones & Tilford (2001), Thorogood & Coombes (2004), Tones & Green (2004), Nutbeam & Bauman (2006) and Green & South (2007). Finally, the National Social Marketing Centre also provides a planning model (see Chapter

---

BOX 5.1   Action plans

A **key events plan** drawn up by a health promoter who plans to set up a health stall in a local supermarket could look like this:
1. *Discuss with my manager* at October meeting.
2. *Identify support from colleagues* by November.
3. *Approach supermarket manager* (before Christmas rush); agree space and times.
4. *Convene planning group* of colleagues in January to sort out who will do what and when, and evaluate plans, and identify the resources required.
5. *Set up first stall* in March.

A brief **milestone plan** for the early stages of setting up a community health project could be like this, in a framework of 3-monthly 'milestones':

January–March 2003	Steering group agrees job description for community health worker. Job advertised.
By end of June 2003	Interviews; appointment made. Community worker takes up post.
By end of September 2003	Community worker induction programme completed.
By end of December 2003	First progress report to Steering Group.

EXERCISE 5.3 Ideas into action: planning a health promotion project

Work alone or in a small group.

Think of an area of health promotion where there is an identified need, and it is within the remit of your job to meet that need. It could be an established area of work such as antenatal education, smoking cessation, teaching food hygiene, or an area of new work you would like to tackle. If you are not currently in a job which involves health promotion, think of a health-related project you would like to tackle in your personal life, or a project for any voluntary/community group you are associated with, or just imagine what you would like to do if you had the opportunity.

Work through the following stages of the planning cycle. Start by writing each of the following headings at the top of a separate large sheet of paper, and then work through them:

1. **Aims and objectives**
   Ask yourself 'What am I trying to achieve?' Identify your broad aim, or aims, then be more specific and identify your objectives.

2. **The best way of achieving my aims**
   Think of all the ways in which you could achieve your aims and identify the best way.

3. **Resources**
   Identify the resources you already have available and any extra ones you will need.

4. **Evaluation**
   Ask yourself 'How will I know if I am succeeding?' Identify how you will evaluate both the process and outcome of your work.

5. **Action plan**
   Identify who will do what, with what resources, and by when.

Be aware that when you are thinking about one section, it may have implications for the others, so you may find yourself going back to modify and refine what you have already written.

---

3) and tools for planning on their website (http://www.nsms.org.uk).

PRACTICE POINTS

- Health promotion work benefits from being planned and evaluated in a systematic way.
- A planning cycle should ensure that needs and priorities are identified, aims and objectives are clearly set and methods for achieving aims and objectives are carefully considered in the context of available resources.
- Evaluation is an important component of the planning process and evaluation methods should be formative and measure the process, and summative, measuring the outcome of health promotion interventions.

References

Department of Health 2001 Better prevention, better services, better sexual health – the national strategy for sexual health and HIV. London, The Stationery Office.

Department of Health 2004 Choosing health: making healthier choices easier. London, The Stationery Office.

Department of Health 2005 Delivering choosing health: making healthier choices easier. London, The Stationery Office.

Green J, South J 2007 Evaluation. Berkshire, Open University Press.

Medical Foundation for AIDS and Sexual Health 2008 Progress and priorities – working together for higher quality sexual health. London, MedFASH.

Nutbeam D, Bauman A 2006 Evaluation in a nutshell: a practical guide to the evaluation of health promotion programs. Maidenhead, McGraw-Hill Medical.

Parry-Langdon N, Bloor M, Audrey S, Holliday J 2003 Process evaluation of health promotion interventions. Policy & Politics 31(2): 207–216.

Rootman I, Goodstadt M, Hyndman B et al (eds) 2001 Evaluation in health promotion: principles and perspectives. WHO Regional Publications, European Series, No 92. Denmark, World Health Organization.

Thorogood M, Coombes Y 2004 Evaluating health promotion: practice and methods. Oxford, Oxford University Press.

Tones K, Green J 2004 Health
  promotion: planning and strategies.
  London, Sage.
Tones K, Tilford S 2001 Health
  promotion – effectiveness, efficiency
  and equity, 3rd edn. Cheltenham,
  Nelson Thornes.

Websites

http://www.cochrane.org/reviews
http://www.dh.gov.uk/en/
  Healthcare/DH_082787
http://www.nice.org.uk
http://www.nsms.org.uk
http://www.who.int

Chapter 6

Identifying health promotion needs and priorities

CHAPTER CONTENTS

SUMMARY

This chapter begins with an analysis of the concept of need. This is accompanied by an overview of essential factors for you to consider when identifying health promotion needs. These include the scope and boundaries of professional remits; the difference between reactive and proactive choices and the importance of placing the people who are the targets and users of health promotion at the centre of the needs identification process. This discussion is supplemented with an exercise on the user friendliness of services. In the next section on finding and using health information, types and sources of information are identified and exercises included on gathering and applying information. This is followed by a framework for assessing health promotion needs, with a case study and an exercise. In the final section there is a focus on priority setting, with exercises on analysing the reasons for health promotion priorities and on setting priorities.

Many organisations at different levels have a role in identifying public health needs, including those needs that can be addressed by health promotion interventions. These range from international agencies, such as the World Health Organization (WHO), national organisations, such as government departments, to organisations at local level, such as primary care trusts (PCTs).

See Chapter 4 for information on the range of agencies with a public health and health promotion role, Chapter 7 for national and local health strategies, and Chapter

16 for making and implementing national and local health strategies.

The focus in this chapter is on the need for interventions undertaken by health promoters working with individual clients, families, groups and communities.

Identifying the people who are intended to benefit from health promotion activities (sometimes called target groups) is a complex process. These people may be referred to as *users*, which imply they use health promotion services such as smoking cessation groups. In some cases people receive help that they may or may not use, for example receiving advice and information leaflets. Alternatively, people may be called *consumers, customers, clients* or *patients* if they are receiving their health promotion via medical services, such as a coronary rehabilitation service. Positive action may be necessary to ensure that everyone has equal access to services and can benefit from them.

Going one stage further and identifying and prioritising people's needs is also a complex and difficult process. Needs may exceed the finite resources available to meet them so difficult choices may have to be made.

Before looking further at how the needs of the users and receivers of health promotion can be met, it is worth considering what is understood by a need.

CONCEPTS OF NEED

It is useful to think of need in terms of:

- the kinds of health problems which people experience or are at risk from
- the requirements for a particular kind of health promotion response
- the relationship between health problems and the health promotion responses available.

Bradshaw's (1972) taxonomy of need was established many years ago but it is still very useful in distinguishing between four different kinds of need.

1. NORMATIVE NEED – DEFINED BY THE EXPERT

Normative need is a need defined by experts or professionals according to their own standards; falling short of those standards means that there is a need. For example, a dietitian may identify a certain level of nutritional knowledge as the desirable standard for her client and defines a need for nutrition education if her client's knowledge does not reach that standard. This normative need is based on the judgements of professional experts, which may lead to problems. One is that expert opinion may vary over what is the acceptable standard, and the values and standards of the experts may be different from those of their clients.

Some normative needs are prescribed by law, such as food hygiene regulations (see Food Standards Agency 2006), or by national policy and related guidelines and targets (see, for example, Department of Health (DoH) 2009a).

2. FELT NEED – WANTS

Felt need is the need that people feel; it is what they *want*. For example, a pregnant woman may feel the need for (and want) information about childbirth. Felt needs may be limited or inflated by people's awareness and knowledge about what could be available: for example, people will not feel the need to know their blood cholesterol level if they have never heard that such a thing is possible or know about the potential risk of high blood cholesterol levels to health.

3. EXPRESSED NEED – DEMANDS

Expressed need is what people say they need; it is felt need that has been turned into an expressed request or demand. Commercial weight-control groups and exercise classes are examples of expressed need; they are provided in response to demand.

Not all felt need is turned into expressed need or demand. Lack of opportunity, motivation or assertiveness could all prevent the expression of a felt need. Lack of demand, therefore, should not be equated with lack of felt need.

Expressed needs may conflict with a professional's normative needs. For example, a patient may express a need for a course of individual professional counselling as a result of experiencing a mental heath problem, but the resources may not be available for this type of health promoting service and normative needs and priorities may be focused on other types of interventions to promote mental health.

4. COMPARATIVE NEED

Comparative need for health promotion is defined by comparison between similar groups of clients, some in receipt of health promotion and some not. Those who are not are then defined as being in need. For example, if Company A has an employee health policy covering stress at work and the provision of healthy food choices in the staff canteen and Company B does not, it could be said that there is a comparative need for health promotion in Company B. This assumes that the health promotion in Company A is desirable and ideal, which of course it may not be.

NEED, DEMAND AND SUPPLY

Over time, there has been debate over need, demand, supply and quality of health services and other public sector services that relate to health promotion, such as education. Levels and quality of service can vary across the country, and between GPs and hospitals even in the same neighbourhood, resulting in what has been termed as a postcode lottery (Kiss 2006). The need for services may be similar or different, but supply is unevenly distributed and this results in significant health inequalities (see, for example, Jaffa (2003) in relation to mental health services, Cockcroft (2007) in relation to cancer care, and the BBC (2009) reporting variation in health visitor provision).

If demand outstrips supply it means that people do not always get the access to the health services they want, or that health professionals believe they need. This issue of uneven provision also applies to health promotion services, with different levels of provision in different geographical areas (Scriven 2002, DoH/WAG 2005). The Institute of Healthcare Improvement (IHI) has a range of tools to ensure that demand matches supply (http://www.ihi.org), but nonetheless the problem arises because the health services and other public bodies have a finite pot of money to spend, so they have to prioritise. This can result in rationing (Campbell 2007, Klein 2007). To overcome the problems associated with rationing, the 2008 *NHS Next Stage Review* (DoH 2008a) endorsed NHS funding within personal health budgets. This new initiative of giving personal health budgets to the general population (for more detail see DoH 2009b) coincides with an NHS Confederation report *Personal Health Budgets: the*

Shape of Things to Come (NHS Confederation 2009) which suggests that direct payments could result in enhanced health outcomes and positively change the nature of the patient–professional relationship. The scheme is currently in a pilot phase so its effect on the supply and demand for health promotion services is not yet known.

Measures to address the uneven supply and quality of health services have also included publication of national standards, in the form of the national service frameworks (NSFs) that set out the pattern and level of service which should be provided for major care areas such as mental health and disease groups such as cancer (http://www.dh.gov.uk). Local services are required to work towards these standards. National bodies also have a role in ensuring that the best value-for-money services and treatment are provided fairly wherever people live. The Care Quality Commission (http://www.cqc.org.uk) is responsible for ensuring good-quality services in the NHS, and the National Institute for Health and Clinical Excellence (http://www.nice.org.uk) provides the evidence for clinical practice and health promotion.

IDENTIFYING HEALTH PROMOTION NEEDS

How does a health promoter set about identifying people's needs? There are three key areas it is useful to think about first: the scope and boundaries of your job; the balance between being reactive and proactive in your work; and the extent to which you are putting your clients first. Each of these is addressed in turn.

THE SCOPE

For some practitioners the task of identifying needs has already taken place. For example, dental hygienists working in a dental surgery with individual patients already have the clearly identified task of educating patients in oral hygiene. But they may want to think carefully about how they can make their service as person centred and user friendly as possible. And they will certainly have to identify and respond to the individual needs of each patient.

Other workers, however, have more choice and scope in the range of health promotion activities they can undertake. Health visitors and community workers may have considerable scope, but the degree of autonomy they have will vary according to the policy of their managers and the resources available. All health promoters will need some competency in being responsive to the health promotion needs of their clients, and will need to be clear about the boundaries of their work: which health promotion activities are within their remit to undertake and which are not, however desirable they may be. For example, a family planning nurse may be asked to undertake sex education with young people in schools, but is this within the boundaries of her job?

REACTIVE OR PROACTIVE?

It is useful to make an initial distinction between being *reactive* and being *proactive* when identifying needs. Being reactive means responding or reacting to the needs and demands that other people make. Pressure from vested interest groups and the media may introduce bias into how needs are perceived, and produce pressure to react. Being proactive means taking the initiative and deciding on the area of work to be done. It may include rejecting the demands of other people if these do not fit existing policies and priorities.

> See Chapter 3, section on analysing your aims and values: five approaches.

Being reactive or proactive can be related to the approaches to health promotion, which were discussed in Chapter 3. Using a client-directed approach means being reactive to consumers' expressed needs, whereas using a medical or behaviour change approach probably means being proactive. This is particularly true of preventive medical interventions such as immunisation campaigns. In practice, there is usually a balance to be struck between being reactive and proactive.

PUTTING USERS' NEEDS FIRST

It is important to ask the questions about whose needs should come first, the users or the providers of health promotion. There may be conflict between the two: for example, users may want a family planning service to be open on Saturdays to improve access but providers are unable to supply this

service because of difficulties in getting staff to work at weekends. However, numerous international policy directives, such as the seminal *Ottawa Charter* (WHO 1986), and national strategies such as *Choosing Health* (DoH 2004), have emphasised the need for more people-centred health promotion.

The core values that would be embedded in people-centred health promotion are:

● empowerment
● participation
● the central role of the individuals, family and community in any process of health development
● equity and nondiscrimination.

The implications of these values are clear. People have the right to participate in making decisions about their health and should be enabled to do so. The needs, wants and expectations of individuals, families and communities should be respected by health promoters and influence priority setting and the delivery of health promotion services. You can measure how user friendly your services are by undertaking Exercise 6.1.

These values suggest that key characteristics of people-centred health promotion might include the following:

For individuals, communities and population groups:

● Access to clear, concise and intelligible health information and education that increase health literacy and enable needs to be expressed.
● Equitable access to health including treatments, and psychosocial support.
● Development of personal skills which allow control over health and engagement with healthcare systems: communication, mutual collaboration and respect, goal setting, decision making, problem solving, self-care.
● Supported involvement in health decision making, including health policy.

For health promotion practitioners and specialists:

● Holistic understanding and approach to health improvement.
● Respect for people and their decisions.
● Recognition of the needs of people seeking to improve their health.
● Professional and personal skills to meet these needs: competence in promoting health, communication, mutual collaboration and respect, empathy, responsiveness, sensitivity.

EXERCISE 6.1   Using services that promote health or prevent ill health: user views

Find out about some services available locally, designed for the public, staff and/or health students (whichever is relevant to you) that aim to promote health or prevent ill health. The public library, human resources department of your employer, NHS trust or local council, for example, may be able to provide information about what services are available. These could include swimming facilities, exercise classes, the resources and information service of your local Public Health and Health Promotion Departments or an NHS walk-in centre.

Select one of these, appropriate and acceptable to you, and visit it. Make notes about what happens and how to make a service responsive to its users.

See also the section on working for quality in Chapter 8 for information on quality in health promotion services.

■ Is it easy to find out that the service exists?
■ Is it easy to locate, with clear signposting where needed?

■ Is public transport easily available/is there easy access for parking your car?
■ Are the opening times convenient to you?
■ If there is a charge for the service, is it affordable and good value for money?
■ How are you welcomed at reception? Are you given all the information you need? Do you feel at ease? Are the staff friendly?
■ What do you think about the environment – is it safe, clean and comfortable?
■ What do you think about the quality of the service you received? Do you have any ideas about how it could be improved? Will you use this service again?
■ What have you learnt as a service user which you can now apply to health promotion practice?

- Commitment and adherence to quality, evidence-based and ethical practice.
- Team work, collaboration and partnership across disciplines and with clients.

(Adjusted from http://www.wpro.who.int)

Let us now return to the central question: how are needs for health promotion identified?

FINDING AND USING INFORMATION

The starting point for defining health promotion needs is information of various kinds from a range of sources. If you are gathering information on a local area for the first time, it would be helpful to share the work, and the findings, with colleagues. For example, health visitors may have done a neighbourhood profile as part of their training; the public health department in the local PCT will probably have health data on the local population. Gathering and updating all these different kinds of information is an ongoing project for every health promoter and sharing the task is a more efficient use of time. Working with colleagues needs to done in conjunction with establishing links with local people, in order to ensure the active participation of users and receivers.

There are a number of different kinds of information you can access when identifying need.

EPIDEMIOLOGICAL DATA

Epidemiology is the study of the distribution and determinants of disease in communities. Epidemiological data indicate how many people are affected by a health problem, how many people die from a particular health problem, and who are most at risk within sex, age, ethnic, socioeconomic, occupational or geographical groupings or perhaps by taking account of factors such as weight, smoking or physical activity levels.

Detailed discussion of the sources and limitations of epidemiological data is outside the scope of this book, but for excellent texts on epidemiology see Bonita et al (2007) and Gordis (2008). The important point to make here is that epidemiological data provide essential information on the health of the population, the causes and risk factors related to ill health and in doing this, the potential for prevention and health promotion.

Mortality and morbidity data are collected nationally, and some data are also available on a regional and local basis. Mortality data are concerned with causes of death; morbidity data with types of illness and disability. Mortality data are derived from death certificates; morbidity data from a wide range of sources, including medical records, sickness absence certificates, child health records, returns of notifiable diseases, disability registers and many others. In addition, surveys such as the government's General Household Survey (GHS) (http://www.statistics.gov.uk) and those carried out for research purposes provide a considerable amount of health information.

Your local NHS organisation, such as a PCT, may have information about the local population including mortality and morbidity data (such as hospital admission rates for particular conditions). This may be broken down to the level of the population of smaller areas such as electoral wards. It might be helpful to compare data for the whole population and electoral ward data (for a neighbourhood) on, for example:

- the major causes of death
- the key causes of childhood admission to hospital
- the main conditions for which adults are admitted to hospital.

Exercise 6.2 is designed to enable you to find out about local health information.

LIFESTYLE DATA

An increasing amount of information about people's health-related behaviour and lifestyle, such as physical activity, sexual behaviour, smoking and drinking, is available on a national basis from survey data. See, for example, the SHEU surveys (http://www.sheu.org.uk) which have up-to-date data on the lifestyle of young people at school. There are active surveys that date back 32 years and therefore act as valuable benchmarks. You may also find that a local or regional NHS organisation has done a lifestyle survey of your local population, and published the findings (see, for example, Jones & Tocque 2005).

SOCIOECONOMIC DATA

The planning or information departments of local councils should be able to help with information about housing, employment, social class and social/leisure/recreation/shopping facilities. Many produce summaries of census data. It might be helpful to compare district/borough/city and

---

EXERCISE 6.2   Gathering local public health information

Ask your local NHS organisation, such as your local PCT (or equivalent in Scotland, Wales and Northern Ireland), for reports or data on the health status of your local population. They may have information available on the Internet. Some local data may also be available on national websites, such as http://www.dh.gov.uk, http://www.statistics.gov.uk or http://www.ons.gov.uk. Browse through the data and see if you can find out, for your local population:

- What are the major causes of death?
- What are the major reasons for people to be admitted to hospital?
- What are the major risk factors for ill health? For example, is there information on what percentage of people smoke in your local population?
- How many people have had communicable diseases (diseases caught from other people) such as measles or sexually transmitted infections?
- Which neighbourhoods or communities have the poorest health?
- What steps are being taken to prevent ill health and promote good health?

Can you find information on anything else to help you in your health promotion work?

---

electoral ward data on social and economic factors, such as:

- unemployment
- household amenities
- income
- ethnicity.

It is advisable to ask for figures that are as full and recent as possible. Much information is obtained from the national census, which takes place every 10 years. The last one was in 2001; information from the analysis of the data is available at the Office of National Statistics (ONS). The ONS has an online facility which will allow you to search for detailed information online (http://www.neighbourhood.statistics.gov.uk). The next national census is planned for 2011.

By setting illness data alongside social and economic data, you may be able to see patterns that might inform your needs identification and priority setting process. You may want, for example, to determine if areas where people with less financial and other resources live are also likely to be the areas of poorest health.

PROFESSIONAL VIEWS

The views of the wider public health workforce reflect experience and perceptions accumulated over the years, which it would be foolish to ignore. What do other workers in your area, such as teachers, youth workers, social workers, GPs, health visitors, district nurses, environmental health officers, police officers, community workers and religious leaders consider the major health concerns?

PUBLIC VIEWS

Public sector organisations are now charged with the responsibility of seeking the views of the communities that they serve, but some organisations have developed good practice in this area over a number of years. Try contacting the local government in your area for information on this type of work, such as Citizens' Panels, which are representative samples of residents who give their views on local services, priorities and plans (for an example of the work of Citizens' Panels see Bristol City Council website (http://www.bristol.gov.uk) or perhaps look at your own local council website).

There is more about research methods for finding out people's views in Chapter 7, section on doing your own small-scale research.

There are several methods of obtaining the views of the public at large, from informal discussions/ interviews to large-scale surveys using questionnaires or in-depth interview techniques. Identifying priority groups and thinking clearly about them will influence the choice of methods used to contact and involve them.

It is best to start with the characteristics of the groups and then design the best approach. For instance, how large are the relevant groups? Do they have particular age, class or ethnic structures? What makes it a group (geography, membership, current use of services and facilities)? Are the members of the group mobile? Do they have easy access to transport? What times of day are they likely to be available for meetings? Be absolutely clear about what sort of relationship you are pro-posing to have with local groups and individuals. For example, if you plan simply to establish consultation mechanisms, there may be hostility if local people have played a stronger partnership role in the past.

Public consultation and involvement are discussed in detail in Chapter 15.

The groups involved may include patient and public involvement forums (DoH 2008b) and patient advice and liaison services (PALS; http://www.pals.nhs.uk), local voluntary organisations and community groups such as self-help groups, black and minority ethnic groups, pensioners' clubs, tenants' associations, and a variety of local advisory groups or planning subcommittees, in addition to groups of key clients such as parents. Gathering views informally is useful but there are problems in ensuring accuracy and that subjective information is representative. However, these subjective data can usefully feed into the wider picture.

You might want to consider undertaking some first-hand research but first think about how much time and money it will take. Will the results justify the costs? If you still think it is worth doing, who could do it? If it is very small scale you could perhaps undertake it yourself, maybe in collaboration with some colleagues.

LOCAL MEDIA

The opinions and data collected from local media will provide you with a picture at a particular point in time. Monitoring local radio, TV and newspapers will give a view of any major changes in the community. All this adds to the profile of needs you are building up, providing a basis for planning health promotion.

ASSESSING HEALTH PROMOTION NEEDS

The assessment of health promotion needs can be approached systematically by asking a series of key questions. The answers will help you to decide whether you should respond to a particular need, and if so, how.

1. WHAT TYPE OF NEED IS IT?

Is this a normative, felt, expressed or comparative need?

In a sex education class in a school, for example, what kind of need is being met: the normative needs decided by the school nurse; the personal, social and health education (PSHE) teaching team and the school governors; or the felt or expressed needs of the school pupils; or the comparative needs decided after looking at what was being made available on the PSHE curriculum in other schools; or what the comparative need for particular types of sexual health education, such as high teenage pregnancy rates, in a local area are compared to national figures suggesting a need for more work on contraception advise?

2. WHO DECIDED THAT THERE IS A NEED?

Whose decision is it: the health promoter's, the individual or group, or both?

Sometimes the answer to this question is not immediately obvious, because the need has emerged after discussion between the health promoter and their clients. People do not always know what they need or want, because their awareness and knowledge of the possibilities are limited. The health promoter may help by raising awareness and knowledge of health issues; in this way she may create a demand (an expressed need) for health promotion. For example, the public's demand for nonsmoking in restaurants came only after health promoters had raised awareness of the hazards of passive smoking, which motivated people to express their need for a smoke-free environment in eateries. An ideal situation is when there is a synergy between clients' and health promoters' needs.

3. WHAT ARE THE GROUNDS FOR DECIDING THAT THERE IS A NEED?

Is there any evidence of need in the form of objective data, such as facts and figures? If local data are not available, has the information been collected in other localities and is it reasonable to assume that the same conditions will apply? Be aware that gathering data can be a delaying tactic to avoid doing something about an obvious problem. For example, surveys have shown that elderly people without cars find it difficult to get to hospitals if public transport is poor. It is reasonable to assume

that this applies in most localities with poor public transport. So, collect information only if the answer to a question is really not known. Have the views of the clients been sought? Do they see this as a need?

4. WHAT ARE THE AIMS AND THE APPROPRIATE RESPONSE TO THE NEED?

> See the section on setting aims and objectives in Chapter 5 for a more detailed look at setting aims and objectives and identifying appropriate ways of achieving them.

Health promotion cannot solve all problems or meet all health needs. You should be clear on what the need is, then what your aims are for meeting that need, then the appropriate way to meet it. For example, there may be an identified normative need to increase the uptake of immunisation and aim to achieve an 80% uptake rate. You then have to decide the appropriate way to achieve your aim. It would be all too easy in this case to say that there is a need for a health education campaign to get parents to have their children immunised because messages about attending immunisation clinics may be seen to be the answer. But this may make no difference because the appropriate response is to educate the health professionals who are being too cautious and withholding immunisation wrongly when a child has only a mild contraindication, or to move the time and/or location of the clinics so that working parents, and those without cars, are able to bring their children.

Case studies 6.1 and 6.2 offer examples of how need for health promotion is assessed, applying the four assessment questions. Exercise 6.3 asks you to think about assessing a need in your own area of work.

SETTING HEALTH PROMOTION PRIORITIES

You may have a large number of health promotion needs that you feel should be met, but there are always constraints on resources, such as time and finance. Concentrating effort on priority areas is essential to ensure quality and effectiveness.

Before attempting to set priorities it is helpful to analyse current practice and recognise the wide range of criteria that will affect decisions about

CASE STUDY 6.1 IMPROVING UPTAKE OF TB SCREENING SERVICES

Background

TB incidence has varied over the years across north-east central London, and in Camden is relatively high compared to other PCT areas. Targeted work was required with the community to improve uptake and information about TB screening services.

1. What sort of need is it?

The need to increase community knowledge and uptake of TB screening services was both normative (based on policy directives and professional opinion) and comparative (based on activities in other PCT regions).

2. Who decided that there was a need?

The local public health specialists and practitioners acting on national policy directives decided there was a need for this initiative.

3. What are the grounds for deciding there is a need?

The grounds for deciding there is a need was based on the above average TB incident rate per 100 000 in Camden and the existence of national policy stating TB information should be available for all newcomers in a community. Prior to this scheme there was a lack of any form of recruitment into screening other than through port health and GP/hospital appointments.

4. What are the aims and the appropriate response to the need?

The project aims were to encourage individuals from new migrant communities to engage with health screening services available in the borough, with a particular focus on TB.

NHS Camden is now implementing the following interventions, based on the primary research results:

- TB posters, leaflets and information cards.
- Welcome pack for new migrant or those new to health services in Camden.
- Stakeholder toolkit.
- Stakeholder training around screening pathways in the borough and target audience insights.
- Peer-to-peer activity.

In addition to this, stakeholders identified that sustained outreach work and more peer-to-peer education was needed in relation to accessing screening services within the borough. It was also thought that there needed to be deeper engagement work with Somali, Bengali and homeless groups.

(Case study prepared by Aideen Dunne, Health Promotion Specialist, NHS Camden.)

EXERCISE 6.3   Assessing a health promotion need

Use the following questions to assess a health promotion need that you have identified in your own work, or one which you are likely to meet in the future.
1. What type of need is it?
2. Who decided that there is a need?
3. What are the grounds for deciding that there is a need?
4. What are the aims and appropriate response to the need?

---

health promotion interventions. Undertaking Exercise 6.5 enables you to focus on these factors.

The need to prioritise is vital, but one difficult issue to consider is how to approach work with people whose health experience is poor. It is automatic to consider that these people should be top priority, but it is important to consider whether focusing all health promotion effort on those most at risk will, in the end, be of greatest benefit.

When reducing the incidence of coronary heart disease, for example, two broad approaches can be used: the *high-risk* and the *whole population* approaches. The high-risk approach identifies people particularly at risk, such as smokers, people who are obese or who have high blood pressure, and develops interventions with these people to change lifestyle factors and treat their raised blood pressure, for example. But there may be poor return for effort, as these groups could include addictive smokers with poor diets who have no intention of changing, or people so overwhelmed with social and/or psychological issues in their lives that tackling smoking and eating habits is the last thing on their minds even if they would like to make changes.

The whole population approach works at community rather than individual level, with, for

CASE STUDY 6.2 A PHYSICAL ACTIVITY SCHEME TO IMPROVE ACTIVITY LEVELS IN LOW INCOME HOUSEHOLDS

Background

In 2008 Pro-Active Camden commissioned a Physical Activity Needs Analysis which surveyed Camden residents. This survey had a particular focus in the four priority wards of Camden, which has the highest rates of all-cause mortality. The findings showed that insufficient time and cost were the two main reasons for not participating in physical activity. When asked where they would most like to undertake physical activity, the majority of residents stated a leisure/sports centre. Camden has a number of gyms spread out across the borough that can provide access to swimming, gym equipment and fitness classes in one location.

1. What sort of need is it?

The need for low-cost physical activity is an expressed need by Camden residents.

Low physical activity levels and the need for physical activity intervention is a comparative need as the target group for this scheme had lower activity levels than the general Camden population. The leisure providers also felt that low cost was a need.

2. Who decided that there is a need?

The public health team at NHS Camden made the decision to explore barriers to physical activity based on national policy directives to increase physical activity levels; however the scheme was in response to an expressed community need.

3. What are the grounds for deciding there is a need?

Analysis of the community survey, consultation with local leisure providers and comparison of local health statistics provided the rationale for targeting this need with the methods employed.

4. What are the aims and the appropriate response to the need?

The aim of this project was to increase access to physical activity among Camden's low-income population by offering free access to specific leisure centres situated across the borough. All Camden residents who qualified (in receipt of a specific set of benefits) received free access to a local leisure centre for a month. Those who attended five or more times during that month then qualified for 6 months funded membership. This strategy removed cost as a barrier but participants paid through effort by attending five or more times.

A marketing strategy to raise awareness of the scheme was put in place: this included a direct mail to Camden residents registered as unemployed or in receipt of certain benefits, advertisement in local newspapers and media packs mailed to community amenities (including post offices, job centres, housing offices and healthy living centres).

(Case study prepared by Aideen Dunne, Health Promotion Specialist, NHS Camden and Nick Pahl, Public Health Strategist, Screening, NHS Camden.)

---

example, strategies to improve access to cheap healthy food, increase skills and confidence in producing healthy meals for families, and community development approaches to build up social support. At the same time, supporting changes at a wider population level, such as reducing the underage sales of cigarettes, and lobbying for increased income support, could result in better health gain across whole populations.

Generally, both approaches need to be taken (not necessarily by the same health promoters), as they complement each other. This is why developing partnership working is so important as it allows different aspects of the same issue to be addressed by the health promoters who are best placed to tackle a particular aspect at a particular time, thus achieving greater impact.

There can be no exact method for setting priorities because they ultimately depend upon the normative judgements and the available resources of the health promoters involved. But it may be helpful to work through the checklist in Exercise 6.4.

EXERCISE 6.4 Setting priorities for health promotion

1. Health promotion issues, approaches and activities

Do you define your priorities in terms of:

■ Issues that have an influence on health (the wider determinants such as poverty, unemployment, racism, ageism, inequalities)?
■ Health promotion approaches (such as medical, behaviour change, social marketing, educational, client centred, societal/environmental change)?
■ Health promotion activities (preventive health services, community-based work, organisational development, economic and regulatory activities, environmental measures, health education programmes, healthy public policies)?
■ Health problems (such as heart disease, food poisoning, cancers, HIV/AIDS, obesity, mental illness)?

Why?

2. Consumer groups

Who are the people your health promotion is aimed at?

■ Policy makers and planners?
■ Individual clients or service users?
■ Families?
■ Selected target groups?
■ The whole community? If so, how do you define your community?

Why?

3. Age groups

Do you define your priority consumer groups further in terms of age: children, young people, parents, older people, etc.?
  Why?

4. At-risk groups

■ Do you define your priority consumer groups further in terms of high-risk categories such as smokers, people with high blood pressure, the unemployed or those living on low incomes? If so, why? Have you examined the evidence leading to the identification of these at-risk groups?
■ If your group includes people with highest health needs, for example people living in areas of social deprivation with many health and social needs, do

you know whether there is evidence that work focusing on specific issues will be successful? Would you get more health gain for your effort if you focused on whole populations rather than those most in need?

5. Effectiveness

■ Have you any evidence that health promotion in your priority areas is likely to be effective?

See Chapter 7 for information on how to collect evidence.

■ Have you any evidence that it will provide value for money?
■ How could such evidence be collected?

6. Feasibility

■ Is it feasible for you to spend time with your priority groups?
■ Do you have access to these groups?
■ Do you have credibility with these groups?
■ Do you have the skills and resources to work with these groups?

7. Working with others

■ Do you know what work is already being done with your priority groups, by other health promoters, community groups and voluntary organisations?
■ Are you sure that your work will complement any other work that is going on and not be seen as duplication or interference?
■ Does your work fit in with existing local strategies and plans for health promotion?
■ Are there any local partnership groups already set up to address the needs of your priority group?

8. Ethics

■ Are there ethical aspects to your work which you need to consider?
■ Is your work ethically acceptable to you?
■ Will it be acceptable to your consumer groups?
■ Will it be congruent with their values?
■ How may the desired outcome affect their lives?

9. Add anything else you feel it is important to consider

Now identify your top priority and add any other priorities.

EXERCISE 6.5   Analysing the reasons for health promotion priorities

Identify a health promotion activity which has a high priority in your work. This could be work that you undertake with a number of clients (such as a smoking cessation programme) or just one (for example, a health visitor talking to a mother about maintaining breastfeeding); it could be part of your usual work or a special event such as a campaign. It will be especially helpful for the purposes of this exercise if you can identify an area of work that has recently become a priority.

   Now work through the following tasks.

1. Identify who it was who decided that this work should take priority (e.g. you? your seniors? your clients? all three?).
2. List all the possible reasons why this work has priority – include the reasons that you are sure about as well as any that are speculation.

Your reasons could include any of the following and probably many more:

- I feel that it's important.
- It is the established policy of senior managers.
- We have always done it and see no reason to change.
- There was pressure from the public.
- It was in response to a crisis.
- We had to be seen to be doing something.
- There is new evidence of need.
- There is evidence that the work has been effective in a similar area.
- It was the current national/local theme (e.g. World AIDS Day).
- We had a new staff member with special expertise, which we wanted to use.
- We had to economise and be more efficient.
- It was politically expedient.
- There was a change in national policy.

3. Identify what you think the most important reasons are. Do you think that they are sound reasons for setting priorities?

PRACTICE POINTS

- You will have some scope for making choices about the range of health promotion activities you undertake. These choices must be based on a careful assessment of health promotion needs. The starting point is to undertake a needs identification process.
- The views of users and receivers of services are paramount, therefore developing skills in gathering information directly from them is especially important.
- You can assess health promotion needs systematically by asking four key questions: What kind of need is it? Who decided that there was a need? What is the evidence for deciding that there is a need? What is the appropriate response to the need?
- Like all health promoters, you have a duty to reassess priorities regularly, through analysing whether your activities are targeted effectively, are feasible, complement the work of other practitioners and are acceptable to local people.
- Priorities depend ultimately on the normative judgments of those involved. Best practice involves in-depth discussion on priority setting with other health promotion practitioners and local people.

References

BBC 2009 Health visitor 'postcode lottery'. http://news.bbc.co.uk/1/hi/health/8027111.stm.

Bonita R, Beaglehole R, Kjellstrom T 2007 Epidemiology, 2nd edn. Geneva, World Health Organization.

Bradshaw J 1972 A taxonomy of social need. New Society March: 640–643.

Campbell D 2007 Doctors admit: NHS treatments must be rationed. The Observer, Sunday 6 May. http://www.guardian.co.uk/uk/2007/may/06/health.politics.

Cockcroft L 2007 Figures reveal cancer care 'postcode lottery'. http://www.telegraph.co.uk/news/uknews/1570535/Figures-reveal-cancer-care-postcode-lottery.html.

Department of Health 2004 Choosing health: making healthy choices easier. London, The Stationery Office.

Department of Health 2008a High quality care for all: NHS next stage review final report. London, The Stationery Office.

Department of Health 2008b Patient and public involvement forums. http://www.dh.gov.uk/en/Managingyourorganisation/

PatientAndPublicinvolvement/ DH_4074577.

Department of Health 2009a The coronary heart disease national service framework: building on excellence, maintaining progress – progress report for 2008. London, The Stationery Office.

Department of Health 2009b Personal health budgets: first steps. London, The Stationery Office.

Department of Health and the Welsh Assembly Government 2005 Shaping the future of health: promoting health in the NHS. London, The Stationery Office.

Food Standards Agency 2006 The food hygiene (England) regulations 2006. http://www.food.gov.uk/ foodindustry/regulation/ europeleg/eufoodhygieneleg/ foodhygregeng.

Gordis L 2008 Epidemiology, 4th edn. London, Elsevier.

Jaffa T 2003 Distribution and characteristics of in-patient child and adolescent mental health services in England and Wales. The British Journal of Psychiatry 183: 547–551.

Jones A, Tocque K 2005 North west public health observatory synthesis report 4: lifestyle surveys – developing a local and regional picture. Liverpool, North West Public Health Observatory, Centre for Public Health, Liverpool, John Moores University.

Kiss J 2006 Channel 4 to launch NHS postcode lottery. http://www. guardian.co.uk/society/2006/ nov/23/health.newmedia.

Klein R 2007 Editorials. Rationing in the NHS: the BMA asks the right questions but answering them will be difficult. British Medical Journal 334: 1068–1069.

NHS Confederation 2009 Personal health budgets: the shape of things to come? London, NHS Confederation. http://www. nhsconfed.org/Publications/ Documents/personal_health_ budgets160109.pdf.

Scriven A 2002 Report of the survey into the impact of recent national heath policies on specialist health promotion services in England. London, Brunel University.

World Health Organization 1986 The Ottawa charter for health promotion. Geneva, WHO.

Websites

http://www.bristol.gov.uk/ccm/ navigation/council-and-democracy/councillors–democracy-and-elections/citizen-panels

http://www.cqc.org.uk

http://www.dh.gov.uk/ en/Healthcare/ NationalServiceFrameworks/ DH_081639

http://www.ihi.org/IHI/Topics/ OfficePractices/Access/Changes/ MeasureandUnderstandSupplyand Demand.htm

http://www.neighbourhood.statistics. gov.uk/dissemination

http://www.nice.org.uk

http://www.ons.gov.uk

http://www.pals.nhs.uk

http://www.sheu.org.uk

http://www.statistics.gov.uk/ssd/ surveys/general_household_ survey.asp

http://www.wpro.who.int/sites/pci/ health_care.htm

Chapter 7

Evidence and research in health promotion

CHAPTER CONTENTS

SUMMARY

This chapter covers particular aspects of knowledge and skills that enable you to draw on evidence, undertake research and use various techniques to inform and prioritise your health promotion work. These include linking your work into broader national and local health promotion plans and strategies, basing your work on evidence of effectiveness, using published research, doing your own small-scale research, getting value for money, audit and health impact assessment.

The role of the NHS and local government in planning health strategies is outlined in Chapter 4. How local policy is made and implemented is discussed in Chapter 16.

International (such as the World Health Organization (WHO) 2006) and national health strategies focus efforts on agreed priorities, and provide the framework for setting objectives and monitoring progress towards their achievement. A health promoter at a local level *contributes* to these broader strategies and *complements* work of other health promoters. Fig. 7.1 illustrates how health promoters from different local agencies complement each other's efforts in contributing to national goals of increasing physical activity in the population.

The role of the WHO and other international bodies is discussed in Chapters 1, 4 and 16.

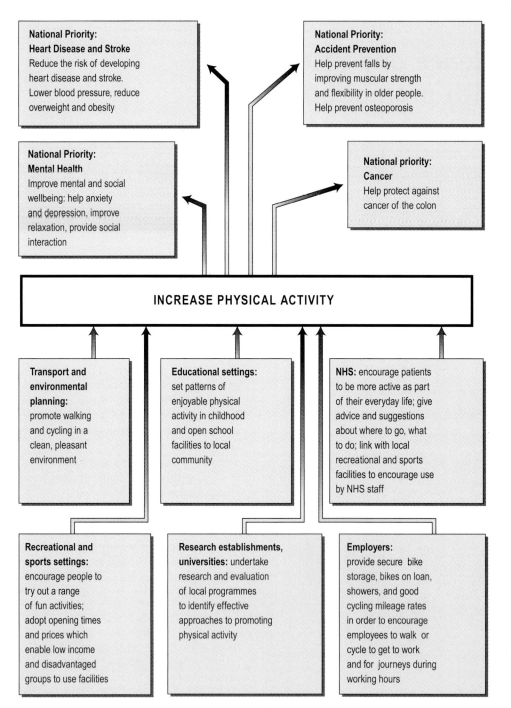

Fig. 7.1 Contributing to priorities in national strategies. Local complementary contributions to promoting physical activity. Heart disease and stroke, accidents, cancer and mental health feature as priorities in national strategies for health in England, Scotland, Wales and Northern Ireland.

NATIONAL PUBLIC HEALTH STRATEGIES

The first national health improvement strategy in England was *The Health of the Nation* (Department of Health (DoH) 1992). There were comparable strategies for Wales, Scotland and Northern Ireland.

See also Chapter 1, section on national initiatives.

The National Audit Office (1996) reporting on *The Health of the Nation* targets concluded that, while the initiative was making an impact, progress was uneven and slow. Deaths from heart disease, strokes and certain cancers were being reduced but there were rising levels of obesity, alcohol consumption by women and smoking by children which threatened to undermine health gains.

In the areas where targets were being reached, it was difficult to determine how far this was due to health promotion efforts (Appleby 1997). For example, there was a decrease in the rate of accidental deaths (many due to road accidents) in children. But this could have been because of improved education about accident prevention or a safer environment, such as more traffic calming schemes. Or it could have been because more injured children were saved from dying with better or quicker treatment, or maybe even because parents were informed of the risks of letting their children out to play, walk to school or cycle on the roads, so that their exposure to life-threatening risks was reduced.

A final assessment of *The Health of the Nation* (DoH 1998) concluded that, although the strategy was widely welcomed, it did not realise its full potential and was not seen to be as important as other health service priorities, such as waiting lists. Some key findings were that the strategy made little impact on local policy making, caused only a slight increase in health promotion spending, did not impact on primary care practitioners or hospital services, and was generally disliked by local authorities because of its disease-led targets. On the positive side, the evaluation indicated that the strategy enabled coordinated health promotion efforts, providing a focus for organisations outside the NHS to be involved and a spur to multiagency action where previous joint work had not existed.

The report made useful recommendations for the success of future health promotion strategies, calling for more evidence-based practice and evaluation and performance management.

New national strategies were introduced in the late 1990s and then again in the 21st century:

- England: *Saving Lives: Our Healthier Nation* (DoH 1999) and *Choosing Health: Making Healthy Choices Easier* (DoH 2004). The key principle of *Choosing Health: Making Healthy Choices Easier* is to support the public in making healthier and more informed choices in regards to their health. The Government pledged to provide information and practical support to get people motivated and improve emotional wellbeing and access to services so that healthy choices are easier to make.

- Northern Ireland: *Health and Wellbeing: Into the Next Millennium* (Department of Health and Social Services (DHSS) 1997), *Investing for Health* (Department of Health, Social Services and Public Safety 2002). *Investing for Health* presents a cross-departmental, multisectoral framework for action to improve health and wellbeing. The strategy recognises the important contribution to be made by members of statutory and nonstatutory groups, community and voluntary groups. The principles and values that should guide the improvement of health are identified and the costs of poor health are highlighted. The aims are to address a broad range of economic, social and environmental determinants of health and wellbeing.

- Scotland: *Towards a Healthier Scotland* (Scottish Office (SO) 1999). *Better Health, Better Care: Action Plan* (SO 2007). *Better Health, Better Care* has central themes of patient participation, improved healthcare access, and improving health and tackling health inequalities. This action plan sets out to help people to take more control of their health, especially in disadvantaged communities, ensuring better, local and faster access to health care. The three main components of health improvement, tackling health inequality and improving the quality of health care are set within a comprehensive programme of targeted action.

- Wales: *Promoting Health and Wellbeing: Implementing the National Health Promotion Strategy* (National Assembly for Wales (NAW) 2001a) and the associated *Improving Health in Wales: a Plan for the NHS and it's Partners* (NAW 2001b). *Promoting Health and Wellbeing: Implementing the National Health Promotion Strategy* sets out key elements of helping communities through local health alliances, health promoting schools, community health development, reaching young adults and developing a healthy workforce. There are targeted programmes covering a wide range of public health action. Other elements of the plan cover improving the skills and knowledge of health promoters, better communication of health information, health impact assessment, and research and evaluation.

Health promoters need to take account of these strategies and their emphasis on individual responsibility for health, the need to address the wider determinants and the importance of partnership working.

See Chapter 1, section on national initiatives, for more about inequalities targets.

LOCAL HEALTH STRATEGIES AND INITIATIVES

There are many government-initiated local health programmes that provide sources of funding for health promotion. Local strategies were given new impetus with the development of health improvement programmes, later known as health improvement and modernisation plans (HIMPs). These required more coordination between local agencies at both a strategic and operational level than had previously been the case. HIMPs for action were based on local needs that cover prevention and health promotion as well as treatment and care services. They emphasised reducing inequalities and developing partnerships to address locally identified needs and national health strategy priorities. To explore the impact they had on health promotion see Abbott & Gillam (2001).

See also Chapter 4 for the role of the health service and local government in promoting health.

Others local strategies include the following.

Local strategic partnerships

At a local level the NHS is involved in local strategic partnerships (LSPs), has oversight of the community plan (see below) and in areas of deprivation is responsible for developing a local strategy for neighbourhood renewal (see http://www.neighbourhood.gov.uk for links to local websites

for LSPs and http://www.idea.gov.uk for information on local area agreements and LSPs).

Community strategies

Local authorities have powers to promote or improve local economic, social and environmental wellbeing. They are required to prepare community strategies (or plans) and to coordinate these activities (see Darlow et al 2008) and associated partnerships across a wide range of agencies (see, for example, LutonForum 2005).

Neighbourhood renewal strategy

The Neighbourhood Renewal Strategy and Fund was launched in 2001 (Social Exclusion Unit 2001) and set out a joined-up approach to tackling the social and economic determinants of health in the most deprived local authority areas.

Healthy living centres

The Healthy Living Centres (HLCs) Initiative was launched in 1999, funded from the National Lottery to develop a network of HLCs across the UK. This funding is usually used for programmes of activity rather than a physical building. For examples of the work of HLCs see Rankin et al (2006) and for an evaluation of the whole scheme see Hills et al (2005). HLCs are not mentioned in recent policy, but the intention at the outset was that HLCs would become sustainable and there is evidence that this is happening (see, for example, Chesterfield Borough Council 2009).

Health action zones

The first wave of health action zones (HAZs) was set up in 1997 with special government funding to improve health outcomes and reduce health inequalities (Health Development Agency 2004). HAZs have pioneered new ways of tackling health inequalities through partnership working between the NHS, local authorities, community groups, the voluntary and private sectors; linking health, regeneration, education, housing and anti-poverty initiatives. A central aim for HAZs was integrating the services and approaches they develop into mainstream activity, and some made considerable progress and had an impact on local health improvement (Barnes et al 2005, Bauld and MacKenzie

2007). Where HAZs still exist they have been incorporated into mainstream agencies, for example, Northern Neighbourhoods Health Action Zone (http://www.nnhaz.co.uk).

The New Deal for Communities (NDC)

The NDC programme involved funding to poorest neighbourhoods in the country for 10 years to support plans that bring together local people, community and voluntary organisations, public agencies and local business in an attempt to make lasting improvements to health, employment, education and the physical environment. It was the intention that these improvements would be delivered in a way that could be sustained beyond government funding and into the long term. The government has issued various guidance notes which relate to succession, but Healey (2009) argues that it is too early to make an assessment of the contribution that guidance and shared good practice from the NDC programme is making to the development of local sustainability plans in NDC areas. For an example of how NDCs function see Newcastle New Deal for Communities (http://www.newcastlendc.co.uk).

Sure Start

This is a government scheme which aims to support parents and children under 4 years in areas of high health need (see Gidley 2007 for a more detailed discussion of the Sure Start programme and http://www.dcsf.gov.uk for publications relating to recent Sure Start funding and other initiatives).

Exercise 7.1 aims to help you find out about national and local health strategies relevant to your work.

EVIDENCE-BASED HEALTH PROMOTION

Delivering evidence-based health promotion is a key goal within the international, national and local strategies outlined above (Jones & Scriven 2005, Scriven 2008) Health promoters are required to know how to assess the evidence and apply the assessment to practice.

This requires competencies in:

- Critically appraising primary and secondary research.

EXERCISE 7.1 Finding out about national and local health promotion strategies

1. Have a look at the national strategy for health in your country (see section on National Health Strategies above to find out about yours). Try the Internet, libraries at educational institutions or at work, colleagues in health promotion or planning at your place of work, or contact the public health department of your local NHS organisation.
2. What do you think are the good and not-so-good points about your national strategy?
3. How does your own health promotion work contribute to the aims set out in the national strategy?
4. If you work in the NHS or local authority, list your local health plans and strategies and assess:
   - What are the good and not-so-good points about your local plans?
   - How do the local plans relate to your national strategy?
   - How does your own health promotion work contribute to the aims set out in your local plans?

- Knowledge of the hierarchy of evidence.
- Assessment of evidence of effectiveness of services, programmes and interventions, which impact on health.
- Conducting a literature review, which includes the use of electronic databases, defining a search strategy and summarizing results.
- Applying research evidence, evidence of effectiveness, outcome measures, evaluation and audit to influence health promotion programme interventions, services or development of practice guidelines.
- Interpreting and balancing evidence of effectiveness from a range of sources to inform decision making.

See Chapter 2 for more information on competencies in health promotion.

An evidence-based approach provides a defense against the indiscriminate use of practices in situations which have no research-based legitimacy. Evidence-based health promotion requires a culture where you openly share your experience and write up and publish your work, which enables others to learn from your successes and failures. It uses the skills of reflective practice, thinking about what you do and questioning whether it is the right approach in your situation.

HOW DO YOU KNOW WHAT WORKS?

There can be a gap between evidence and practice. It is not always easy for practitioners to keep up-to-date with new research findings, or to apply research findings in their own particular situation. Attention needs to be given to how research findings can best influence and also emerge from practice, and the processes of disseminating and implementing health promotion research.

There are many published research studies that help to show which health promotion interventions work best. These are easily accessible on the Internet at such sites as Cochrane (http://www. cochrane.org); the International Union of Health Promotion and Health Education (IUHPE) data source (http://www.hp-source.net) and the main evidence-based Internet site for health promotion in England, the National Institute for Health and Clinical Evidence (NICE) (http://www.nice.org.uk).

Health promotion is complex and it is sometimes difficult to provide evidence of effectiveness for single interventions. Often it is not one intervention that produces results, but a combination of activities, of which you may be involved in just one, as Fig. 7.1 demonstrates. Another example is preventing childhood obesity, where the evidence is that a multifaceted approach is the most effective. A combination of interventions range from targeting antenatal education, to working with parents and ensuring they have access to buying affordable healthy foods, to increasing children's physical activity levels, through the targets set by the Schools Sports Strategy (OFSTED 2006) and ensuring healthy food consumption while children are at school using the new standards, which cover all food sold or served in schools (Department for Children, Schools and Families 2005).

Research shows that for many health promotion issues a more comprehensive, integrated approach that focuses both on attitudes and behaviours and changes to such things as the environment and legislative and fiscal policies is the most effective (see, for example, National Audit Office et al 2006).

Evidence may also not exist. The particular piece of work you plan to undertake may not have been done before, and indeed the particular set of circumstances in which you are working may be unique. So the best that can be done is to be aware of what the published research in *related* areas of work tells you, and to reflect on how what was learned might apply to your circumstances. Where evidence is not available, it is vital to ensure that you evaluate your work in order to add to the evidence base by drawing the evidence from your practice and disseminating the results.

It also helps to think carefully about what constitutes *evidence* (for a useful discussion on these issues see Kelly et al 2004). Evidence can be drawn informally, with the views of local people and your own experience also constituting evidence. Your job as a health promoter is to use your judgement to decide whether the evidence available applies to your clients and circumstances and, if so, how. GPs, for example, may quote a number of factors which they believe provide evidence that health promotion is effective, including changes in the health or health behaviour of their patients over time.

However, formal sources of evidence are generally regarded as the most reliable, so you should plan carefully and evaluate or audit what you do. In this way you will be building up your own body of knowledge about what is effective.

Audit is discussed later in this chapter.

Finally, it is also important to bear in mind that your decision about whether to do a particular piece of health promotion work should also be based on ethical considerations. You could decide that it is your responsibility to intervene, even though you have little or no information about what might work. Health promotion is driven by both values and evidence, which are often intertwined. So there are two key questions: *Do we think this ought to be done*? and *Will it work*?

See Chapter 3 for more about values and ethics in health promotion.

USING PUBLISHED RESEARCH

Health promoters need to be well informed about published research and also how to *use* their knowledge of research findings to improve their practice. Familiarity with research findings can also give you arguments on which to base a case for more, or different and better, health promotion. Keeping abreast of current evidence should be part of your everyday working practice.

HOW TO SEARCH THE LITERATURE

You may sometimes wish to find out about research on a particular topic, perhaps because you are proposing to introduce new health promotion work and want to know what has been shown to work best. For example, imagine you are a nurse working in cancer care and you are considering introducing a counselling service for women who are undergoing mastectomy (surgery to remove a breast, usually because of breast cancer). You want to know if research shows what the health promotion needs of these women are and how best to meet them. Where do you start?

First you need to establish a research question. It pays to take time to discuss this with colleagues and you could also discuss it with someone who has recently had a mastectomy. What did she find helpful, and what was unhelpful?

Once you are clear about what you want to find out, list no more than six key words that feature in your question. The cancer care nurse might include the words mastectomy, needs and counselling in her list. Then write words that mean the same thing, or are similar in meaning, by each key word. For example, you might put breast removal as an alternative to mastectomy, and advice as an alternative to counselling. These key words and their synonyms/alternatives will be helpful when you go to the library or search on the Internet (for excellent guides to doing your literature search and finding information online, see Aveyard (2007) and Dochartaigh (2007)). In addition, many journal articles include a list of key words after the title, which will help you to know whether the article is likely to be of interest to you. When you have found a few references, you can start by reading the most recent one. This will provide you with more references. Once you are under way, the next problem is to avoid being swamped by information. Here again, your key words should be useful in stopping you from being side-tracked and in keeping your research question in mind.

It is important to keep records of what you read. There is computer software designed to help you store and retrieve references (see for a comparison of the different software http://en.wikipedia.org). For a book, you need to record:

- author's (or editor's) surname and initials
- year published
- title and subtitle

- edition, if not the first
- chapter, or numbers of pages, if you are only going to refer to part of the book
- place of publication
- publisher.

For articles in journals you need to record:

- author's surname and initials
- year of publication
- title and subtitles of article
- journal title
- volume and part numbers
- the inclusive page numbers of the article
- date of publication.

If you are gathering research evidence that will be used to inform a health promotion decision or action, then the first thing you need to know when reading an article is whether it is a report of actual research or just a knowledgeable account of facts and opinions. The *abstract*, the summary paragraph at the start of an article, will quickly inform you why a study was done and the main findings. Research reports usually have the following format:

- Introduction – background to the study.
- Literature review – critical summary of previous and related research.
- Method – a description of how the study was carried out.
- Results – the findings of the study.
- Discussion – a discussion of the findings.
- Conclusions – the implications of the findings.
- References – all the studies and books referred to in the article.

You need to read research articles critically, using the following questions:

When was the research carried out? Although the article is recent, it could be reporting on research that was carried out some years previously and has been superseded by more up-to-date research.

Why was the research undertaken? Do you see the need for this research? Will it contribute new knowledge on the subject? Will this knowledge be useful in practice?

How was the research carried out? Did it use methods and tools that were likely to provide answers to the questions posed by the researchers? What type of research was carried out? For example, if the researchers wanted to find out what works in changing the behaviour of sedentary people with angina to cause them to take more exercise, then *experimental research* would be required. This is research that establishes a relationship between cause and effect, often through studying subgroups of people, where the *experimental* subgroup experiences the intervention under consideration, and the *control* subgroup does not. Another type of research is *action research*. This is used to find out exactly how to implement changes, or solve problems, in a specific situation through watching and documenting in a systematic manner how the changes are introduced. (See Bowling (2009) for an excellent and detailed overview of research methods and methodological considerations.)

Does the researcher draw reasonable conclusions from the results? This can be a difficult question to answer, especially if, for example, it is quantitative research and you are unfamiliar with statistics. If you are not sure that you understand, it is important that you read more on critiquing research, particularly if you are going to be implementing the findings. (See Caughlan et al 2007 and Ryan et al 2007 for more detail on critiquing research articles.)

How could or should this research affect health promotion practice or policy? Even if the research was not carried out in your specialty or particular area of work, it could have implications for them. For example, findings about how best to communicate with patients who are very anxious after a heart attack could be used to help improve communication with patients who have cancer.

Through asking these, and other, questions you should be able to come to a judgement about whether a piece of research is reliable. It should have:

- been carried out by competent researchers
- used appropriate research design
- contained sound baseline data
- used a research instrument (such as a questionnaire) that has been piloted (tried and tested first to identify and correct any problems) and validated (tested to show that it really does measure what it was supposed to measure).

DOING YOUR OWN SMALL-SCALE RESEARCH

While you can improve your effectiveness through examining research findings and considering whether and how they apply to your work, in certain situations you may wish to carry out research yourself. For example, you and a group of colleagues may have uncovered an unmet health promotion need and your manager has agreed to fund a study to look in more detail at the need and how it could best be met.

What is defined as *research* here is a planned, systematic gathering of information for the purpose of increasing the total body of knowledge. If you are inexperienced, it is important for you to read extensively and try to elicit help from an experienced researcher. The following information should help to guide you in your reading and also introduce you to the process of undertaking small-scale research.

The research process involves carrying out some specific tasks, which are set out in Box 7.1. Although the tasks will tend to be carried out in the sequence set out in the box, this is not always the case, for example, you may write parts of the research report incrementally, as you go through each research task. You may have a much clearer idea about the purpose of the research *after* you have read the literature on other investigations in your area of interest.

The most important task in this list is the first one, as the kind of question you want to answer will form the basis of the whole project. For example, suppose you set the question 'What is the best way to encourage a group of university undergraduate students to engage in safer sex practices and to use condoms?' This question is concerned with ways of motivating and perhaps changing attitudes in order to encourage health-enhancing behaviour. The experts in this field are psychologists, so it is to the body of psychological research literature that you will turn to for soundly based principles. However,

---

BOX 7.1   Research tasks

1. Define the purpose of the research.
2. Review the literature.
3. Plan the study and the method(s) of investigation.
4. Test the method by carrying out a pilot study.
5. Collect the information.
6. Analyse the information.
7. Draw conclusions based on the findings of the analysis.
8. Compile the research report.

you may instead be concerned to know which of a number of alternative effective ways to motivate students to use more condoms is best value for money. If so, you will want to look at cost-effectiveness studies and make use of the work of health economists. It is vital that you are clear about the practical reasons for engaging in this research. If you are very sure about why you are doing it, who will use the findings and for what purposes, then you are likely to come up with some useful answers. If you are distracted by interesting but irrelevant information, your research could be confused and therefore flawed.

Time spent on task 3, planning, is a good investment. If you are going to apply for funding, your planning must include investigating sources of funding and the particular interests of different potential funders. Many tasks can take longer than the initial estimate and you will need to allow plenty of time for consulting people; for example, to arrange interviews if this is part of the research. Ethical issues and the need to apply for permission from ethical committees if you are using human subjects must also be taken in to account. Ethics committees in the NHS will evaluate the research proposal and will require additional information about issues such as confidentiality (for a useful discussion on the complexities of gaining ethical approval see Jamrozik 2004).

You will also need to consider ways of collecting the information you need. Any information collected needs to be *valid* and *reliable*. *Validity* means actually measuring what you purport to measure. For example, if you are attempting to measure the success of health education in encouraging a group of people to take more physical exercise, a valid measure would be directly to observe whether or not they spend more time on physical activities. Asking them to complete a written questionnaire may not give valid responses because research shows that people often respond to questions and questionnaires in ways they think the experts want them to. *Reliability* means that if the research is repeated using the same research instruments, it will give the same results (for examples of how to test reliability and validity see Elley et al 2003).

BASIC TOOLS OF RESEARCH

There are a number of basic tools used in health promotion research.

Questionnaires

These are useful when you want to collect information from relatively large numbers of people. Questionnaires should be kept as simple as possible, but this does not mean that they are easy to design. A great deal of care is needed in the formulation of questions to ensure that valid conclusions can be drawn from the answers. Questionnaires are most useful for collecting information that is quantifiable, such as factual knowledge. Advantages of questionnaires include: they can be answered anonymously, and respondents may therefore be more truthful, and they can be given to a whole group of people at the same time, so using respondents' and researcher's time effectively.

The questionnaire should always first be piloted on a small sample of people from the group for which it is intended. You will then be able to identify and redesign any questions that have been misinterpreted.

The response rate to questionnaires can be low, and you may need to think about the implications of this; for example, will the results really reflect the views of the target population? Also, some people may not want to complete the questionnaire and even if they fill one in they may do so casually, without giving it careful thought.

You need to consider right from the start how the information collected will be analysed. Decisions about whether computer software programmes, such as SPSS (see Pallant 2007), will be needed to analyse the information may affect the design of the questionnaire. Consultation with a statistician and/or an experienced researcher may be helpful at this point.

You have to put a lot of thought into the design of quantitative questionnaires by clarifying closed questions with defined ways of responding (such as tick boxes), so that they will give accurate results. Qualitative questionnaires with open questions can be more complicated to analyse.

See Chapter 10, section on asking questions and getting feedback, for more about open and closed questions.

Personal interviews

With face-to-face interviews you can develop rapport and encourage people to talk more openly. You may find out things that you did not think to ask about, but which are very relevant. The main advantage of personal interviews is that there is more scope for initiative by the interviewee. For example, the interviewee can seek clarification, and may be able to express views and opinions more easily verbally than in writing. The disadvantage is that, unless you are very skilled, you may bias the response, that is, you may get the responses you want to get or expect to get. For example, asking 'You do feel better, don't you?' biases the answer towards 'Yes', whereas 'Do you feel better?' removes some of this bias.

Interviews can be one-to-one or with groups, face-to-face or by telephone. They can be organised through using pre-prepared questions (a *structured interview*) or allowed to flow more freely. At one extreme, you could design an interview schedule that looks like a questionnaire; at the other extreme, you might simply have three or four broad headings which you wish to discuss (a *semistructured interview*). Box 7.2 is an example of a telephone interview schedule. Special interview groups, such as focus groups, concentrate on a particular issue through focusing on pre-determined questions (see Saks & Allsop 2007 and Bowling 2009 for more details on survey design, interviewing and conducting focus groups).

Participant and nonparticipant observation

Observation can include observing behaviour, such as how well a person performs an exercise routine, and physiological observations, such as monitoring weight. *Participant observation* happens when the researcher is also actively involved in what is being observed, such as actively contributing to discussions in a meeting. *Non-participant observation* means that the researcher takes no part in what is being observed.

Advantages of participant observation are that the researcher may be more aware of what is going on, including less tangible things such as the mood of a group of people. However, the researcher could have difficulty in making objective observations and may find it difficult to record what is happening, so that information could be lost. The non-participant researcher may find it easier to make objective observations, and may be able to plan and record observations more easily. On the other hand, having an observer who does not participate can seem threatening; people might not open up or may not behave as they normally do. This could have a big effect on what is observed, and invalidate the research (see Cooper et al 2004 for an example of the use of participant and nonparticipant observation in health research).

Sampling

If it is too expensive or time-consuming to collect information from the whole population or group you are interested in, then you need to select individuals so that you avoid getting a biased response. There are a number of sampling techniques which can be used to ensure that the sample is representative of the whole population.

Random sampling. This involves identifying people at random from the whole group. For example, imagine you are a practice nurse. Using the practice age–sex register you could decide at random on a number between 1 and 10 (say 5) and send out questionnaires to the 5th, 15th, 25th, 35th (and so on) person on the list.

Quota sampling. This uses your knowledge of a particular group to help set criteria about who to include in the sample. Criteria you might use include age, sex and ethnicity. Once the group has been divided into segments, using your criteria you can use a proportion from each segment for your sample. This ensures that people with certain characteristics are not over- or under-represented.

Convenience sampling. This means that researchers question the people they can get hold of at the time. This is biased but, accepting that it is very difficult to avoid bias altogether, it is important to decide whether the particular bias that has been

---

BOX 7.2	Patient satisfaction with health education and information: telephone survey schedule

- When you were in hospital, what information were you given about your illness?
- Do you now feel you have sufficient information about what was wrong with you?
- Were you able to discuss your anxieties with anyone while you were in hospital?
- Who did you prefer to discuss things with? *Prompt: Was it a nurse, a doctor, another professional or a domestic helper?*
- Did you have sufficient privacy to feel able to talk openly? *Prompt: Did you have access to a comfortable, private room for private conversations?*

introduced is acceptable. Bias should be discussed in any dissemination of the research (see Bowling, 2005, 2009 for further details on sampling and research bias).

THE RESEARCH REPORT

See also the section on report writing in Chapter 8, and the section on written communication in Chapter 10.

The final stage of your research will be to produce a written report, which will disseminate your findings. People who read the report may be interested in assessing the validity of the findings for themselves, in repeating the research in similar circumstances and avoiding any pitfalls, or in applying the research findings in the context of commissioning or providing health promotion services. So the report should be written with the objective of helping readers to use it in these ways. You may need to consider producing more than one version of the report for different groups of readers; for example, a two-page summary for community groups, and a full report for your health promotion professional and managers.

The contents of your research report may include the information set out in Box 7.3, although not every point will be applicable to a particular report, which should be written with the needs of the readers in mind.

Finally, a warning: in a field like health promotion, interpretation of research data is a complex matter, often because of underlying differences of opinion on what is health and what constitutes success. It is therefore all too easy for the sceptical to dismiss research findings. So it is extremely important that any health promotion research is

of good quality. Poor research is worse than no research because it wastes resources and misleads.

VALUE FOR MONEY

You need to think not only about evidence but also the question of whether you are getting value for money. Health economics is a discipline that provides a way of thinking about value for money and making efficient use of scarce resources. It is not about doing things more cheaply, but about choosing priorities and making the best choices with the resources available. The health economist focuses on costs and outcomes. *Costs* involve much more than money: they may include people, equipment, buildings and intangible costs, such as distress. *Outcomes* include length of life and things that are more difficult to measure, such as quality of life. There are a number of national centres of excellence in health economics which provide a wide range of useful resources, such as the one in York (http://www.york.ac.uk).

Opportunity cost

This is an important concept. Resources are finite and prioritising one intervention or service means giving up the potential benefits of another. So, for example, money devoted to a drugs mass media campaign takes money away from drug education in schools. All health promotion activities involve the use of resources that are expected to produce benefits, but at the same time incur opportunity costs in the form of benefits that will be forgone. It

---

BOX 7.3   Checklist of the contents of a research report

- **Abstract** (concise summary of the research).
- **Background** (statement about the purpose of the research, the background, the reasons for carrying out the research and the questions to be answered).
- **Literature review** (critiquing other research in the field).
- **Methods**:
  A description of the methods used for collecting the information and the reasons for selecting these methods.
  A description of the population sample studied, the sampling methods and response rates.

A discussion of the ethical implications.
Data analysis methods and the reasons for selecting these methods.
A description of the pilot study and any changes that were made as a result.
- **Results** (all appropriate data displayed clearly).
- **Discussion** (analysis of the findings, stating clearly the limitations of the study).
- **Conclusion** (with recommendations for further research).
- **References** (listing source material).

is often a matter, in practice, of getting the right *balance* between alternative activities; for example, in health education about smoking, getting a balance between national advertising and local facilities to help people stop smoking.

Cost–benefit analysis

This is the process of comparing benefits with costs. Failing the cost–benefit test does not mean that an activity is not worth investing in, but it does mean that the cost of pursuing these benefits, in terms of other benefits that will have to be forgone, cannot be justified. Formal cost–benefit analysis is a complex process, not least because it is difficult to decide how different benefits should be measured and valued. Nevertheless, it can be useful to apply the basic concepts of analysing the costs and the benefits when you are allocating resources and evaluating results. (See Mason et al 2008 for an account of the difficulties of applying cost–benefit analysis to heath promotion interventions at the community level.)

Cost-effectiveness analysis

This means comparing the costs and outcomes of alternative activities to achieve the same goal (see Vijgen et al 2007 for an example of a cost-effectiveness analysis of smoking cessation programmes in schools). It can be used when it is possible to measure the outcomes of alternative activities in the same unit of measurement, such as measuring blood pressure. For example, supposing that research had shown that exercise, drugs and diet (or a combination of these) were effective in lowering high blood pressure, these interventions could then be costed to see which ones were the most cost-effective. This approach is used in considering alternative health interventions.

At a national level, NICE, funded by the Department of Health, undertakes this kind analysis.

AUDIT

Audit is the systematic examination of the operations of a service, followed by the implementation of recommendations to improve quality. Basically, an audit will scrutinise how the service carries out each stage of the planning/evaluation cycle, which we described in Chapter 5.

Strengths and weaknesses will be revealed, and ways of overcoming weaknesses will be identified. Audit can involve either an internal review by the people responsible for delivering a service or scrutiny by an independent external auditor. For examples of clinical audit see the National Clinical Audit Support Programme (NCASP) at the NHS Information Centre (http://www.ic.nhs.uk).

The audit cycle in Fig. 7.2 starts with the specification of standards or criteria, followed by the collection of data, the assessment of performance and the identification of the need for change and implementing the improvements.

It is in the nature of cycles that you can, in practice, start anywhere. So you might start with collecting data on performance, assess performance and recommend the need to specify standards. The difficulty with auditing health promotion practice is that it is often embedded in other work. For example, audit of health promotion in clinical settings may involve scrutinising issues about relationships and communication, all of which are vital to the quality of health promotion work, but may not relate specifically to clinical audit.

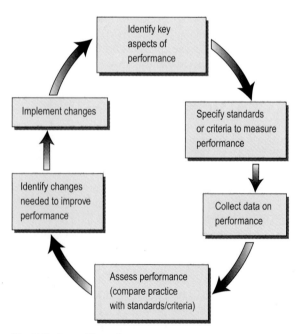

Fig. 7.2 An audit cycle.

For further reading on quality standards see Chapter 8, section on working for quality.

Many of the tools described in the section on research in this chapter can also be used in audit. So, for example, you could use a telephone survey after discharge to study the satisfaction of patients with information and education they received as inpatients. When telephoning patients, you would need to reassure them that participation in the survey is voluntary, and that their comments would be completely confidential. The sort of questions you might like to ask are set out in Box 7.2.

AUDIT, RESEARCH AND EVALUATION

Audit, research and evaluation are complementary activities. Research is concerned with generating new knowledge and new approaches, which can be applied beyond the specific context of the study. Evaluation involves making a judgement about one specific intervention or project, which is the focus of its concern. Audit seeks to improve the performance of a continuing service, such as an environmental health service or a midwifery service, through reviewing its practice. All three are crucial to the pursuit of evidence-based health promotion.

You should not need to do a detailed evaluation of everything you do, because you may be basing what you do on techniques and materials that have already been evaluated by others and form part of the published evidence. What you *should* do is to audit your health promotion practices regularly to check whether what you have planned and the techniques you have chosen are working properly. If you need further training in how to carry out an audit of your health promotion practice, it would be worth finding out about local opportunities for training in clinical audit as the basic concepts can be applied to health promotion. Another area to pursue could be training related to measuring and improving quality or quality assurance. Quality cycles and audit cycles are very closely related and the purpose of audit is to improve quality. You could also discuss, with your manager, local arrangements for performance appraisal (mechanisms for checking on and improving the performance of staff), professional development

plans and supervision, since these are all related to audit.

See the section on working for quality in Chapter 8.

HEALTH IMPACT ASSESSMENT

Health impact assessment (HIA) is a relatively new approach, which accepts that social, economic and environmental factors, as well as genetic make-up and health care, make a difference to people's health. It is a systematic way of assessing what difference a policy, programme or project (often about social, economic or environmental factors) makes to people's health. For example, it has been used when public sector organisations have wanted to understand the effect on people's health of policies on transport, air quality, economic development, regeneration or housing.

The assessment can be carried out before, during or after a policy is implemented, but ideally it is done before, so that the findings can inform decisions about whether and how to implement the policy. Key steps are to:

- Select and analyse policies, programmes or projects for assessment.
- Profile the affected population – who are likely to be affected and their characteristics.
- Identify the potential health impacts by getting information from the range of people who have an interest in the policy, or who are likely to be affected by it.
- Evaluate the importance, scale and likelihood of the potential impacts.
- Report on and make recommendations for managing the impacts.

(See Kemm et al 2004 for discussion of the concepts and principles of HIA and the HIA gateway (http://www.dh.gov.uk) for advice and tools on conducting HIAs including the National Audit Office (2009) guidelines.)

PRACTICE POINTS

■ It is important to identify how your health promotion work contributes to local and national strategies. Your effectiveness depends not only on what you do but also on how well your work complements that of other health promoters.

- All health promoters have a duty to appraise evidence and to base their work on evidence of effectiveness where it exists.
- Doing research involves specialised skills, and you should aim to develop the appropriate competencies that the particular type of research requires.
- You need to consider whether you are getting value for money, through using the ways of thinking developed in health economics.

- All health promoting services should regularly undertake audit: take stock of how they operate and identify how things can be improved.
- If your work involves making or implementing policies that affect people's health, health impact assessment may be a useful tool.

References

Abbot S, Gillam S 2001 Did health improvement programmes improve in their first two years? Health Education Journal 60(4): 354–361.

Appleby J 1997 Feel good factors. Health Service Journal 3: 24–27.

Aveyard H 2007 Doing a literature review in health and social care. Berkshire, Open University Press.

Barnes M, Bauld L, Benzeval M et al 2005 Health action zones: partnerships for health equity. London, Routledge.

Bauld L, MacKenzie M 2007 Health action zones: multi-agency partnerships to improve health. In: Scriven A, Garman G (eds) Public health: social context and action. Berkshire, Open University Press.

Bowling A 2005 handbook of research methods in health: investigation, measurement and analysis. Berkshire, Open University Press.

Bowling A 2009 Research methods in health: investigating health and health services, 3rd edn. Berkshire, Open University Press.

Caughlan M, Cronin P, Ryan M 2007 Step-by-step guide to critiquing research. Part 1: quantitative research. British Journal of Nursing 16(11): 658–663.

Chesterfield Borough Council 2009 Inspired: The Health Living Centre Newsletter. Edition 2 Spring 2009. Chesterfield, Chesterfield Borough Council. www.chesterfield.gov.uk/healthylivingcentre.

Cooper J, Lewis R, Urquhart C 2004 Using participant or non-participant observation to explain information behaviour. Information Research 9(4). http://informationr.net/ir/9-4/paper184.html.

Darlow A, Hawtin M, Jassi S et al 2008 Formative evaluation of community strategies 2004–2007: final report. London, Department of Communities and Local Government.

Department for Children, Schools and Families 2005 Nutritional standards for school lunches and other school food. London, DCSF.

Department of Health 1992 The health of the nation: a strategy for health in England. London, The Stationery Office.

Department of Health 1998 The health of the nation: a policy assessed. London, The Stationery Office.

Department of Health 1999 Saving lives: our healthier nation. London, The Stationery Office.

Department of Health 2004 Choosing health: making healthy choices easier. London, The Stationery Office.

Department of Health and Social Services 1997 Health and wellbeing into the next millennium. Regional strategy for health and social wellbeing 1997–2002. Belfast, DHSS.

Department of Health, Social Services and Public Safety 2002 Investing for health. Belfast, DHSSPS.

Dochartaigh NO 2007 Internet research skills: how to do your literature search and find research information online. London, Sage.

Elley RC, Ngaire KM, Swinburn B et al 2003 Measuring physical activity in primary health care research: validity and reliability of two questionnaires. New Zealand Family Physician 30(3): 171–180.

Gidley B 2007 Sure Start: an upstream approach to reducing health inequalities. In: Scriven A, Garman G (eds) Public health: social context and action. Berkshire, Open University Press.

Healey J 2009 Written answers, Tuesday, 5 May. Communities and Local Government New Deal for Communities. Hansard source. http://www.theyworkforyou.com/wrans/?id=2009-05-05a.271639.h.

Health Development Agency 2004 Lessons from health action zones. London, HDA.

Hills D, Elliot E., Kowarzik U et al 2005 The evaluation of the Big Lottery Fund Healthy Living Centres Programme: fourth annual report of the Bridge Consortium. London, The Big Lottery Fund.

Jamrozik K 2004 Research ethics paperwork: what is the plot we seem to have lost? British Medical Journal 329: 286–287.

Jones C, Scriven A 2005 Where are we headed? The next frontier for evidence of effectiveness in the European Region. Promotion & Education, Special Edition 1.

Kelly M, Speller V, Meyrick J 2004 Getting evidence in to practice in public health. London, Health Development Agency.

Kemm J, Parry J, Palmer S 2004 Health impact assessment. Oxford, Oxford University Press.

LutonForum 2005 Luton's community plan 2002–2012: a better quality of life for the people of Luton: 2005 revision. Luton, LutonForum.

Mason AR, Carr Hill R, Myers LA, Street AD 2008 Establishing the economics of engaging communities in health promotion: what is desirable, what is feasible? Critical Public Health 18(3): 285–297.

National Assembly for Wales 2001a Promoting health and wellbeing: implementing the national health promotion strategy. Cardiff, NAW.

National Assembly for Wales 2001b Improving health in Wales: a plan for the NHS and it's partners. Cardiff, NAW.

National Audit Office 1996 Health of the nation: a progress report. London, The Stationery Office.

National Audit Office 2009 Delivering high quality impact assessments. London, The Stationery Office.

National Audit Office, Healthcare Commission and Audit Commission 2006 Tackling child obesity– first steps. London, The Stationery Office.

OFSTED 2006 School sports partnerships: a survey of good practice. London, HMSO.

Pallant J 2007 SPSS survival manual: a step by step guide to data analysis using SPSS for Windows Version 15. London, Allen and Unwin.

Rankin D, Truman J, Backett-Milburn K et al 2006 The contextual development of healthy living centres services: an examination of food-related initiatives. Health & Place 12(4): 644–655.

Ryan M, Caughlan M, Cronin P 2007 Step-by-step guide to critiquing research. Part 2: qualitative research. British Journal of Nursing 16(12):738–744.

Saks M, Allsop J 2007 Researching health: qualitative, quantitative and mixed methods, 2nd edn. London, Sage.

Scottish Office 1999 Towards a healthier Scotland. Edinburgh, The Stationery Office.

Scottish Office 2007 Better health, better care: action plan. Edinburgh, The Stationery Office.

Scriven A 2008 Developing competencies for evidence based health promotion. In: Tarko K, Barabas B (eds) Egeszsegfejlesztes a Tudomanyokban. Szeged, Hungary, University of Szeged Press: 135–141.

Social Exclusion Unit 2001 A new commitment to neighbourhood renewal: a national strategy and action plan. London, The Cabinet Office.

Vijgen SMC, van Baal PHM, Hoogenveen, RT et al 2007 Cost-effectiveness analyses of health promotion programs: a case study of smoking prevention and cessation among Dutch students. Health Education Research. Advance access published online on August 4, 2007.

World Health Organization 2006 Health for all policy framework for the WHO European region. Geneva, WHO.

Websites

http://www.cochrane.org/reviews
http://www.dcsf.gov.uk/everychildmatters
http://www.dh.gov.uk/en/Publicationsandstatistics/Legislation/Healthassessment/DH_647
http://www.hp-source.net
http://www.ic.nhs.uk/services/national-clinical-audit-support-programme-ncasp
http://www.idea.gov.uk
http://www.neighbourhood.gov.uk/page.asp?id=542
http://www.newcastlendc.co.uk
http://www.nice.org.uk
http://www.nnhaz.co.uk
http://en.wikipedia.org/wiki/Comparison_of_reference_management_software
http://www.york.ac.uk/inst/che

Chapter 8

Skills of personal effectiveness

SUMMARY

This chapter is about developing skills to effectively manage your health promotion work. A number of skills are covered including managing information; report writing; time management; project management; change management; and finally, working for quality. Case studies and practical exercises are included to illustrate and give the context in which health promotion skills are applied.

Working effectively in health promotion requires a clear view of your aims and plans and the necessary competencies to implement your goals.

See also Chapters 5, 6 and 7 for details on planning for health promotion.

MANAGEMENT SKILLS IN HEALTH PROMOTION

It is not easy to define what management is, but in general terms it is about adopting practices which ensure effectiveness and efficiency in your work. *Effectiveness* means producing effects and accomplishing your goals. Being efficient means producing results with little wasted effort. It's the ability to carry out actions quickly. However, by being efficient you may not necessarily be achieving effectiveness, so it is important to establish the correct balance.

A comprehensive introduction to management is beyond the scope of this book, but for further details you may wish to consult Boddy (2005) for general management and Longest (2004) for health service management.

Some aspects of management have already been covered, such as setting priorities and planning. A number of other managerial skills you will need to be effective and efficient as a health promoter are outlined in this chapter. However, it is important to emphasise that possessing these skills will not automatically make you effective and efficient. Other factors also influence this, including:

- How well you integrate ethical principles into your basic everyday work; how you exercise your *responsibility* as a health promoter. 'Response-ability' is your ability to choose your response and is a product of your conscious choice, based on values, rather than a reaction to your circumstances.

  For further reading on ethics and values in health promotion, see Chapter 3.

- The people you work with. Your effectiveness and efficiency are limited or enhanced by the competencies and motivation of those you work with, for example receptionists, secretaries, colleagues and others within and outside your organisation.
- Your organisation. Both the structure and culture of your organisation will influence what you are able to achieve.
- The wider world. The state of the economy, government legislation, the organisation of local government and the impact of social trends are just a few examples of factors in the world outside your organisation that influence how effective you can be.

This book is designed to increase your awareness of these wider influences on your work, as well as to develop your own competencies.

There are some key aspects of personal effectiveness which will help you to manage health promotion.

MANAGING INFORMATION

Whether you keep information on computer and/or a manual filing system it is easy to be swamped by documents and papers, so keep only what is essential and cannot be kept by someone else or in another existing system.

EXERCISE 8.1   What information do you need to store?

Make a list of all the types of information you collect at present and analyse it by asking yourself the following questions about each one.
1. Do I need to keep this information?
2. How easy is it for me to find the information when I need it?
3. Could someone else, or another information system, keep the information for me?
4. Who else might need access to this information? How easy would it be for them to find it?
5. How could this information best be stored?

Think about who else collects information in your workplace and how they store it. Is there a central filing system? Does it work? Which information could and should you keep centrally? Undertake Exercise 8.1 to enable you to identify what information you need to store.

PRINCIPLES OF EFFECTIVE INFORMATION SYSTEMS

When reviewing or setting up your information system, it is useful to keep reminding yourself of three basic principles:

1. Keep it simple! Systems are only as effective as the people who put in and take out the information. The simpler the system the more likely it is that busy people will use it correctly.
2. Do not devise any more systems than are absolutely necessary.
3. Organise systems so that anyone who might want to use them can easily understand them.

WRITING REPORTS

Important information is often conveyed through written reports. For example, you are likely to need to write a report on plans for health promotion, or an evaluation report on a specific project. You may need to write reports for your manager or formal reports for committees. Written reports are likely to be read when you are not there, so there is no immediate feedback about whether the key points have been understood. To reduce the danger of being misunderstood, good skills in preparing and writing reports are essential.

See Chapter 10, section on written communication skills.

Work through the following stages each time you prepare and write a report.

Stage 1: Define the purpose

To help to clarify the purpose, complete the following sentence: 'As a result of reading this report, the reader will ...' What?

The purpose could be to inform, to influence decision making, to initiate a course of action, or to persuade. Whatever it is, keep it clearly in mind throughout all the later stages.

Stage 2: Define the readers

Identify the readers and consider them at all stages. Direct the report to the needs and interests of the readers. What do they already know about the subject? How much time do they have for reading? What kind of style is appropriate, for example, formal or informal?

Stage 3: Prepare the structure

Decide on the structure of the report. A report normally contains the following sections:

- **Title** – this should accurately describe what the report is about.
- **Origins** – for example the author's name, occupation, work base and date.
- **Distribution list** – it is a great help to readers if they know who else has seen the report. They may detect that someone vital has not received a copy.
- **Contents list** – a long report will need a contents list, showing the main sections of the report and the pages on which the reader can find them. This is not necessary for short reports.
- **Summary** – this is vital for all except the very shortest of reports (less than a page or two). It helps the reader if the summary is easy to find at the beginning of the report. Remember that busy people will often read only the summary (and perhaps the conclusions and recommendations), or at least read the summary first in order to decide whether it is worth spending time reading any more. So the summary needs to set out the essence of the report clearly and concisely. It is sometimes referred to as the executive summary.
- **Introduction** – this sets the context for the report, for example why the work was undertaken.
- **The main body of the report** – this will be the bulk of the report. You need to break up the content into sections and subsections, all with clear headings. Headings should be signposts to help the reader to see a route through the document and have an overview just by skimming through the headings. Sections need to be ordered in a way which will be logical for the reader. It may help to organise material into sections by writing all the possible headings and sub headings down, then move them around until you are satisfied that they are in the most logical order. You could use a numbering system for each section, heading and subheading, e.g. 1, 1.1, 1.1.1.
- **Conclusions** – summarises the conclusions which can be clearly drawn from the information in the report.
- **Recommendations** – these relate to the future, and summarise any changes needed.
- **References** – putting any references at the end makes the report easier to read.
- **Appendices** – a misused feature of some reports, to be avoided unless really necessary. Ask yourself 'What information will most of my readers need the first time they read this report?' If they need this information straight away, put it in the main body of the report.

Stage 4: Write the report

Tackle the various sections in the order that makes it easiest. For example, it may be easiest to write the detailed body of the report first, then summarise the information, then discuss the information, then draw your conclusions, then set out your recommendations, then write the summary of the report and lastly finish it off with the title, contents list, origin, distribution list and other essential details.

Stage 5: Review and revision

After the draft report has been produced, review it and revise as necessary. Make sure pages are numbered and check that sections and subsections are correctly numbered. It is a good idea to get a

---

EXERCISE 8.2   Analysing and improving your use of time

1. Devise a recording format that suits you, based on the example below

Then photocopy or print out a supply of the sheets. Use as many sheets as necessary each day. Remember to include any work you do away from your organisation, for example at home.

 If you discover that a particular activity, for example telephone interruptions, is causing you a problem, then make a detailed log of what happens each time. *Do this immediately* – do not leave it till the end of the day. Keep the diary for at least a week. If none of your weeks are typical you will need to keep the log for several weeks.

 Using codes will save you time. For example, you could use M for meetings, I for interruptions, P for phone calls, IP for phone interruptions.

Time diary

Day _____   Date _____   Page no._____

Activity	Time spent	Comments
_____	_____	_____
_____	_____	_____
_____	_____	_____

2. Now analyse how you used your time

Each week, analyse your use of time by answering the following questions:
- How did you actually use your time compared with how you planned to use it?

- How much of your time do you spend on different activities? Does this reflect the importance of the different activities? Important activities are those that help you to achieve your objectives.
- Which jobs did not get done? Does it matter? Did you finish all the *important and urgent* jobs?
- How much time do you lose through interruptions? What sort of interruptions?
- How much of your time is spent on other people's work?
- Do you do the right job at the right time? Most people have a time of day when they work best. Do you use this time for your most important work?

3. Now plan how to improve your time management

Some of the changes you could make will be obvious. For example:
- You discover that jobs started early in the morning tend to get completed quickly. So you decide in future to do your most important work at this time.
- You discover that you spend about 8 hours each week handling interruptions. You decide to experiment with techniques to cut down this time.
- You discover that urgent jobs are generally done but important long-term projects tend to be neglected. You decide to make realistic plans to ensure that these jobs will be done.
- What else can you do?

---

colleague to proofread the report, someone with good report writing skills who will give constructive comments.

Stage 6: Final check

Always do a final check for writing and typing errors, spelling and other mistakes. It can be helpful to ask someone who has not seen the report before to check it for typing and layout errors. For further information on how to write a report consult the online *How To* website (http://www.howtobooks.co.uk).

USING TIME EFFECTIVELY

How well organised and effective are you at your work? The following paragraphs should give you some ideas about how to improve your effectiveness by looking at how you use your time. Time is an expensive resource, and the one that some may find the hardest to manage. First of all, you need to know where your time goes. Exercise 8.2 and the next section are about analysing and improving the use of your time and scheduling your work appropriately.

TIME LOGS AND TIME DIARIES

A time log involves keeping a record of how you spend your time at regular intervals, which may be as often as every 5 or 10 minutes. It is useful if you wish to know exactly how you are using your time on an activity that seems to be taking longer than you think it should, and can help you to pinpoint the source of the problem. But keeping a log is time-consuming itself, so is really worthwhile only if a particular activity is causing you problems.

If you want to know more about how you generally use your time you can keep a time diary. This records how you have spent your time day by day and should take only a few minutes to fill it in at the end of each day. If you have a short memory you might find it better to fill in your diary more frequently, say at the end of the morning and at the end of the afternoon, or at any other convenient break between blocks of work.

SCHEDULING YOUR WORK

See Chapter 6, section on setting health promotion priorities.

Health promoters can find that they have to do far more than their time permits, and that they are faced daily with too many requests and demands. This means that, first and foremost, they must be very clear about their priorities. Second, they must be assertive about saying 'no' to requests to take on nonpriority tasks. Third, they need to develop skills of organising time and scheduling work to ensure that work which should get done actually does get done.

Scheduling work into the time available involves three steps:

1. Identify how long you need to spend on a job. This depends on:
   - The nature of the activity; for example, whether it is possible to reduce the time allowance without endangering people or the outcomes.
   - How important the job is. If it is unimportant it does not merit a large investment of your time. Ask yourself 'What am I employed for? Will doing this job contribute to my main aims and objectives?' If not, it is unimportant. If the job is important it merits a large investment.
2. Identify how soon you need to have the job completed. This depends on how urgent it is. Urgent jobs are ones that have imminent deadlines. If an urgent job can be completed quickly, deal with it right away. That means it will not interfere with you getting on with the most important jobs.
3. Plan when the work will be done. This involves the following steps:
   - Break the job down into manageable parts. If the job is big or difficult, or parts of it are

boring, try setting aside regular, small amounts of time to complete specific bits. Dividing it into manageable segments will help you to see that you are progressing.
   - Estimate how long each part will take to complete. It can be difficult to estimate how long it will take you to complete a particular task, but an informed guess will at least help you to be more realistic in future. Here are some suggestions that may help:
     • use your experience from similar jobs
     • consult colleagues who have experience in doing the job
     • build in some contingency time
     • keep a note of how long the task actually takes, so that you can make a better estimate next time.
   - Schedule in your diary or organiser when the work will be done. You may find that you need to reschedule daily, to take account of changing priorities. The important thing is to ensure that the key tasks you need to undertake are scheduled to allow enough time for their completion. For more tools and tips on effective time management see Evans (2008).

MANAGING PROJECT WORK

Planning and managing a project can be different from other managerial activities. When you are first given responsibility for a project, it can seem rather daunting. You must turn something that does not yet exist into reality, and control its progress so that it delivers effectively and efficiently.

The most obvious thing about a project is that it has a particular (unique) purpose, which may be encapsulated in its name, such as 'Bromley Active Lifestyles Project' or 'Portsmouth Needle Exchange Project'. It is probably most useful to think of a project as an instrument of change, which, when it is successfully completed, will have made an impact as defined in its aims and objectives.

Another key aspect of projects is that they are time-limited: they have clearly identifiable start and finish times. Projects vary enormously in their scope. Small projects can last only a few days and involve activities by a single person; large projects can involve many people (and indeed many agencies) and last for several years.

BOX 8.1   The stages of a project

1. **Start** is the most important stage of any project and covers areas such as setting the overall aims, gaining approval and the allocation of a budget. It will set the foundations for the lifetime of the project.
2. **Specification** involves defining the detailed objectives of the project, i.e. what the outcomes will be and the targets for delivering these outcomes in terms of quantity, quality and timing.
3. **Design** stage is when the 'what' is translated into 'how'. It may take the form of detailed plans.
4. In the **implementation** stage the plans are put into operation. It is important to note that the end of implementation is *not* the end of the project.
5. The **evaluation, review and final completion** stage will be marked by delivery of the final report, which includes evaluation of the findings and the details of a post-implementation review. This review should take place some time after the end of the implementation stage, so that it is possible to include data on the long-term outcomes of the project.

All projects, however, have the same basic underlying structure and go through a number of stages, as set out in Box 8.1.

These stages are, of course, very similar to the basic planning and evaluation cycle that was described in Chapter 5, and you should read the present section in conjunction with Chapter 5. The difference is that when you are delivering an ongoing service, rather than a one-off project, the cycle repeats itself over and over again.

See Chapter 5, Planning and evaluating health promotion.

Because projects vary so much in terms of their scale and length of life it is particularly important that they are planned systematically. It is also vital to understand how the project contributes to the wider strategic plans of the organisation concerned.

See Chapter 7, section on linking your work into broader health promotion plans and strategies.

STARTING A HEALTH PROMOTION PROJECT

A project will start with a proposal or written document, which can take a number of forms, such as 'terms of reference' or 'report of a feasibility study'. The key elements that must be described in this document include the following:

- Who is proposing to carry out the project, for example, a primary care trust or voluntary organisation.
- Who is the purchaser or commissioner of the project, for example the local authority.
- The aims and outcomes of the project.
- The scope of the project, for example who will use or receive it, the setting in which it will be delivered, which departments, agencies and people will be affected.
- The costs of the project, in terms of staffing, buildings, equipment and other resources.
- The project stages or milestones with timescales.
- Methods and standards: the use of any particular techniques or methods and the adoption of any recognised quality standards.
- Roles and responsibilities of participants in the project (especially important when the project is commissioned by a partnership of a number of agencies).

DETAILED PLANNING

For anything but the very smallest of projects, you will need to develop a detailed plan of each stage immediately before you enter it. Typically, one of the last tasks in the planning of a stage will be planning the next stage. The Gantt chart, named after Henry Gantt, the man credited with its invention (http://www.ganttchart.com), is the primary tool to use for planning, scheduling and monitoring project tasks.

The Gantt chart is made up of a task information side (on the left) and a task bar side (on the right) (See Fig. 8.1 for an example). The task information side sets out the nature of each task and the person or people responsible for it. The task bar is a line that represents the period during which the task will be carried out. The precise content of a Gantt chart should be determined by the intended use. Such a chart is easy to draw and presents the plan in a visual form, which is easily understood by most people (see http://www.ganttchart.com for examples of Gantt charts and available software).

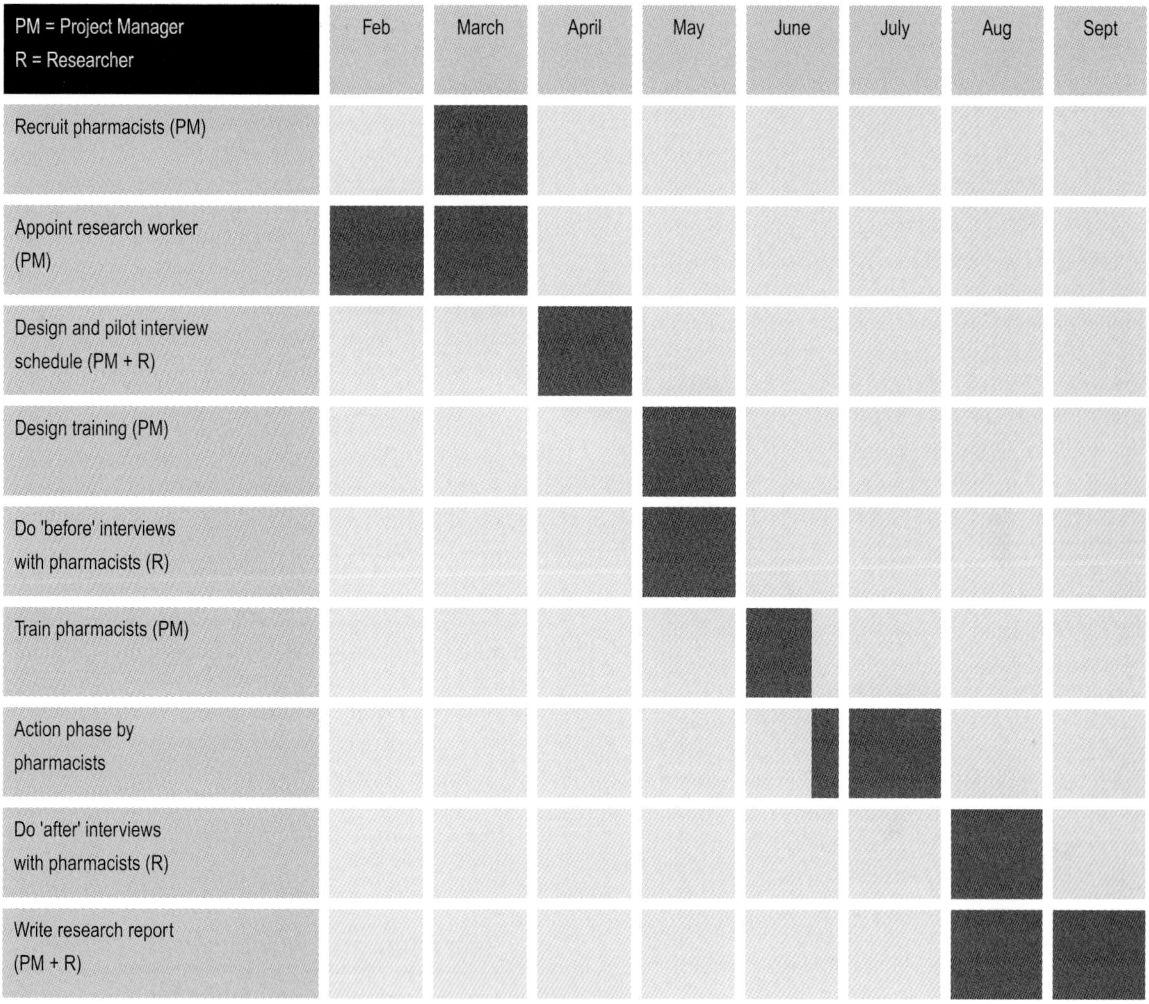

PM = Project Manager R = Researcher	Feb	March	April	May	June	July	Aug	Sept
Recruit pharmacists (PM)		■						
Appoint research worker (PM)	■	■						
Design and pilot interview schedule (PM + R)			■					
Design training (PM)				■				
Do 'before' interviews with pharmacists (R)				■				
Train pharmacists (PM)					■			
Action phase by pharmacists					■	■		
Do 'after' interviews with pharmacists (R)							■	
Write research report (PM + R)							■	■

Fig. 8.1 An example of a Gantt chart (see also Case Study 8.1).

The chart can be used at every level in the planning process, from initial outline planning down to the detailed planning of individual tasks. For complex projects any single bar on the master chart for the whole project might have to be represented by a more detailed bar for that particular task or stage.

One major benefit of Gantt charts is that they highlight critical points, for example where progress in X is dependent on Y already being completed.

Planning tools such as Gantt charts are only aids to help you to achieve your purpose. Sticking to your plan will not necessarily bring success; you may have to make adjustments because of unforeseen circumstances. However, without systematic planning you are unlikely to be able to keep your project on course at all. Case study 8.1 describes the use of the Gantt chart in Fig. 8.1.

CONTROLLING IMPLEMENTATION

In addition to detailed plans, a project needs to have built-in control procedures. Controlling projects is about identifying problems as soon as they arise, working out what needs to be done to ameliorate them, and then doing it. Things that need to be controlled include time, the budget (costs) and quality. Methods for control include progress reports and one-to-one and group progress meetings. Large projects will need to use all of these methods. Progress reports can sometimes be best

CASE STUDY 8.1 USING A GANTT CHART IN PROJECT PLANNING

This small pilot 8-month project aimed to explore the feasibility of using community pharmacists to promote physical activity with customers. Its objectives included identifying barriers and opportunities, and seeing whether training helped.

The plan was to recruit 10 volunteer pharmacists, interview them to ascertain their attitudes towards promoting physical activity with customers and their current practice, and then work with them in a training session. After the training, the pharmacists had a 6-week period to implement the training, followed by another interview to see if their attitudes and actions had changed.

A project manager had responsibility for planning and managing the project; a researcher was employed to design and carry out the interviews and help with the final report.

Fig. 8.1 shows the Gantt chart drawn up by the project manager. It was useful for clarifying what needed to be done when, and for seeing when possible timing difficulties could arise. For example, would pharmacists' or researchers' holidays interfere with the schedule? Were there too many tasks to be completed at one time (for example, recruiting pharmacists and appointing the research worker in February and March)? The Gantt chart also showed which stages required the research worker, so that the project manager could negotiate the appropriate numbers of hours worked at appropriate stages.

presented in a standardised form, which compares progress with the project plan.

> For more about quality, see section on working for quality later in this chapter.

Some problems will be outside the immediate control of the project. For example, a project could be influenced by the training policies of an organisation or other factors deeply embedded in the structure and culture of an organisation. In these cases project managers should do what they can to reduce the impact of these issues on the project, but should also remember that they have a duty to highlight these issues in reports. There are many books on project management that offer detailed advice for those managing a project for the first time. A good example is Lock (2007).

MANAGING CHANGE

Health promoters may experience change in two ways. One is being a part of an organisation that is undergoing change, hence finding yourself being reorganised. The second way is by being a change agent, by initiating and implementing changes in health promotion policy or practice.

The first way, experiencing organisational change, is common in statutory agencies as modernisation and reorganisation affect the NHS and local authorities in particular. Understanding and surviving organisational change is outside the scope of this book (see Baker 2007 for an overview). However, understanding how to implement change successfully is a fundamental part of a health promoter's role.

IMPLEMENTING CHANGE

You may want to introduce a change in your public health practice, such as a different way of running health promotion programmes, introducing a health-related policy at your place of work or starting off new health promotion activities. Implementing change can be very challenging, and it will help to spend some time thinking through your strategy.

KEY FACTORS FOR SUCCESSFUL CHANGE

The key to gaining commitment to change, and overcoming resistance to change, lies in understanding the motivation of all the people who could be affected by the change and how they feel about it. Overall, do they feel positive or negative about the proposed change? The balance between positive and negative factors can be expressed in the change equation in Box 8.2 (Gleicher 1990) developed as a tool to help analyse the key factors involved.

The basis of the equation is the simple assumption that people are rarely interested in change unless the factors supporting change outweigh the costs. As a change agent your job is either to reduce D (the perceived costs) or to increase the sum of A, B and C:

A: Dissatisfaction with the way things are. If you are dissatisfied, you may wrongly assume that others are too. If people are comfortable with the way things are they are unlikely to support change.

B: *A shared vision of a better future.* If a vision of a better future does not exist, or is unclear, people will not strive to achieve it. If there are several competing visions, energy will be dissipated in arguments. Few people would buy into a vision that threatens their livelihood or other cherished aspects of their lives. A vision that threatens important aspects of an individual's or a group's life is almost bound to fail.

C: *An acceptable, safe first step.* The size of the change and the risks involved can seem overwhelming. Many of us could share a common view of what better health for all would mean. But where do we begin? First steps are acceptable if they are small, are likely to be successful or, if they fail, do not cause too much damage and the situation is retrievable.

D: *The costs to the individual or group.* What is important here is how people *perceive* the costs. There will always be costs and change can be perceived as difficult or unfair. Costs can be tangible things like time, money, resources, or more intangible costs like stress or loss of status (see Case study 8.2 for an example of A–D reflected in a change in practice).

BOX 8.2   The change equation

A = the individual's or group's level of dissatisfaction with things as they are now.

B = the individual's or group's shared vision of a better future.

C = the existence of an acceptable, safe first step.

D = the costs to the individual or group.

Change is likely to be viewed positively, and be implemented successfully, *if*: A + B + C is greater than D.

CASE STUDY 8.2 CHANGE IN A LOCAL HEALTH CENTRE

An example of significant change originating from a few people started with a physiotherapist working in a local health centre. Many of her patients were elderly and suffering from arthritis. She found that, in addition to giving instructions verbally, it was useful to write down instructions for the people she saw who needed to comply with exercises at home. She enlisted the help of a friend who was a graphic designer in designing and printing some leaflets based on her advice and instructions. A second physiotherapist had begun to collect a small library of books, such as those produced by the Arthritis and Rheumatism Council, which were left in the waiting room. A list of recommended books was added to the leaflet. Meanwhile, the receptionist had taken another initiative. A friend had told her about a local support group for arthritis sufferers, and she pinned up a poster, giving information about it, in the waiting area.

The practice manager encouraged the staff to share their ideas. As a result a strategy to improve the provision of information to patients was launched, and patients were asked about their needs and preferences.

Other health centres heard about the venture and expressed interest. As a result, a number of other initiatives took place to improve patient information. Plans are now underway for a Patient Education Centre to be located in the foyer of the health centre which will include a computer for online access to specific websites that are recommended by the practice staff.

This case study illustrates the factors in the change equation:

A. The individual's or group's level of dissatisfaction with things as they are now: two of the physiotherapists and the receptionist, and through them the practice manager, saw that there was room for improvement.

B. The individual's or group's shared vision of a better future: the idea of improved help for patients was shared and spread through an increasing number of people in the health centre and other health centres locally.

C. The existence of an acceptable, safe first step: this change was built on a number of small successes, and did not present any major hurdles which could have induced resistance. If the *first step* had been to propose a Patient Education Centre, people may well have perceived major difficulties.

D. The costs to the individual or group were small in the first instance; just a little time and effort. By the time major investment was required for the Patient Education Centre, everybody was committed.

REASONS FOR RESISTANCE TO CHANGE

People react differently to change. While one person may passively resist a change, another may actively try to sabotage it, whereas a third may actually embrace change. Whether you are campaigning for a change, or implementing a change in policy or practice in your work, you will need to deal with the fact that many people will have reasons to resist change, including the following.

Self interest. While a change may be in the interest of most people, it may not be in everyone's best interest. For example, while most people, including some smokers, may support a smoking policy, others may see it as an infringement of personal liberty.

Misunderstanding. The change being proposed may be misunderstood. For example, some may think that an alcohol policy is allowing people with drinking problems to have different standards of work performance and behaviour than the rest of the workforce. Misunderstandings are particularly frequent in organisations where there is a lack of trust between the managers and the workforce.

Belief that a change is not in the interest of the people it is intended to benefit. People may believe that the costs of a change will outweigh the benefits, not only to themselves but also to others or a whole organisation. For example, people may feel that the introduction of ethnic monitoring as part of an equal opportunities policy could actually increase discrimination against black and minority ethnic groups.

Awareness of these opinions is important for the policy maker, because they may be based on knowledge of what goes on in parts of the organisation with which the policy maker has little contact. Policy formation must be based on an accurate analysis of the situation; this is particularly relevant in large organisations, like the health service and local councils.

Low tolerance for change. People may resist change because they are anxious about new demands that will be made of them. Organisational change can require people to change too much, or fail to provide them with the time and support they need.

METHODS FOR OVERCOMING RESISTANCE TO CHANGE

In order to overcome resistance to change it is vital to select the best approach, or combination of approaches, for the situation and the people involved. Five possible options are given below.

1. Education and communication. This involves educating people about a change before it happens and communicating with them in a variety of ways, including one-to-one, group discussion and written documents. An educational and communication approach is indicated when resistance to change is based on inadequate or inaccurate information. The limitation is that it can be time-consuming, especially if a lot of people are involved.

2. Participation and involvement. Resistance to change may be forestalled if those initiating the change identify the people that they think will be resistant, and actively involve them in the process of designing and implementing the change. The initiators of the change must genuinely be prepared to listen and learn. A token effort is liable to provoke more resistance, because people will feel let down if their contribution is not taken seriously.

Participation and involvement are necessary when full commitment to a policy change is needed in order to make it work; policies work when people feel ownership for them because they have been involved in their development. This approach is also useful when the initiators do not have full information about the implications of the change for certain groups of people or certain departments. It could also be the preferred option where the initiators of change have little power, because it harnesses the power of others as a force for change.

Nevertheless, this approach does have limitations. It is very time-consuming and demands a high degree of coordination. It can lead to a poor outcome if an attempt is made to accommodate everyone's needs.

3. Facilitation and support. This involves helping people to identify what changes are required and providing them with support to plan and manage the change themselves. This could be done, for example, by providing time for people to reflect on the situation, and to identify their own objectives and how to meet them. Support could include emotional support to cope with the stress of change, and the development of mentoring schemes, where more experienced people help others with their managerial or professional development. This approach works best where anxiety and fear lie at the heart of resistance. The limitation of this approach is that it, too, can be time-consuming and expensive (for example, if it is necessary to employ counsellors for a large workforce).

4. Negotiation and agreement. This involves offering incentives to actual or potential resisters, for example, through negotiating with trade unions about the effects of the change on working conditions. This is particularly appropriate when it is obvious that some people will lose out as a consequence of the changes. It can be effective if there are specific pockets of resistance, but could be expensive if everyone argues that they are also losing out.

5. Political influencing. This approach can be useful where one, or a few, powerful individuals are the source of resistance. It can be relatively quick, but has the drawback that it can lead to problems in the future if people feel that they have been manipulated.

See also Chapter 16, section on the politics of influence.

WORKING FOR QUALITY

Working for quality involves examining the nature of the service and assessing how good it is when judged against a number of criteria.

CRITERIA FOR QUALITY

What are the criteria for quality in health promotion work? The checklist in Box 8.3 may be helpful in identifying aspects of quality in your health promotion work. The checklist can be applied to your work overall, or to a particular health promotion programme.

IMPROVING QUALITY

Initiatives to improve quality are usually successful if people work together to pool ideas. This could be a group of people authorised by management to examine a particular issue or problem, such as improving the quality of patient information literature, the way in which antenatal advice is being given to prospective parents, or the way a GP practice is helping patients to stop smoking.

Sometimes such groups are called *quality circles*. These are work groups of between three and 12 employees who do the same (or similar) work, who meet regularly to address work-related problems. The issues to tackle are selected by the group itself and the outcomes are presented to management. In many cases the group is also involved in

---

BOX 8.3   Checklist: Criteria for quality in health promotion

1. **Appropriateness:** is it relevant and acceptable to clients – the individual, group or community concerned?
2. **Effectiveness:** does it achieve the aims and objectives you set?
3. **Social justice:** does it produce health improvement for all concerned, not for some people at the expense of others? In other words, is it 'fair'?
4. **Equity and access:** is it provided to all people whatever their racial, cultural or social background on the basis of equal access for equal need? (This may mean, for example, unconventional clinic times, wheelchair access, leaflets in Braille and ethnic minority languages, information on audio and video cassettes, etc.)
5. **Dignity and choice:** does it treat all groups of people with dignity and recognise the rights of people to choose for themselves how they live their lives? Is it nonjudgemental, accepting that people have the right to withdraw from, or reject, health promotion if they so wish?
6. **Environment:** does it ensure an environment conducive to people's health, safety and wellbeing? Does it recognise that people feel at home in different environments, and may feel uncomfortable or intimidated in some settings? Is the social environment friendly and welcoming?
7. **Participant satisfaction:** does it satisfy all those with an interest in the outcomes of the health promotion work, such as commissioners, managers, clients and other interest groups, acknowledging that the views of clients should be paramount?
8. **Involvement:** does it involve all those with an interest, including clients, in planning, design and implementation? Does it avoid 'tokenism', with clients' views genuinely sought and incorporated in a nonpatronising way?
9. **Efficiency:** does it achieve the best possible use of the resources available, and provide value for money?

implementing the solutions. Management commitment to taking account of the outcomes and implementing recommended changes is crucial to success.

Typically, a quality circle will:

- Begin by drawing up a list of issues for consideration, using techniques such as brainstorming.
- Select the issue to be addressed.
- Gather information about the nature of the problem, and analyse the causes.
- Generate a range of solutions, and establish the best options or combination of options.
- Prepare a report on their findings for management decision.

An example of a quality circle might be a group of nurses working in a coronary care unit looking at how to improve the quality of the patient education programmes which are run for discharged patients. The activities of such a group are described in Case study 8.3.

DEVELOPING QUALITY STANDARDS

It may be helpful to look at improving quality by setting specific quality standards, which are an agreed level of performance negotiated within available resources.

Examples of standards that relate to public health and health promotion are available on the National Institute for Health and Clinical Excellence (NICE) website (http://www.evidence.nhs.uk). Quality standards in health promotion work have been developed (see, for example, Health Development Agency 2004) and can be set for health promotion materials (see, for example, Hawthorne et al 2009). The criteria listed below could be used as a list of quality standards for health education leaflets (see also Children, Youth and Women's Health Service 2006):

- Appropriate for achieving your health promotion aims.
- Content consistent with the values of health promotion.
- Relevant and easily understood by the people for whom the leaflets are intended.
- Involved the target audience to ensure it meets their needs.
- Not racist or sexist.

- Accurate, up-to-date information informed by evidence.
- Free of inappropriate advertising.

See section on guidelines for selecting and producing health promotion resources in Chapter 11.

A further challenge is to develop standards that are *quantifiable* in some way. This is a difficult task, but you could, for example, develop a five-point scale for assessing the quality of your leaflets, so that you score them out of five for the extent to which they fulfill each quality standard. Another example could be that you decide that a quality management issue is to respond quickly to requests from your clients. You could develop this by setting a standard such as returning telephone calls within 24 hours, and written requests within 3 days.

Setting, monitoring and reviewing quality standards can involve a great deal of time and effort. The benefit comes from seeing clearly identified improvements in service.

PRACTICE POINTS

- To implement health promotion work successfully you need to develop management skills that include information management, report writing, time management, project management, managing change and developing quality.
- Managing information involves storing in the simplest way the paperwork and electronic files that are essential and that cannot be kept in another information-retrieval system.
- Writing a report involves being clear about the report's purpose and following a coherent and logical structure. Always get your report checked prior to publication.
- Managing time involves monitoring your time through using time logs and diaries and scheduling tasks appropriately.
- Project work involves detailed and systematic planning. A Gantt chart is a useful tool.
- Managing change requires an effective change strategy and is more likely to be successful if people have a shared vision and believe that the factors in favour of the change outweigh the costs.
- Working for quality is best achieved collaboratively. Management support and involvement are essential for success.

CASE STUDY 8.3 BLOGGSVILLE ROYAL HOSPITAL: CORONARY CARE UNIT

Improving the quality of patient education

A group of four nurses in the coronary care unit have been meeting regularly as a quality circle, and have decided to investigate how to improve the quality of education for discharged patients. At present a course of six group sessions is provided for patients after discharge, and nurses take turns to organise and run the courses.

The group first looked at the data for attendance at the group sessions. They discovered that, over the last year, 60% of discharged patients attended at least one session, but of these, only 20% attended three or more sessions.

They conducted a series of interviews with discharged patients to investigate the reasons for attendance or nonattendance, and to find out patients' preferences about how they would like the education to be provided. They discovered that some patients do not like attending a group under any circumstances, and some strongly dislike coming back into the hospital environment. But some of these would like one-to-one opportunities for guidance from specialists such as a dietitian (on healthy eating), a physiotherapist (on exercise and fitness) and a psychologist (on how to stop smoking, stress management and relaxation).

Other patients would prefer to have written information, audiotapes (for relaxation and self-hypnosis) and videotapes (of appropriate exercise routines), rather than come back to the hospital. Others would like more information about community groups and facilities for exercise tailored to their needs: for example, free trials of fitness classes, swimming sessions for elderly people. Others are interested in knowing if there are self-help or voluntary groups they could join, such as clubs for people who are being rehabilitated following heart disease. Some patients, especially those who are socially isolated, have particularly valued the opportunity to meet as a group and to exchange experiences.

After analysing these findings, the group of nurses produced a report for their manager recommending that a range of educational opportunities is provided for the education of discharged patients including:

■ Putting patients in touch with local self-help and cardiac rehabilitation schemes.

■ Setting up a video and audiotape library providing appropriate material for discharged patients on free loan.
■ Offering opportunities for counselling by specialists (dietitian, physiotherapist, psychologist) before discharge.
■ Selecting or producing appropriate written material, and making it available to patients before discharge.
■ Inviting all patients to return for an open evening, with information and demonstrations about facilities and activities available locally. This would include local authority exercise and leisure facilities, alternative medicine practitioners, community and self-help groups and commercial leisure organisations.

The report includes a financial breakdown, which demonstrates that the recommendations will have additional costs, primarily related to the proposed services to be provided by the professions allied to medicine. However, savings will be made on the nursing staff time currently devoted to running the courses and through financial sponsorship of written material by approved 'ethical' commercial sponsors.

This case study shows how the quality of the patient education programme could be improved on a number of criteria:

■ **Appropriateness:** clients would find the new approach more acceptable and relevant.
■ **Effectiveness:** more clients would gain from the programme.
■ **Equity and access:** clients could access advice and help in different ways, and those who disliked group meetings, or found attendance difficult, would have their needs met in other ways.
■ **Environment:** it was recognised that some people disliked the hospital environment.
■ **Participant satisfaction:** clients and nurses would be more satisfied with the results.
■ **Involvement:** clients were involved in redesigning the programme, with their views taken into account.
■ **Efficiency:** it would be a better use of resources because it would reach the people intended, and avoid wasting resources on a programme that reached very few.

References

Baker D 2007 Strategic change management in public sector organisations: a guide for public sector and not-for-profit organizations. Oxford, Chandos.

Boddy D 2005 Management: an introduction, 3rd edn. Essex, Financial Times/Prentice Hall.

Children, Youth and Women's Health Service 2006 Developing quality consumer health information. Adelaide, Government of South Australia. http://www.chdf.org.au/Content.aspx?p=133.

Evans C 2008 Time management for dummies. Chichester, John Wiley & Sons.

Gleicher D 1990 Open Business School/Institute of Health Services Management/NHS Training Authority managing health services. Milton Keynes, The Open University Book 9: 36–37, Managing Change.

Hawthorne K, Robles Y, Cannings-John R, Edwards AGK 2009 Culturally appropriate health education for type 2 diabetes mellitus in ethnic minority groups. Cochrane Database of Systematic Reviews, Issue 3. Art. No.: CD006424. DOI: 10.1002/14651858.CD006424.pub2.

Health Development Agency 2004 Promoting children and young people's participation through the National Healthy School Standard. http://www.evidence.nhs.uk/ Details.aspx?ci=http%3a%2f%2fwww.wiredforhealth.gov.uk%2fPDF%2fNHSS_participation_briefing.pdf.

Lock D 2007 Project management, 9th edn. London, Gower.

Longest BB 2004 Managing health programmes and projects. New York, Jossey Bass.

Websites

http://www.evidence.nhs.uk/Search.aspx?t=quality+standards&m=ain.Public%2bHealth&ps=10&pa=2&s=Relevance

http://www.ganttchart.com

http://www.howtobooks.co.uk/business/reports

Chapter 9

Working effectively with other people

SUMMARY

This chapter focuses on developing skills of working effectively with other people and organisations in order to plan and implement health promotion. The following key aspects are discussed: communicating with colleagues; coordination and teamwork; participating in meetings; effective committee work; working in local partnerships for health with other agencies. Practical exercises and a case study are included.

Some health promoters plan and undertake their health promotion work entirely on their own, but most are likely to be working with other people from the wide range of professional backgrounds that make up the multidisciplinary workforce that promotes health:

- Colleagues, who may be peers, managers or people you manage.
- Colleagues in other parts of your own organisation.
- People drawn from the community and/or from different agencies (local, national or international) who are working with you on a health promotion activity of mutual interest and importance.

A key aspect of success will be how well you work with other people, and this chapter discusses the knowledge and skills needed for interprofessional communication and collaborative working.

COMMUNICATING WITH COLLEAGUES

Some fundamentals of effective face-to-face and written communication are dealt with in Chapter 10. While these are presented primarily with client contact in mind, they are also applicable to contact between health promotion colleagues. The following factors are particularly important to ensure effective working relationships:

See Chapter 10.

- Working in a team which recognises and builds on the strengths of other team members.
- Actively listening to the people you are working with, so that you understand clearly their opinions, ideas and feelings.

A considerable proportion of your time may be taken up by communications with working colleagues, including telephone conversations, face-to-face discussions and written communications on paper and via e-mail. Try Exercise 9.1 to help increase your awareness of how you communicate with colleagues, and how your communication might be improved.

COORDINATION AND TEAMWORK

Health promotion often involves multiagency and multidisciplinary working, therefore effective coordination and teamwork are required.

Poor coordination can result in losses in efficiency and effectiveness of programmes; it is especially difficult when big bureaucracies like the NHS and local authorities are working together. There are several ways of coordinating, and it is important to use the one best suited to the situation.

APPOINTING A COORDINATOR

A potential problem for coordinators is that they may not directly manage the people they are trying

---

EXERCISE 9.1   How you communicate with colleagues

Record all the types of communication with colleagues that you carry out over one working day, by making a tally of all the occasions in four categories, as set out below. Then add up your total for each category, and your grand total for the day.

You might like to compare your results with those of your colleagues.

Face-to-face verbal	Telephone	Paper: letters and memos	Electronic: e-mail, Web cam/computer conferencing
_____	_____	_____	_____
_____	_____	_____	_____
_____	_____	_____	_____
_____	_____	_____	_____
_____	_____	_____	_____
_____	_____	_____	_____
_____	_____	_____	_____
TOTALS _____	_____	_____	_____

Think about whether there is anything you would like to change or improve; for example:
- If you spend a lot of time on the telephone, could you improve your telephone skills?
- Could you use your time more efficiently if you used less time-consuming methods of communications (for example, phone or e-mail) instead of writing letters or having meetings?
- Are there ways that you can use technology to communicate more effectively and efficiently with colleagues?
- Do you need to selectively spend more time face-to-face in order to understand colleagues and establish a closer working relationship?

to coordinate and therefore cannot control them in the same way as a manager. They must convince people that any requests they make are legitimate. Coordinators can be at a low level in a hierarchical organisation. A diabetic nurse trying to coordinate the production of a patient information leaflet, for example, might find it difficult to obtain the commitment of a consultant. The very word *coordinator* may provoke resistance to being organised in some people.

There are several tactics that can help to overcome resistance.

Using your reputation

People will find it difficult to turn down any reasonable requests if your work is well known and well regarded and you are respected by those who work with you. So you need to publicise your work and seek to establish a good reputation.

Establishing good relationships

Building and maintaining good relationships requires effort and is an essential investment for every coordinator.

Bargaining

It may be possible to bargain with individual people or departments: could you offer them something in return for their cooperation?

Out-ranking

This should be used only as a last resort. It requires a senior manager from your hierarchy to request cooperation through the other person's manager. While the other tactics build trust, this one endangers it and may result in a lack of goodwill.

Discussion and negotiation

Talking to all involved could result in clarification of responsibilities and improved mutual understanding, leading to the group giving you more legitimate authority. This could mean first discussing the issue with individuals, and later convening a meeting when you have got sufficient commitment to solving the problem. Undertake Exercise 9.2 to assess how you might improve your coordination and teamworking skills.

> **EXERCISE 9.2   Improving coordination and teamworking**
>
> In the health promotion work you do that involves working with other people, can you think of any ways by which you could improve coordination and teamworking?
> - What steps could you take to enhance the reputation of your health promotion work?
> - With whom could you build a better relationship to improve coordination or teamwork?
> - What have you got to offer if you are bargaining?
> - Can you think of any health promotion activities that you undertake routinely together with other people which could be more efficient with a set procedure?
> - Are there any ways by which you could develop stronger links with other staff at your level in different departments or agencies, to facilitate joint working in health promotion?
> - Have you any opportunities for joint objective setting or joint planning that could help to coordinate health promotion in your situation?
> - Can you think of anything else? Discuss this with colleagues who are also involved in health promotion.

POLICIES, PROCEDURES AND PROTOCOLS

> Making and implementing policies is discussed in Chapter 16.

Policies are increasingly important in coordinating health promotion work. Using *set procedures* are ways of coordinating routine tasks. *Protocols* are agreed written procedures that everyone follows, ensuring that everyone carries out a particular task in the same way. For example, there may be a smoking cessation protocol in a GP surgery about how to help a patient to stop smoking. The protocol ensures that whoever is dealing with the patient (the doctor, the practice nurse, the district nurse or the health visitor) will offer the same range of help and follow the same follow-up procedures (for an excellent example of a smoking cessation protocol see http://www.alhcc.scot.nhs.uk).

JOINT PLANNING

In this approach the parties involved not only agree objectives but also meet regularly to develop and implement a joint plan. This may minimise the need for one individual to be given the job of coordinator and prevent the problem of one agency or department being perceived as controlling the agenda. However, it can be very difficult to get all the people involved together on a regular basis, and to ensure that communications are always clear to all those involved.

JOINT WORKING THROUGH CREATING TEAMS

An autonomous team is given the authority, training, money, staff, premises and equipment to carry out the health promotion programme. There is no need for a coordinator, since the whole team is working together from the same base. Joint working of this kind is usually not suitable for short-term programmes, but can be excellent for long-term projects such as those involving community development.

CREATION OF LATERAL RELATIONS

This type of coordination depends on strengthening relationships between individuals in broadly equivalent jobs in different departments or agencies. Setting up project teams, which are dissolved once the particular project is completed, can do this. It could also be done by forming interdepartmental or multidisciplinary teams or partnerships, which are given more authority for making decisions, without having to refer them up the different hierarchies. However, this can lead to conflict with the existing vertical lines of command, and works best where there are good links between the various managers.

CHARACTERISTICS OF SUCCESSFUL TEAMS

There are different sorts of teams. The teams of relevance here are associations of people with a common work purpose, for example a primary healthcare team. Successful teams have the characteristics set out in Box 9.1. If you experience a team that does not seem to be working well, it can be helpful for the team to consider this list together, to identify the roots of the difficulties (for more information on how to develop successful team working see Jelphs & Dickenson 2008).

BOX 9.1   Characteristics of successful teams

- A team consists of a group of identified people.
- The team has a common purpose and shared objectives, which are known and agreed by all members.
- Members are selected because they have relevant expertise.
- Members know and agree their own role and know the roles of the other members.
- Members support each other in achieving the common purpose.
- Members trust each other, and communicate with each other in an open, honest way.
- The team has a leader, whose authority is accepted by all members.

PARTICIPATING IN MEETINGS

The detailed planning and organisation of meetings are beyond the scope of this book (see Barker 2006 and Hadler 2006 for useful guidance on running meetings). The guidance below is an aid to how to be an effective participant at meetings. As a participant there are a number of constructive things you can do:

- Encourage the Chair into good practices: for example, ask for clarification on the purpose of the meeting, and ask for a summary of what has been agreed at the end.
- Come prepared and arrive on time.
- Acknowledge the authority of the Chair.
- Agree what to do about taking notes: does each person take their own, or does one person take them and circulate a copy to everyone else? Do you want detailed notes of everything you discussed, or just action points?
- Actively contribute to the meeting, express your views succinctly, keep an open mind and listen to other people's opinions.
- Encourage everyone to participate by referring to members' relevant experience or expertise.
- Only make commitments that you are genuinely able to fulfill, and make sure you fulfill them on time. Say 'no' clearly and nondefensively if you are unable or unwilling to take on a task.
- Remember that discussion and debate about ideas will help decision making but personal rivalries will not.

EFFECTIVE COMMITTEE WORK

A committee is a group of people appointed for a specific purpose accountable to a larger group or organisation: examples are the management committee of a voluntary organisation or the health committee of a local authority. There are many common routines and procedures that help facilitate committees, and it is useful to be familiar with them. The details will vary from committee to committee, although the principles remain the same. Some committees start their life with recommendations from a steering group, which include proposals for the interim committee rules. These are then approved at the first committee meeting. After review and modification, a set of rules will be agreed which become the accepted rules for the committee.

OFFICERS

The officers are servants of the committee and carry out its instructions. Committees have key officers, usually the Chair, the Secretary and the Treasurer, but larger committees may have additional appointments, for example, a Minutes Secretary.

Chair

Much of the work of the Chair may be done between meetings, but it is at the meetings when the Chair is most visible, and has responsibility for ensuring that the committee successfully completes its tasks. It is vital for the Chair to be heard clearly during meetings, so that all the committee can be involved. Good Chairs delegate as much as possible, to ensure active involvement of all members. The Chair also has the responsibility of preparing the next Chair and must ensure that opportunities are provided for the Vice Chair to develop.

Secretary

The Secretary is responsible for all the nonfinancial papers and reports, for general planning and organisation (often in collaboration with the other officers) and for seeing that the committee's work is coordinated and nothing is forgotten. Good organisation, coordination and computing skills are needed. There are a number of software programmes (such as SharePoint – see Samson 2008) that can help with this work.

The Secretary is responsible for compiling the agenda for the committee meetings. This is the list of things to be done or agreed during the meeting. It will often include standard items such as 'apologies for absence', 'minutes of the previous meeting', 'matters arising from the previous meeting' and 'any other business'. The important point is that the agenda acts as an advance organiser for everyone attending the meeting, so that they are able to prepare. The committee members need to receive the agenda and associated papers in good time before the meeting, usually a week in advance.

The Secretary is also responsible for the final version of the minutes, and for agreeing these with the Chair, even if a Minutes Secretary takes the notes at the meetings. Minutes are accurate records of the meeting, and should always identify precisely who has responsibility for what action, by what date, and when a report back will be made to the committee.

Treasurer

A Treasurer will only be necessary if the committee is responsible for any financial matters. Treasurers are expected to report on the financial position quickly and precisely at any time by recording and summarising every transaction, so that it is easy to see the current situation. At the end of the financial year all financial transactions are summarised in an annual statement, a clear one-page summary.

Quorum

It is unlikely that all committee members will be able to attend all meetings. The rules usually state the minimum number of members who must be present for the meeting to be considered representative of members' views and to have the authority to make decisions. This is called a quorum and is usually one-third or one-half of the total voting membership.

COMMITTEE BEHAVIOUR

Committees can be informal, but there are reasons for various formal behaviours. For example, the rule that only one person speaks at a time and is not interrupted is meant to ensure a fair hearing for everyone. The Chair should not allow a vociferous few to dominate the meeting.

The rule of everyone speaking by addressing the meeting through the Chair helps to prevent a number of sub-discussions developing at the same time. On the other hand, it may seem more natural and helpful to address another committee member directly. Ultimately it is the job of the Chair to set a tone that encourages all members to participate while keeping the meeting under control.

UNDERSTANDING CONFLICT

In itself, conflict is not bad. Conflict is inevitable at times in any group because of differences in needs, objectives or values. The results of conflict will be positive or negative depending on how it is handled. Handled well, conflict can be a creative source of new ideas and can help a group to change and develop. It can also strengthen the ability of group members to work together. Conflict is badly handled when it is either ignored so that negative feelings develop, or approached on a win/lose basis rather than a compromise or a win/win position. Undertake Exercise 9.3 to assess your conflict resolution style.

WORKING IN PARTNERSHIP WITH OTHER ORGANISATIONS

See Chapter 4, section on primary care trusts for more on local strategic partnerships.

Health promotion programmes and projects often require people from different organisations to work together; it is an established way of working in health promotion. Health promotion partnerships may be formally structured, with partners or members at different levels from chief executives to field workers. There may be a written constitution and terms of reference, or arrangements may be fairly informal. They may be long term, or set up for a time-limited period to work on a specific project (see Scriven 2007 for a detailed examination of partnership working).

The main reasons for setting up local partnerships are:

- to harness a range of complementary skills and resources to work towards common goals
- to avoid duplication and fragmentation of effort
- to avoid gaps in services or programmes.

See Chapter 4, Fig. 4.1 for an overview of the organisations working for public health.

Recent UK government health reforms have created the opportunity for new styles of partnerships (Glasby & Dickenson 2009). Public health work often involves health services and local authorities pooling their budgets for joint initiatives and forming partnerships for planning, commissioning and delivering services. These new-style partnerships are genuine joint enterprises with local authorities and others. Case study 9.1 is

---

EXERCISE 9.3   Your conflict resolution style

When confronted with conflict in a group you work in, which of these styles do you use?

Style	Characteristic behaviour
Avoidance	Ignores the problem; avoids raising the issue; denies that there is a problem
Accommodating	Attempts to cooperate with everyone, even at the expense of not meeting personal or team objectives
Win/lose	Fights to win at any cost, even if it means alienating colleagues or causing the rest of the team to fail in meeting their objectives
Compromising	Suggests a compromise that would meet everyone's basic needs and maintain good relationships
Problem-solving	Openly confronts the problem and encourages everyone to face the disagreements and to express fully their opinions and ideas. Searches for a new solution which meets everyone's needs as fully as possible

Review this chart with other members of groups you work in. Can you think of situations in which these different approaches to conflict resolution were used? Discuss what worked and what did not. What could have been done differently to improve the outcome?

What's your conflict resolution style?

CASE STUDY 9.1 HEALTHY LIVING IN THE NEIGHBOURHOOD: A CASE STUDY ON COMMUNITY DEVELOPMENT AND PARTNERSHIP WORKING

Healthy Living in the Neighbourhood was initiated by Featherstone High School and the South Southall Extended Schools Partnership with support from Ealing Healthy Schools and statutory and voluntary partners, such as Ealing City Learning Centre and Ealing Primary Care Trust. It is a schools and community partnership project designed to encourage peer education and community support in the healthy living changes being made in schools. Interactive learning and a multimedia extravaganza allowed young people to share their learning experiences with the wider community and increase long-term uptake of healthy living messages.

Rationale

Schools in South Southall reacted quickly and creatively to government initiatives on healthy living. Young people are well informed on healthy living but the uptake of healthier choice outside the school is slow. The general consensus among students is that the banning of certain foods and changes to their school lunch menus have been top down. Schools have recognised that the impetus for change rests with the students, and that their decision to embrace healthy living will break down barriers of resistance at home with their families.

Process

Healthy Living in the Neighbourhood endeavoured to cater to needs of the nine schools in an extended schools partnership, through devising workshops in both healthy living and media/IT/creative technologies.
Key steps were:

- Identification of schools to participate from the extended schools partnership.
- Catering to individual schools' needs through consultation.
- Developing and delivering after school, in the holidays and during noncurriculum time a series of participatory multimedia workshops for young people on health themes.
- Implementing training for staff on multimedia skills, thereby building skills in the community.
- Filming a documentary of year 11 students' healthy living efforts.
- Compiling a DVD documenting the work of the project.

Workshops and training

Students explored a broad range of healthy living issues and were given the opportunity to create websites, blogs, video diaries, documentaries, music, animation, photo journalism, newsletters and more. The skills learnt in the various workshops have been made sustainable by teacher and peer training, and the work produced was shared with peers, family and community via the schools' and extended schools' websites. During the termly extended schools partnership meetings, any concerns were raised and the project was evaluated on an ongoing basis to determine the effect it's impact on participating schools.

The documentary

Three year 11 students from Featherstone High School were filmed in a 20-minute documentary, Good Attitude, following their efforts to change their health behaviour. They had 8 weeks to learn to eat well and exercise and to discover how changes might make a big difference to what they may achieve in their lives. This documentary was the focus of the overall DVD resource produced by and for the schools. The DVD is provided to all primary and high schools in Ealing and includes lesson plans for Key Stage 3 that relates to the Ealing Scheme of Work for personal, social and health education (PSHE) and Healthy Schools programme. In addition, the DVD includes the Family Recipe Book produced by the partnership and used in parent cookery classes, a selection of the work produced over the course of the project and other materials requested by participating schools.

Outcomes

- Featherstone High School students were trained in blogging and podcasting during a summer workshop and recorded their experiences on a healthy living plan throughout the Autumn term. Teacher training was implemented during a 2-week period where the teaching timetable is disbanded and students participate in a range of outings, educational visits and educational workshops.
- 'Healthy Living at Three Bridges Primary': a year 5 class at Three Bridges Primary School was trained in video making at the Ealing City Learning Centre and they used their skills to produce a short film, produced by South Southall Extended Schools. The class shares their healthy living experiences creatively with the school and wider community.
- 'We Like to Be Healthy': a song performed and written by the children at Greenfields Children's

Continued

CASE STUDY 9.1 HEALTHY LIVING IN THE NEIGHBOURHOOD: A CASE STUDY ON COMMUNITY DEVELOPMENT AND PARTNERSHIP WORKING – cont'd

Centre produced by South Southall Extended Schools in partnership with Featherstone High School.

■ A year 5 class at Featherstone Primary was trained in blogging during a holiday activity workshop and recorded their experiences while on a healthy living plan. Teacher training and peer training were implemented during the Autumn term.

■ The holiday programme of activities focused on the healthy living theme and, open to all pupils from the South Southall Extended Schools Partnership, included music production, journalism, design and photography, blogging and podcasting.

Points learnt from Healthy Living in the Neighbourhood experience

■ Keep ideas realistic and ensure projects are small scale. Schools have increasing workloads and a growing number of priorities, therefore it is essential to work on achievable partnership projects. Initial ideas were for projects on a larger

scale, before realising the practicalities and limitations of time, resources and manpower.

■ Community partnership projects can take longer than anticipated. Building trust and relationships and getting schools on board takes time.

■ Cater for schools expressed needs at all times. Schools need to see that their involvement is relevant to their priorities.

■ A community partnership project needs strong coordination and leadership to drive the project forward. All partners need to be committed to the initiatives, carrying out the actions and ensuring skills learnt are sustained and not forgotten.

The South Southall Extended Schools Partnership includes Clifton Primary, Dairy Meadow Primary, Featherstone High School, Featherstone Primary, Greenfields Childrens Centre, Havelock Primary, St Anselm's Primary, Three Bridges Primary, Wolf Fields Primary.

(Case study produced by Natalie Shepping, South Southall Extended Schools Coordinator, London.)

---

an interesting example of partnership working. Neighbourhood renewal strategies are also leading the way in breaking down organisational barriers and engaging members of communities in partnership arrangements.

> See Chapter 4, sections on primary care trusts and local authorities, for information on health action zones and neighbourhood renewal strategies. Also see Chapter 6, section on local strategies and initiatives.

In general, partnerships can take different forms, and vary in terms of how closely members work together. It is useful to think of three main ways of working, spanning a range of degrees of involvement between partners:

Networking – Cooperating – Joint working

Networking

Networking means coming together with other people from different agencies, and exchanging information and ideas on activities and plans. This is useful for coordinating activities, avoiding

duplication and sharing knowledge of mutual interest. Members meet and talk, but they do not actually work together. Networking has the lowest degree of involvement between organisations.

Cooperating

Cooperating means that member agencies help each other in ways that are compatible with their own goals. They meet, talk and agree to participate in each other's work when this is helpful for their own work plans. For example, in an accident prevention partnership, people who work in the accident and emergency (A&E) department of a hospital may cooperate with a local alcohol advisory service (a voluntary organisation) to ensure that patients brought in with a drink problem know that they can go to the alcohol agency for help. This cooperation helps the alcohol agency to reach needy potential clients, and helps the A&E department to fulfill its role of helping patients with longer term health needs. This way of working in partnership means a moderate degree of involvement between partners.

Joint working

Joint working means coming together to agree a mutually acceptable plan, and working together to carry it out. This necessitates a high degree of involvement between partners. For example, the police, the probation service, road safety officers from the local authority and a local alcohol advisory service may all work together to plan, implement and evaluate a joint programme of work to reduce drink-driving levels.

Partnerships can operate in one, two or all of these ways. Sometimes joint working is thought to be the most effective, but networking and cooperating can be useful when it is not always feasible or worthwhile to aim for full joint working.

FACTORS FOR SUCCESSFUL PARTNERSHIP WORKING

Successful partnerships are usually the result of investing a considerable amount of resources, skill and time to enable members to work well together (Markwell et al 2003). The Verona Benchmark, a partnership benchmarking tool, is useful in informing and assessing partnership processes and outputs (see the special edition of *Promotion and Education* 2000 7(2), for a series of articles on Verona Benchmarking and specifically Watson et al 2000). Key factors for success are:

- All partners need to be working towards a shared vision of what the partnership should achieve, with an agenda and goals to which all partners concur.
- There must be an agreed approach. All partners need to feel a sense of ownership with no one partner dominating.
- Commitment from the highest level of member organisations is vital to ensure that belonging to the partnership fits in with the organisation's strategic aims and that there will be management support for input of time and other resources.
- There must be commitment of sufficient time and resources and realistic expectations. Partnership working is time-consuming, and it may take months or years to develop a shared understanding and joint plans, or achieve outcomes from joint health promotion activities. There must, however, be demonstrable achievements, otherwise the partnership will be regarded as ineffective.

- Someone acceptable to all partners needs to take responsibility for running the partnership (for example setting up, chairing and servicing meetings) and coordinating action. A full-time coordinator can be extremely helpful.
- There must be mutual respect between partners; all partners need to feel that others value their input.
- Working relationships need to be characterised by openness and trust. Partners need to recognise and resolve potential areas of conflict.
- There must be an agreed framework for reviewing the partnership, changing the way of working if necessary, and even bringing it to an end if it has outlived its usefulness or is unproductive.
- Awareness and understanding of partner organisations should be promoted through joint training programmes and incentives to work across organisational boundaries.
- Partnership arrangements need to be regularly reviewed and adapted to reflect the lessons learned from experience.

See also earlier sections in this chapter on coordination and teamwork.

POTENTIAL DIFFICULTIES WITH PARTNERSHIP WORKING

Partnership working can result in many difficulties. Major problems are:

- Organisational change, which blights long-term commitment and planning.
- Competition between member agencies for funding, for example between different voluntary organisations who are seeking funding from the same source.
- Lack of resources, both money and person-power.
- Lack of top-level commitment from members of the partnership.
- Domination by an individual.
- An imbalance of input from different agencies, which can lead to resentment and issues about ownership of joint activities and who takes the credit for success.
- Professional jealousy and unwillingness to share expertise and information.

- Differences between agencies and individuals in terms of different goals and values; different organisational cultures and ways of working; different levels of expertise and experience.

It is worth bearing in mind that not all partnerships are successful. Many fade out or are wound up. Partnership working is not an end in itself; it is a means to an end, and there are circumstances where the end is better achieved by an organisation working alone.

PRACTICE POINTS

- A key aspect of successfully implemented health promotion programmes is how well you and other health promoters work together.
- You need to think about how you communicate with colleagues: the channels you use, how well you use them and the quality of your professional relationships.
- Health promotion often involves different professionals and disciplines working together; there is a range of ways in which you can encourage good teamwork and coordination.
- For effective meetings and committee work, you require knowledge of and competencies in the roles and responsibilities of committee members.
- Health partnerships between two or more organisations work at varying levels of involvement with each other, from networking at a local or national level to full joint working and from local partnerships to strategic partnership. Think about the many factors that contribute to success, and the potential pitfalls to avoid.

References

Barker A 2006 Creating success: how to manage meetings, 2nd edn. London, Kogan Page.

Glasby J, Dickinson H 2009 Partnership working in health and social care. Bristol, Policy Press.

Hadler G 2006 Meetings – how to organize and run meetings more effectively. http://www.articlesbase.com/leadership-articles/meetings-how-to-organize-a-run-meetings-more-effectively-74847.html.

Jelphs K, Dickenson H 2008 Working in teams: better partnership working. Bristol, Policy Press.

Markwell S, Watson J, Spellar V et al 2003 The working partnership: book 1, introduction. London, Health Development Agency.

Samson M 2008 Seamless teamwork: using Microsoft® SharePoint® technologies to collaborate, innovate, and drive business in new ways. Reading, Microsoft Press.

Scriven A 2007 Developing local alliance partnerships through community collaboration and participation. In: Handsley S, Lloyd CE, Douglas J et al (eds) Policy and practice in promoting public health. London, Sage.

Watson J, Speller V, Markwell S, Platt S 2000 The Verona Benchmark: applying evidence to improve the quality of partnership. Promotion & Education 7(2): 16–23.

Websites

http://www.alhcc.scot.nhs.uk/N&L%20for%20PM/Protocols%20Policies%20Documents/Clinical/SMOKING%20CESSATION%20PROTOCOL.doc

PART 3

Developing competence in health promotion

PART CONTENTS

PART SUMMARY

Part 3 aims to provide you with guidance in how to assess, develop and improve your competencies in health promotion.

Competencies are the combinations of knowledge, attitudes and skills needed to plan, implement and evaluate health promotion activities in a range of settings. You will also need to develop other core competencies of health promotion, such as communicating and educating, marketing and publicising, facilitating and networking and influencing policy and practice. Some chapters of Part 3 will be more important to some professions or disciplines than others. So you may wish to start by studying the chapters most relevant to you, rather than going through them in sequence. Cross-referencing is provided to help you to identify which sections of other chapters may also be relevant to your particular needs.

In Chapter 10 the fundamentals of communication are addressed, including establishing relationships, and the links with promoting self-esteem and assertiveness. Four basic communication skills are identified and guidance provided on how to improve them. Communication and language barriers, nonverbal communication and written communication are discussed.

In Chapter 11 some principles governing the choice of communication tools in health promotion are covered. The advantages and limitations of a variety of teaching and learning resources are considered and guidance provided on how to produce and use displays, written materials and statistical information. The use of mass media in health promotion is explored, including practical help about working with the local press, radio and television. There is a section included on the use of information technology in health promotion.

In Chapter 12 the principles of adult learning are outlined. How you can enable people to learn and evaluate the learning outcome is described, along with guidelines on giving talks, and on patient health education.

Chapter 13 covers the health promotion competencies required to work effectively with groups, covering how to lead groups and how to understand group behaviour.

Chapter 14 concentrates on how to enable people to change their behaviour towards healthier living, including information on models of the process of changing health-related behaviour. Strategies that can be used, such as working with a client's own motivation and counselling to help people to make decisions are discussed alongside the principles that help with using these approaches.

In Chapter 15 the focus is community-based work in health promotion, including community participation, community development and community health projects.

Chapter 16 is about how local and national policies, programmes, plans and strategies are made and how they can be influenced. The methods that health promoters can use to challenge health damaging policies, and develop, implement and evaluate health promotion policies are outlined, including sections on the principles and the planning of campaigns.

Chapter **10**

Fundamentals of communication

SUMMARY

This chapter starts with an exploration of client/
professional relationships and a discussion of the
links between self-esteem, self-confidence and
communication, accompanied by a case study
on relationship skills. Discussion on four basic
communication skills (listening, helping people to talk,
asking questions and getting feedback) is followed by
consideration of communication and language barriers
and nonverbal communication. The chapter ends with
a section on written communication. Exercises are
provided on overcoming communication barriers and
on each basic communication skill.

See also Chapter 12, which discusses communication
and education between health promoters and patients.

Effective communication in a range of contexts is
fundamental to success in health promotion (See
Corcoran 2007 for details on communicating for
health promotion in different contexts). Communication should be clear, unambiguous and without
distortion of the message.

This chapter discusses some fundamentals of
relationships with clients, communication barriers
and basic communication skills (see Hartley 2004
for an interesting assessment of possible verbal and
nonverbal communication barriers). These skills
will often be applied in one-to-one situations,
though they may apply when working with groups,
running workshops, as well as in more formal
situations.

EXPLORING RELATIONSHIPS WITH CLIENTS

Health promoters should ask themselves some fundamental (and possibly uncomfortable) questions. For example, what is your basic attitude towards the people to whom your health promotion is directed? Do you accept them on their own terms or do you judge them by your own standards? Do you aim to enable people to be independent, make their own decisions, take control of their health and solve their own health problems? Or are you actually encouraging dependency, solving their problems for them and thereby decreasing their own ability and confidence to take responsibility for their health? It may be useful to work through the following questions, thinking about how you relate to your clients.

ACCEPTING OR JUDGING?

Accepting people is demonstrated by:

- Recognising that clients knowledge and beliefs emerge from their life experience, whereas your own have been modified and extended by professional education and experience.
- Understanding your own knowledge, beliefs, values and standards.
- Understanding your clients' knowledge, beliefs, values and standards from their point of view.
- Recognising that you and your clients may differ in your knowledge, beliefs, values and standards.
- Recognising that these differences do not suggest that you, the professional health promoter, are a person of greater worth than your clients.

Judging people is demonstrated by:

- Equating people's intrinsic worth with their knowledge, beliefs, values, standards and behaviour. For example, saying that someone who drinks beyond safe limits is foolish both judges and condemns that person, and takes no account of life experience and cultural background. Saying that drinking beyond safe levels may damage health does not judge the person in the same way.
- Ranking knowledge and behaviour. For example, 'I'm the expert so I know better than you' is judgemental; 'I know a considerable amount about this particular health issue' is a statement of fact. 'My standards are higher than yours' is judgemental; 'My standards are different from yours' is not.

AUTONOMY OR DEPENDENCY?

There are a number of ways in which you can help clients to take more control over their health.

Autonomy can be enabled by:

- Encouraging people to think things through and make their own health decisions, resisting the urge to dominate the decision-making process.
- Respecting any unusual ideas they may have.

Autonomy can be hindered if:

- You impose your own solution on your clients' health problems.
- You tell them what to do because they are taking too long to think it through for themselves.
- You tell them that their ideas are not good and won't work, without giving an adequate explanation or an opportunity to try them out.

An aim which is compatible with health promotion principles and ethical practice is to work towards as much autonomy as possible. By doing this, you are helping people to increase control over their own health. Obviously, there are times when working towards autonomy may not be feasible. For example, it is more demanding of resources and clients may be dependent on a health promoter because they are ill, or uninformed or likely to put themselves or other people in danger.

A PARTNERSHIP OR A ONE-WAY PROCESS?

Do you think of yourself as working in partnership with people in pursuit of health promotion aims, or do you see health promotion as your sole responsibility, with yourself as the expert?

A partnership means:

- There is an atmosphere of trust and openness between yourself and your clients, so that they are not intimidated.
- You ask people for their views and opinions, which you accept and respect even if you disagree with them.
- You tell people when you learn something from them.
- You use informal, participative methods when you are involved in health promotion, drawing

on the experience and knowledge that clients bring with them.

- You encourage clients to share their knowledge and experience with each other. People do this all the time, of course (for example, knowledge and experience are discussed between participants on a smoking cessation programme and parents in a baby clinic), but do you actively foster and encourage this?

A one-way process means:

- You do not encourage clients to ask questions and discuss health needs.
- You imply that you do not expect to learn anything from your clients (and if you do learn, you don't say so).
- You do not find out people's health knowledge and experience.
- You do not encourage people to learn from each other.
- You use formal health promotion approaches rather than participative methods.

CLIENTS' FEELINGS – POSITIVE OR NEGATIVE?

A change in people's health knowledge, attitudes and actions will be helped if they feel good about themselves. It will rarely be helped if they are full of self-doubt, anxiety or guilt.

Clients will feel better about themselves if:

- You praise their progress, achievements, strengths and efforts, however small.
- The consequences of unhealthy behaviour such as smoking are discussed without implying that the behaviour is morally bad.
- Time is spent exploring how to overcome difficulties, such as practical strategies to help a client stop smoking. This will help to minimise feelings of helplessness.

Clients will feel bad about themselves if:

- You ignore their strengths and concentrate on their weaknesses.
- You ignore or belittle their efforts.
- You attempt to motivate them by raising guilt and anxiety (such as 'if you don't stop smoking you'll damage your baby').

To sum up, the health promotion aim of enabling people to take control over and improve their health is best achieved by unconditional positive regard and working in nonjudgemental partnerships

(Freshwater 2003). This should seek to build on people's existing knowledge and experience, move them towards autonomy, empower them to take responsibility for their health and help them to feel positive about themselves.

SELF-ESTEEM, SELF-CONFIDENCE AND COMMUNICATION

The ability to communicate is closely linked to how people feel about themselves. People with a low sense of self-esteem tend to be over-critical of themselves and to underestimate their abilities (Allen et al 2002). This lack of self-confidence is reflected in their ability to communicate. For example, they may lack assertiveness and thus may either fail to speak up for themselves or react with inappropriate anger and even violence.

Assertiveness means saying what you think and asking for what you want openly, clearly and honestly. It does not mean being aggressive or bullying, but it is in contrast with hiding what you really feel, saying what you don't really mean or trying to manipulate people into doing what you want.

Assertiveness helps people to create win–win situations (situations where everyone involved feels that they have achieved a reasonable outcome) through direct and open communication and through avoiding aggressive behaviour (which can result in win–lose situations, where one party feels that they have won and the other party feels they have lost) or manipulation (lose–lose situations, where, for example, one party in a negotiation walks out). It builds the self-esteem of all concerned. Successful negotiation is a good example of how assertiveness can work. In a successful negotiation both parties are more likely to come away with the following thoughts:

- This is an agreement which, while not ideal, is good enough for both of us to support.
- Both of us made some compromises and sacrifices.
- We will be able to have successful negotiations with each other in future.

Many clients with low self-esteem will need to learn how to feel better about themselves before they can communicate effectively with health promoters (Emler 2001). Although Emler (2001) reports that most programmes to raise self-esteem had not been successful, people with low self-esteem require key life skills in order to take control of their health. These skills include how to communicate and relate to others in a morally responsible manner, and with respect and sensitivity towards the needs and views of others. Unfortunately, the nonstatutory status and the time allotted to personal and social education in schools may be insufficient for young people to develop these skills (King 2005).

Case study 10.1 illustrates how parents can learn to develop the self-esteem of their children and ensure that their children understand the rights of other people. While the case study refers to parents and children, the same principles can be used by health promoters with their clients.

So, when working with clients with low self-esteem, you may find it helpful to:

● Be aware of the client's feelings.
● Recognise the opportunity to help the client to learn about how to handle difficult feelings.

● Listen and acknowledge that you have these feelings too.
● Label the feelings.
● Set limits for the interaction while exploring strategies to solve the problem.

LISTENING

As a health promoter, you need to develop skills of effective listening so that you can help people to talk and identify their needs and feelings.

Listening is an active process. It is not the same as merely hearing words. It involves a conscious effort to listen to words, to the way they are said, to be aware of the feelings shown and of attempts to hide feelings. It means taking note of the non-verbal communication as well as the spoken words. The listener needs to concentrate on giving the

---

CASE STUDY 10.1 RELATING SKILLS – LORRAINE AND JACK

Lorraine is late for work and tries to coax her 3-year-old son, Jack, into his coat so that she can take him to nursery school. Jack starts to cry. Lorraine hugs him but tells him that he's got to go to school. She is at a loss about what else to do, and when she reaches nursery school Jack is still crying. One of the nursery nurses notices his distress and manages to calm him. When Jack has recovered, the nurse talks to Lorraine about what she's learnt from a book by Gottman & Declaire (1997) and about five steps to better parenting. Lorraine learns that children whose parents consistently practise these five steps have better physical health and score higher academically than children whose parents do not. They also relate better with friends, have fewer behaviour problems and are less prone to acts of violence.

A week later in a similar situation Lorraine tries out what the nurse suggested. She starts in the same way as before, by empathising with Jack, but this time she goes further and provides him with guidance on what to do with his uncomfortable feelings. The conversation goes something like this:

Jack: 'It's not fair. I don't want to go to school'. (Starts to cry.)
Lorraine: 'Come here Jack'. (Takes him on her knee.) 'I'm sorry but we can't stay at home. I have lots to do at work. Does that make you feel sad?'

Jack: (nodding) 'Yes'.
Lorraine: 'I feel a bit sad too. It's OK for you to cry'. (Hugs him while he cries.) 'I know what. Let's think about what to do on Saturday when I don't have to go to work and you don't have to go to school. Can you think of anything special you would like to do on Saturday?'
Jack: 'Can we go to the park and feed the ducks?'
Lorraine: 'Yes. That would be great'.
Jack: 'Can Nick come too?'
Lorraine: 'Perhaps. We'll have to ask his Mum. But right now it's time to get going'.
Jack: 'OK'.

Lorraine has gone through five steps:
1. She becomes aware of Jack's feelings.
2. She recognises the opportunity for helping Jack to learn about how to handle emotions.
3. She listens to Jack, tries to understand his feelings and lets him know it is OK to feel bad and upset sometimes, and that she has these feelings too.
4. She helps Jack to find the words to label the emotion he is having.
5. She sets limits while exploring strategies to solve the problem.

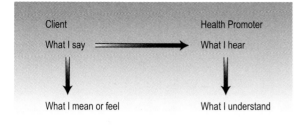

Client	Health Promoter
What I say →	What I hear
↓	↓
What I mean or feel	What I understand

Fig. 10.1 The listening process. *(Figure adapted from Rollnick et al 1999).*

speaker full attention, being on the same level physically as the speaker and adopting a nonthreatening posture.

Fig. 10.1 illustrates that active listening involves searching for an understanding of the underlying meaning behind the words used by the client. It shows how the meaning conveyed by the client can become distorted if the client cannot express exactly what he or she means. At the second step it shows that the health promoter may not hear what is being said. Third, the health promoter may hear the words accurately, but interpret them in a different way from that which the client intended.

When listening, it is easy to allow attention to wander. Some of the things you may find yourself doing instead of listening are planning what to say next, thinking about a similar experience, interrupting, agreeing or disagreeing, judging, blaming or criticising, interpreting what the speaker says, thinking about the next job to be done or just plain daydreaming.

The task of a listener is to encourage people to talk about their situation unhurriedly and without interruption, enabling them to express their feelings, views and opinions, and to explore their knowledge, values and attitudes. This reinforces the speakers' responsibility for themselves and is essential for helping them towards greater responsibility for their own health choices. To practise listening skills work on Exercise 10.1.

ENABLING PEOPLE TO TALK

The main task of the listener is to encourage and enable someone to talk. There are several useful techniques, as follows.

See also Chapter 14, section on strategies for decision making, which discusses counselling skills.

EXERCISE 10.1   Learning to listen

Work in groups of three to six people. Appoint someone as a timekeeper.
1. Person A speaks for 2 minutes, without interruption, on a subject of her choice to do with work or other interests (for example, sensible drinking guidelines, keeping fit and active, pets, holidays). Everyone else in the group listens, without interrupting or taking notes.
2. Person B repeats as much as she can remember, without anyone else interrupting. Person B may not:
   – add anything extra to what A said
   – give interpretations (for example 'It's obvious from what she said that ...')
   – give comments (for example 'She's just like me ...').
3. A, and the rest of the group, identify what was inaccurate, forgotten or added.
4. Repeat, with a different topic, until everyone has had a turn at being A and B.
5. Discuss the following questions:
   – What helped me to listen?
   – What helped me to remember?
   – What hindered my listening?
   – What hindered my remembering?
   – What did I learn about myself as a listener?

Giving an invitation to talk

To get someone started it may be helpful to give out a specific invitation to talk. Examples are:

'You don't seem to be your usual self today. Is something on your mind?'

'Can we talk some more about that matter you raised briefly at yesterday's meeting?'

'You look worried – are you?'

Giving attention

This means listening closely to what is being said, and being fully aware of all the channels of communication, including nonverbal behaviour. It requires effort and concentration to listen hard and give full, undivided attention.

Encouraging

This means making the occasional intervention to encourage someone to carry on talking. It tells the speaker that you really are listening, and want to hear more. Such interventions include noises like 'mm mm', words such as 'yes …' and short phrases such as 'I see …' or 'And then …?' or 'Go on …'.

Another useful intervention is the repetition of a key word which the speaker has just used. For example, if the speaker says 'I am worried by my weight gain', you could repeat the word 'weight …?'

Paraphrasing

This means responding to the speaker using your own words to state the essence of what the speaker has been saying. Use key words and phrases, for example, 'So you're not sure whether to have the baby vaccinated or not?' or 'So you are feeling unhappy because you are overweight and being unhappy triggers overeating?'

Reflecting feelings

This involves mirroring back to the speaker, in verbal statements, the feeling he is communicating. To do this it helps to listen for words about feelings, and to observe body language. Examples are 'You seem pleased' or 'You are obviously upset about this'.

Reflecting meanings

This means joining feelings and content in one succinct response, to get a reflection of meaning:

'You feel … because …'
'You are … because …'
'You're … about …'

For example:

'You feel pleased about your progress.'
'You're depressed because your children have grown up and left home.'
'You're angry about all the rubbish left on the streets of your neighbourhood.'

Summing up

This is a brief re-statement of the main content and feelings which have been expressed throughout a conversation. Check back with the speaker to ensure that the statement is accurate. For example, say 'It seems to me that the main things you've been saying are … Does that cover it?'

Exercise 10.2 gives you the opportunity to practise skills in enabling people to talk.

ASKING QUESTIONS AND GETTING FEEDBACK

Skilful questioning will help people to give clear, full and honest replies. It is useful to distinguish different types of questions.

TYPES OF QUESTIONS

Closed questions are questions that require short, factual answers, often only one word. Examples are:

'What is your name?'
'Is this address correct?'
'Are you able to see me again next Tuesday?'

Closed questions are appropriate when brief, factual information is required. They are not appropriate when the aim is to encourage talking at more length. So 'Did you get on OK with your healthy eating plan last week?', which could be answered by 'yes' or 'no', is not the best way to encourage people to express their experiences of trying to change what they eat. A better question would be 'How did you get on with your healthy eating plan last week?' This is an open question.

Open questions give an opportunity for full answers. Examples are:

'How did you get on at the meeting yesterday?'
'What situations do you feel trigger overeating?'
'What do you think about trying to take a short brisk walk every day?'

Note that words like 'how', 'what', 'feel' and 'think' are useful for encouraging a full response.

Biased questions indicate the answer the questioner wants to hear, or expects to hear. In other words, biased questions are likely to bias the response by leading the person who answers in a particular direction. Examples are:

'You're feeling better today, aren't you?' (This is biased because it would be easier to answer 'yes' than 'no'.)
'You have been doing what we discussed last time, haven't you?'
'Surely you aren't going to do that, are you?'

Multiple questions contain more than one question. Multiple questions are likely to confuse,

---

EXERCISE 10.2   Helping people to talk

Work in pairs. Each person chooses a topic she feels strongly about (which might be a personal experience or topic of general concern such as sex education, traffic jams, cuts in the health service or violence on television). Stay with the same topic for all three stages of the exercise. (The whole exercise takes about 45 minutes.)

Stage 1. Giving attention

One person speaks for 2 minutes, and the other listens, giving only nonverbal feedback. Then swap roles. After both of you have had your turn, spend 10 minutes discussing these questions:

When you were listening:
- What did you find difficult about listening?
- Did your mind wander?
- Did you maintain eye contact?
- What did you notice about the speaker's nonverbal communication?

When you were speaking:
- What did the listener do which helped you to talk?
- Did the listener do anything that made it difficult for you to talk?

Stage 2. Encouraging

One person speaks for 2 minutes. The other listens and gives encouraging interventions (such as 'mm mm'), words ('yes ...') and nondirective comments ('I see ...') or repeats key words. Swap roles. Then spend 5 minutes discussing these questions:

When you were listening:
- What sort of interventions did you make?
- How did you feel about making them?

When you were speaking:
- What interventions did you notice?
- Did you find them helpful?

Stage 3. Paraphrasing, reflecting back and summing up

One person speaks for 5 minutes and the other listens. The listener makes encouraging interventions as in Stage 2, but *also* paraphrases, reflects feelings and reflects meaning when she feels it is appropriate. At the end, she makes a brief statement summing up the main content and feelings of the speaker, checking with the speaker that her summing up is accurate. Exchange roles. Then spend 10 minutes discussing these questions:

When you were listening:
- What sort of interventions did you make?
- How did you feel about making them?

When you were speaking:
- What interventions did you notice?
- Did you find them helpful?

---

because the listener will not know which question to answer, and probably will not remember all of them. Examples are:

'Is this a serious problem for you – when did it start?'

'Does your store have a policy on promoting healthy foods – do you stock low-alcohol drinks and did you promote displays of low-fat products during the special campaign last September?'

'What are you going to do to get the Council to take all this rubbish away and are you going to get more bottle banks and newspaper recycling bins?'

'Are you sure you know what to do or would you like me to explain it again?'

Exercise 10.3 is an opportunity to practise asking appropriate questions.

GETTING FEEDBACK

After people have been given some information, or have been taught a skill, it is very important to check to make sure that they really have understood what was said, and remembered it, or mastered the skill. This is especially important when there is any doubt about how much has been understood, perhaps because, for example, someone is in a state of anxiety or has a limited command of English. There are two key points to note about getting feedback.

1. *It is your responsibility to ensure that the communication has been received and understood.* It is not the fault of the listener if they tried but did not understand.

It can be helpful to ask a question in a way which shows that it is your responsibility as a health promoter to be understood. For example, say 'May I check to make sure I've covered everything – could

---

EXERCISE 10.3 Asking questions

Work in groups of about 10 people.

Decide on a topic on which it is easy to think of questions – such as pets, holidays, my job, my family.

- Person A volunteers to answer questions.
- Person B observes the length of A's response to questions.
- Person C observes A's nonverbal behaviour (body language).
- Everyone else has the task of asking questions.

First, everyone in turn asks a *closed* question on the topic.

Second, everyone in turn asks an *open* question on the topic.

Third, everyone asks *biased* questions on the topic. After these three rounds of questions:

- Person A says how she felt about having to answer the three different kinds of questions (e.g. clear? muddled? irritated? angry? confused?).
- Person B says what she observed about the length of A's responses to the three kinds of questions.
- Person C says what she observed about A's nonverbal behaviour when answering the three different kinds of questions.

Discuss the application of what you found out to your work.

---

you just recap what you understand so far?' Avoid questions such as 'Let's see if you've learnt it yet, could you show me?' or 'I don't think you've totally understood, tell me what you think the main points are'.

2. Ask open questions. Closed questions such as 'Do you understand?' are not an adequate way of getting feedback. People may answer 'yes' because they are embarrassed, intimidated or afraid of making a fool of themselves by admitting that they do not understand. Or they might just want to draw the conversation to a quick conclusion. Ask open questions, such as 'Could you please tell me what you're going to do …'

COMMUNICATION BARRIERS

As a health promoter you may encounter numerous difficulties in communicating. Recognising that communication barriers exist is the necessary first stage before work can begin on tackling the problems. There are no easy solutions, but increased awareness and skill can go a long way towards improvement.

Common communication barriers may be categorised into six types.

1. Social and cultural gaps

A number of factors can cause gaps, among which are:

- different ethnic or social groups, which may be apparent in dress, language or accent
- different cultural or religious beliefs, for example about hygiene, nutrition or contraception
- different values, reflected in a different emphasis on the importance of health issues
- different gender or sexual orientation, reflected in different approaches, interests or values.

2. Limited receptiveness

You might want to communicate, but the reverse is not always true: people might not want to be communicated with. They may be unreceptive for many reasons, including:

- learning difficulty or confusion
- illness, tiredness or pain
- emotional distress
- being too busy, distracted or preoccupied
- not valuing themselves, or not believing that their health is important.

3. Negative attitude to the health promoter

Some people may be resistant to you, even before you have met. This may be caused by:

- previous negative experiences
- lack of trust in anyone seen as an authority figure
- lack of credibility of the health promoter (perhaps you set a poor example of good health yourself?)
- perceiving you as a threat, coming to criticise or pass judgement
- thinking that they already have the knowledge and skills

- believing that advice will be given which they cannot comply with because of financial or social constraints, or being asked to change a lifestyle or behaviour that they enjoy
- not wishing to confront issues such as personal health problems, or the need to change policies and practices at an organizational level.

4. Limited understanding and memory

There may be difficulties because people:

- understand and/or speak little or no English
- have limited education or learning difficulties, and may be unable to read and write
- are being confronted with technical words, jargon or medical terminology that they do not understand
- have poor or failing memories and cannot remember what was discussed previously.

5. Insufficient emphasis by the health promoter

Communication may fail because you do not give it sufficient time and attention. The reasons may be:

- communication was given a low priority in basic training, so it is given low priority in practice
- lack of confidence, skills and knowledge, which may be the result of inadequate training
- being too busy with other things, and unable to find the time
- managers not being supportive about time spent on health promotion
- reluctance to demystify and share professionally acquired health knowledge.

6. Contradictory messages

Communication barriers are erected when people receive different messages from different people. For example:

- different health professionals give different advice
- family, friends or neighbours contradict health promoters
- health advice changes as evidence is updated.

In order to identify communication barriers in your work undertake Exercise 10.4.

EXERCISE 10.4   Identifying communication barriers

This exercise can be done alone, but it is best carried out in pairs or small groups so that ideas can be shared.

Consider the six types of communication barriers discussed.

1. How many of them can you identify in your own health promotion practice or experience?
2. What other communication barriers can you add to this list?
3. What communication barriers cause you the most problems?
4. What suggestions can you make for helping to break down communication barriers? (Share examples from your own experience and make additional suggestions.)

OVERCOMING LANGUAGE BARRIERS

Language is only one facet of the gulf that may exist between people of different ethnic backgrounds. The root of communication problems may be racism. This is a huge topic, largely outside the scope of this book, but all health promoters should take part in racism awareness training when working with people from different ethnic groups (see Robinson 2002 for more about communication in multiethnic societies)

However, when we focus solely on the question of language barriers, learning a few essential words and phrases in the other person's language may help. Help with learning the language may be available from multicultural education centres run by local education authorities.

When faced with a language barrier, there are some useful guidelines which you can follow to help someone with limited English to understand what is being said. See Box 10.1 and Exercise 10.5.

NONVERBAL COMMUNICATION

Nonverbal communication (NVC) includes the ways people communicate other than by the spoken word. It is sometimes called body language. The main categories of nonverbal communication are as follows.

BOX 10.1   Guidelines for health promotion communication with individuals or small groups who speak little English

If you are engaging in health promotion with individuals of small groups who speak little English, you should attempt to find out whether a translator could be present. If you use a translator, allocate more time for the session. Give information concisely and in stages; this will allow time for the translator to explain to the clients and to translate back information from the clients. Using children or relatives to translate information to clients can be less reliable than using trained translators.

If you do not have a translator, the following points may be helpful:

1. Speak clearly and slowly, and resist raising your voice in an effort to be understood.
2. Repeat a sentence if you have not been understood using the same words. If you use different words you are likely to cause more confusion by introducing even more words which are not understood.
3. Keep it simple. Use simple words and sentences. Use active forms of verbs rather than passive forms, so say 'The nurse will see you' rather than 'You will be seen by the nurse'. Do not try to cover too much information, and stick to one topic at a time.

4. Say things in a logical sequence: the sequence in which they are going to happen. So say 'Eat first, then take the tablet' rather than 'Take the tablet after you eat'. If the listener does not pick up the word 'after' correctly, he will take the tablet first, because that is the order in which he heard the instruction.
5. Be careful of idioms. Being 'fed up', 'popping out' and 'spending a penny' may be totally incomprehensible.
6. Do not attempt to speak pidgin English. It does not help people to learn correct English, and sounds patronising.
7. Use pictures, mime and simple written instructions, which may be read by relatives or friends who understand written English. Be careful of symbols on written material; ticks and crosses, for example, might not convey what you intend.
8. Check to ensure that you have been understood, but avoid asking closed questions that require a one-word answer such as 'Do you understand?' A reply of 'Yes' is no guarantee that your client really has understood.

See section on asking questions and getting feedback earlier in this chapter.

EXERCISE 10.5   Overcoming language barriers

The following five extracts come from the district nurse's side of a conversation with a patient whose English is very limited.

> 'Hello – Oh, we are looking brighter today!'
> 'Have you been visited by the doctor today yet? Did he give you a new prescription?'
> 'I'll see about your insulin after I've seen how your leg's getting on'.
> 'The doctor says you should take one of these tablets three times a day ... I don't think you understand – I'll say that again ... We want you to take one of these tablets three times a day

> ... Oh dear ... (louder) ... DOCTOR SAYS YOU TAKE TABLET THREE TIMES A DAY'.
> 'I'll leave this list of foods for you. There are ticks and crosses on it to show you what you can eat and what you should not eat. Do you understand? Your son can read English, can't he?'

Using the guidelines in points 1–8 in Box 10.1:
- Identify what is unhelpful about the way the district nurse speaks to the patient.
- Suggest better alternatives.

Bodily contact

Bodily contact is people touching each other, how much they touch, and which parts of the body are in contact. Shaking hands, holding hands, or putting an arm around someone's shoulders, for example, all convey a meaning from one person to another.

Some health promoters, such as nurses, obviously touch patients frequently in the course of their work, whereas others, such as environmental health officers, would not. Touching people is governed by rules dictated by cultural expectations and taboos, and by expectations of professional distance, which may be barriers to the positive use of touch. For example, a handshake can say 'I'm glad to see you – welcome' and touching a distressed person can say 'I'm here for you'.

Proximity

Proximity is how close people are to each other. Different messages are conveyed to a patient confined to bed by someone who talks to him from 6 feet away at the foot of the bed and by someone who comes closer and sits on the bed or a chair. However, people vary in the amount of personal space they need, and may feel uncomfortable when others come too close.

Orientation

How individuals position themselves in relation to other people and objects is known as orientation. A useful example is to consider the messages conveyed by the arrangement of a room where a small group of people are meeting. Chairs in rows facing one separate chair (perhaps with a table in front of it) imply that one person will dominate and control the meeting, whereas chairs placed in a circle without a table to act as a barrier imply that everyone is encouraged to join in, and that no one individual is expected to dominate.

Level

This refers to differences in height between people. Generally, communication is more comfortable if people are on the same level; so it feels better to bend down or sit down to talk to a child or a person in a wheelchair, for example. Talking to someone on a different level can leave one or both parties feeling disadvantaged. Sometimes this is done deliberately; for instance, not offering a chair to someone entering an office conveys a message that the visitor is not welcome to stay.

Posture

Posture is how people stand, sit or lie. For example, are they upright or slouched, arms crossed or not? Posture can convey a message of tension and anxiety, for example, by being hunched up with arms crossed, or one of welcome by being upright with arms outstretched.

Physical appearance

All kinds of messages may be conveyed by physical appearance, such as a person's social standing, personality, tidy habits or concern with fashion. Physical appearance can be very important to health promoters because of the messages it conveys. A uniform may convey an impression of professional competence, but may also convey an unwelcome image of authority. Casual dress in a formal committee may convey the impression (perhaps a false one) that the committee's work is not being taken seriously.

Facial expression

Facial expression can obviously indicate feelings, such as sadness, happiness, anger, surprise or puzzlement.

Hand movements and head movements

Movements of the hands and head can be very revealing. Nods and shakes of the head obviously convey agreement and disagreement without the need for words. It is important to note that movements of the head and hands do not convey the same meaning in all cultures. Clenched fists, fidgeting hands (and sometimes tapping feet) reveal stress and tension, whereas still, open hands usually denote a relaxed frame of mind. Mental discomfort, such as confusion or worry, is often shown by putting the hands to the head and playing with the hair, stroking a beard or rubbing the forehead.

Direction of gaze and eye contact

Direct eye contact is significant. As a general rule, a speaker looks away from the listener for most of the time when talking (because they are concentrating on what they are saying), and looks directly at the listener when they wants a response. The general rule is that the listener will look the speaker straight in the eye while they are paying attention to what they say, but will look elsewhere if their attention has wandered. This is particularly important if you work with people on a one-to-one basis: a person who is talking to you will infer that you are not listening if you are looking anywhere other than at them. It is critical when counselling someone in distress; the counsellor needs to be giving the client full attention, and if the client looks up and sees the counsellor gazing elsewhere the implication is that they are not listening (see Bor et al 2008 for more details on the counselling process).

Nonverbal aspects of speech

Consider how many ways a word like 'no' can be said. The way in which it is said can convey meanings such as anger, doubt or surprise. Tone and timing are two nonverbal aspects of speech which convey messages to the listener.

Raised awareness of nonverbal communication can help you to improve communication between you and the people you work with. For example, a person who says 'Yes, I understand' in a doubtful tone of voice, with a puzzled frown, clearly requires further explanation. Words alone are only part of a message, and can be misleading. See Andersen 2007, Knapp & Hall 2007 and Mehrabian 2007 for more information on nonverbal communication and undertake Exercise 10.6 to explore nonverbal communication in your work.

EXERCISE 10.6   Nonverbal communication in your work

Work through the following questions and exercises with a partner.
1. When do you touch people at work, if at all?
   What rules govern when it is acceptable/ unacceptable to touch them?
   Would people you work with be helped if you touched them more?
2. Carry on a conversation with your partner, first standing too close for comfort, then standing too far away.
   What does it feel like? What is the most comfortable distance?
   What implications does this have for your work?
3. When you talk to an individual in the course of your work, where do you sit or stand in relation to that person? For example, is furniture a barrier between you?
   If you talk to people in groups, how do you seat them?
   Do you think communication could be improved by making changes? If so, what changes?
4. Have a conversation with your partner with one of you sitting and the other standing. Both describe your feelings.
   Do you ever communicate with people who are on a physically different level from you?
   What are the implications for your health promotion effectiveness?
5. Practise tense and relaxed postures, then welcoming and rejecting postures.
   Which do you normally adopt with people?
6. Identify a few people you have studied or worked with whom you know fairly well. Think back to your first impressions of these people.

Do you think that your first impressions were right?
What were the important features of their appearance which led to your first impressions?
What is the importance of physical appearance in your health promotion work?
If you wear a uniform, or a white coat, how do you think it affects your relationships with the individuals and groups you work with?
7. Look around at other people in the room.
   What can you infer from their facial expressions, hand and head movements?
   What is the importance of noticing facial expression, hand and head movement in your job?
8. Hold a conversation with your partner while first staring into each other's eyes all the time, and then without looking at each other at all.
   Describe your feelings.
   Watch two people talking.
   Do they look directly at each other or do they frequently look away?
   Do they look more at each other when speaking or listening?
   How important is eye contact in your job?
9. Say 'I don't know' in as many ways as possible, trying to convey a different feeling each time, such as despair, confusion and irritation.
   How important is it for you to pick up on nonverbal aspects of speech in your health promotion work?

(Adapted from teaching materials produced by Habeshaw (undated).)

BOX 10.2   Guidelines on writing

1. The point of writing is clear communication. On the whole, the more simply and briefly you write, the more effective your writing is likely to be.

2. Think about what kind of document you are writing. For example, is it a paper for a formal committee, a memo to your manager or a letter to a client? This will help you to know what style to write in: formal in a set lay out for a committee, brief and to the point for a manager, business-like but friendly to a client.

3. Think about who is reading what you write, and what sort of communication they will welcome: how long should it be, how detailed, how formal or chatty, first person or third person?

4. Use clear, simple language, and avoid long or obscure words if you can find shorter or more familiar ones.

5. Avoid technical terms if you can. If you must use them, explain them in the text or a footnote the first time you use them.

6. Keep sentences short.

7. Break the text up with paragraphs. A paragraph should usually deal with one point and its immediate development. A new point needs a new paragraph. In formal papers and reports use numbering, headings and subheadings to break up the text and guide the reader through.

8. Use active rather than passive verbs where possible, as this is stronger and simpler. For example, write 'the health promoter advised the client on healthy eating' rather than 'the client was advised on healthy eating by the health promoter'.

9. Make sparing use of adjectives and adverbs in order to make your writing more striking. For example, 'the client was really very upset, cried and sobbed a lot and said they would never, ever come back to the smoking cessation programme again' (25 words) could be better expressed as 'the client was distressed and said they would never return to the smoking cessation programme' (15 words).

10. Use language accurately. If in doubt check with a guide to English usage (see, for example, Peters 2004, Seely 2005 and 2007, Cutts 2007).

11. If you have difficulty with spelling and punctuation, use a spell and grammar checker on a word processor or ask someone to check your writing for you.

12. If you have the time, finish a piece of writing and then put it aside for a few days. This gives your subconscious mind a chance to think about it, and you can take a fresh look and edit it. Check for clarity, simplicity and coherent structure.

WRITTEN COMMUNICATION

Writing is a craft, as well as an art, which all health promoters need to develop. The 12-point guidelines in Box 10.2 may help.

See also Chapter 8, section on writing reports.

PRACTICE POINTS

- The quality of your relationships with your clients is at the heart of your health promotion role. It is important to review and consider how your attitudes and values are reflected in your professional stance.

- Good communication is fundamental to health promotion and involves specific skills such as active listening.

- Words, whether verbal or written, are only a small part of communication, and it is important to consider all aspects of communication.

- You are responsible for communicating effectively with your clients, and it helps if you make it clear to them that you accept this responsibility (through asking them to help you by giving you feedback).

- Skills of written communication are important in health promotion, and need to be reviewed and developed.

References

Allen M, Preiss RW, Gayle BM 2002 Interpersonal communication research: advances through meta-analysis. Mahwah, USA, Lawrence Erlbaum Associates.

Andersen P 2007 Nonverbal communication: forms and functions, 2nd edn. Illinois, Waveland Press.

Bor R, Miller R, Gill S, Evans A 2008 Counselling in health care settings. Basingstoke, Palgrave.

Corcoran N (ed.) 2007 Communicating health: strategies for health promotion. London, Sage.

Cutts M 2007 Oxford guide to plain English. Oxford, Oxford University Press.

Emler N 2001 Self-esteem: the cost and causes of low self esteem. London, Joseph Rowntree Foundation.

Freshwater D 2003 Counselling skills for nurses, midwives and health visitors. Berkshire, McGraw-Hill International: 22.

Gottman J, Declaire J 1997 The heart of parenting: how to raise an emotionally intelligent child. London, Bloomsbury.

Hartley S 2004 Bridging the gap between health care professionals and communities. Community Eye Health 17(51): 38–39.

King A 2005 PSHE: should it be mandatory? http://www.teachingexpertise.com/articles/pshe-mandatory-210.

Knapp ML, Hall JA 2007 Nonverbal communication in human interaction, 5th edn. Wadsworth, Thomas Learning.

Mehrabian A 2007 Nonverbal communication. Edison NJ, Transaction.

Peters P 2004 The Cambridge guide to English usage. Cambridge, Cambridge University Press.

Robinson M 2002 Communication and health in a multi-ethnic society. Bristol, Polity Press.

Rollnick S, Mason P, Butler C 1999 Health behaviour change: a guide for practitioners. London, Churchill Livingstone.

Seely J 2005 Oxford guide to effective writing and speaking. Oxford, Oxford University Press.

Seely J 2007 Oxford A–Z of grammar and punctuation. Oxford, Oxford University Press.

Chapter 11

Using communication tools in health promotion practice

SUMMARY

The first part of this chapter offers some principles governing the choice of communication tools and a summary of the uses, advantages and limitations of the main types of health promotion resources. There are guidelines for making the most of display materials, for producing written materials (including guidance on nonsexist writing) and for presenting statistical information. This is followed by a section on mass media, including identifying the key characteristics of mass media, the variety of ways in which mass media are channels for health promotion, what mass media can be expected to achieve and how they can be used effectively. Guidelines are given for working with radio, television and local press. There is a case study on the use of mass media advertising, and exercises on writing plain English, preparing and presenting material on television and radio, writing a press release and writing a letter to the editor. The chapter ends with a section on using information technology for health promotion.

The range of communication tools outlined in Table 11.1 are used extensively by health promoters but may not always be employed with maximum effectiveness. How communication tools are selected and used is as crucial as the quality of the resources themselves.

GUIDELINES FOR SELECTING AND PRODUCING HEALTH PROMOTION RESOURCES

There is a huge range of material available, with a constant turnover as items become out of date or

Table 11.1	Health promotion resources	
TYPE OF RESOURCE	USES AND ADVANTAGES	LIMITATIONS
Leaflets and handouts	Clients can use at their own pace and discuss with other people. Educator and client can work through together. Can be easy and cheap to produce basic written information. Can reinforce points in a talk and add further detailed information	Commercially produced leaflets can be expensive and may contain advertising. Mass-produced leaflets are not tailored to everyone's needs. Not durable, easily lost. Mass distribution can be wasteful
Posters and display charts	Can raise awareness of issues. Can convey information and direct people to other sources (addresses, tel. numbers, 'pick up a leaflet'). Simple posters and information displays can be cheap to produce	High quality is expensive to make or buy. Get tatty quickly unless laminated. Need to ensure any writing is big enough to be read at the distance most people will see it Displays need changing frequently to attract attention
Whiteboards	Good for building up information, explaining particular points. Cheap, reusable	Educator needs to turn back to audience to write on board. Image too small for large groups
Flip-charts	Good for brainstorming and involving groups in producing ideas which can be stuck up round the room for discussion. Useful for recording notes to be written up later. Can be prepared in advance. Useful where no whiteboard available	Educator needs to turn back to audience to write on board. Flip-chart paper easily torn and dog eared
DVDs	Can be used to convey real situations otherwise inaccessible (e.g. childbirth), convey information, pose problems, demonstrate skills, trigger discussion on attitudes and behaviour. Can be used for self-teaching. Can be stopped, started or replayed to allow discussion	Normal TV-size screen too small for large audiences. Educator relies on equipment working properly. Equipment expensive and not easily transported. May need partially darkened room
PowerPoint presentation	Useful in large rooms or lecture theatres with a big screen. Complex information (such as graphs) can be seen clearly	Needs equipment and screen, and blackout
CDs	Good for certain skills development, e.g. relaxation, exercise routines. Equipment cheap, easy to use and transport	Lack of visual material requires extra concentration to hold attention
Health websites	Websites have the potential of reaching a worldwide audience and are useful for raising awareness of health issues, conveying information and delivering self-help materials	There is an enormous amount of health information that can be accessed on the Internet and no control over the quality

out of print and new ones come on the market. You could find yourself with the task of selecting a leaflet, poster, display or DVD from a range of possibilities. Or you may find that there is very little available, and you have to decide whether the one item you have found is suitable.

The guidelines are designed to help you select any kind of material, such as leaflets or audiovisual, and you can also use them as a checklist when producing your own.

Is it appropriate for achieving your aims?

Think about the item in the context in which you intend to use it. For example, if you are working with a group of young smokers who are not motivated to stop, a leaflet or video on how to stop smoking is unlikely to be helpful. Materials to trigger discussion with the aim of challenging attitudes might be better.

See Chapter 14, section on stages of change model.

Is it the most appropriate kind of resource?

Will something else be cheaper and just as effective, such as photographs instead of a DVD? Could you use the real thing, such as parents in person talking about their experiences of a new baby instead of a DVD; actual food instead of pictures or models?

Is it consistent with your values and approach?

If your approach is to work in a nonjudgemental partnership with your clients, the materials you use should reflect your values. You need to avoid material that is patronising, authoritarian, scaremongering or victim-blaming. Resources should not attribute or imply blame to individuals experiencing ill health when that ill health is rooted in their socioeconomic circumstances, for example low income or poor housing.

See section on exploring relationships with clients in Chapter 10.

Is it relevant for your clients?

Does it take account of the values, culture, health concerns, age, ethnic group, sex and socioeconomic circumstances of your clients? Does it reflect local practice and health services available?

Obvious examples of irrelevance are DVDs portraying lifestyles of affluent middle-class families, which are unhelpful if you are working with people in the UK who have limited financial resources. Materials designed for one ethnic group may not be appropriate for another, not just because of language but because some aspects (such as sexual behaviour or attitudes to bereavement) are seen differently in different cultures.

Is it racist or sexist?

All resources should be nonracist and nonsexist. Racist materials stereotype people, attributing certain roles or character attributes based on ethnic group alone. Implicit in this are the assumptions that one ethnic group is superior to another and represents the desired norm. (See Robinson 2002 for information on communicating with ethnic groups.)

Sexist materials stereotype gender roles, behaviours or character attributes. Resources should also not make assumptions about sexual orientation. Guidance on nonsexist writing is provided later in this chapter.

Resources should reflect the fact that we live in a multiracial society where the roles of men and women have changed and continue to do so. Strong, positive messages and images should be provided of people of all ethnic groups and both sexes.

Will it be understood?

Is it written in plain English, which people will readily understand? Are there any incorrect assumptions about the level of literacy or existing knowledge? Does it need to be produced in other languages, to make it accessible to people from minority ethnic groups? Do leaflets need to be produced in other formats so that they are accessible to people with disabilities, such as in large type or Braille, or for DVDs, for example, with sign language or subtitles inserted on the screen?

Is the information reliable?

Is information in the materials accurate, up to date, unbiased and complete? Or does it contain one-sided information on controversial issues, and out-of-date or incomplete messages?

Does it contain advertising?

Commercial companies such as drug companies, baby food manufacturers or makers of safety equipment who produce material will produce leaflets and posters that will carry the name of the company or its products, or include advertisements. Using these resources can imply that you (or your employer) are endorsing the product. It may also damage your image as a credible source of unbiased health information, and lead people to doubt the value of the information.

For these reasons, resources containing company names, products and advertising should be avoided whenever possible. However, the item may be just what you want, and there may be no alternative. In which case:

● The product or service advertised must be ethically acceptable as healthy and environmentally friendly. This excludes tobacco, alcohol and confectionery advertising, for example.
● The advertising content must be low key. The company name on the front or back cover is acceptable, but constant references to named-brand products are not.

THE RANGE OF HEALTH PROMOTION RESOURCES: USES, ADVANTAGES AND LIMITATIONS

Table 11.1 summarises the wide range of resources available for health promotion and the key points about their uses, advantages and limitations. It is also important to note:

● Resources are aids, and should generally not be seen as substitutes for the health promoter. Leaflets should be used in conjunction with face-to-face discussion. DVDs are best presented with an introduction and a follow-up discussion.

● It takes time and practice to become familiar with using all the health promotion resources available.

> See the section on health promotion teaching and learning in Chapter 12.

PRODUCING HEALTH PROMOTION RESOURCES

Most resources, particularly posters, leaflets and audiovisual materials, come ready made, but you might want to work with a community group to help them to produce materials that target their particular need, or produce some yourself.

> See also Chapter 10, section on written communication, and Chapter 12, section on improving patient communication.

This chapter does not offer a comprehensive guide on how to produce materials, but approaching the task in a systematic way using the planning and evaluation flowchart in Chapter 5 may be helpful. If you are producing a resource such as a health promotion leaflet, you will need to consider who will write the draft, who will edit it, whether and how to pilot the draft, what it will cost and whether you need the services of a desktop publisher, designer, illustrator, translator or printer.

Making the most of display materials: posters, charts, display boards and stands

Be brief and to the point. Keep the objective firmly in mind. Do not include material that is irrelevant; it will only distract from the main message.

Emphasis the key point(s). Use size of lettering, style or colour to achieve this. Place the important messages just above the centre of a display, which is the point of maximum visual impact.

Use language the audience understands. Explain any unfamiliar technical terms. If possible, express the message in both pictures and words. Test it out on a few people to ensure that you have no unexpected ambiguities in your message.

Be bold. Words and pictures should be as large as possible.

Make the most of colour. Colour can create continuity; for example, a repetition of background colour can link a series of posters. Colour can be used to identify parts of a diagram or highlight important information. Choose colours with care, because responses to colour are emotional (for example, green is soothing), and because colours may be associated with certain messages, images and places (such as red for danger, purple for funerals, white for clinical cleanliness).

Improve the display site. If all you have is a blank wall or a wall covered with distracting wallpaper, fix a rectangle of coloured card to the wall as a background display board. If a display board has a rough or marked surface, give it a coat of paint or a covering of coloured paper, hessian or felt.

Use the display site to best advantage. Busy corridors can only be useful sites for posters with immediate appeal and few words. More information can be conveyed in a waiting area, and it may be possible to supplement displays with leaflets to take away. Ensure that writing on displays is at eye level and large enough to read without people having to move from the queue or their chair.

Be aware of lighting. Daylight is unreliable; spotlights directed onto a display are ideal.

Making the most of written materials: instruction sheets and cards, leaflets and booklets

Pilot materials on a sample of consumers. Do not assume that you know what they like, want or need: *ask them.*

Use colour, layout and print size to improve clarity. Larger print may be helpful for those people with a visual impairment.

Use plain English. Use everyday words; avoid jargon and explain any technical or medical words. Aim for short sentences of 15–20 words. Use active rather than passive verbs,: for example, say 'Increase your fruit and vegetable consumption …' rather than 'Your fruit and vegetable consumption should be increased …'. Undertake Exercise 11.1 to practise plain English.

Do a readability test on your written materials. Many word-processing packages are able to give readability statistics as well as the average sentence length and the percentage of passive sentences used. They

---

EXERCISE 11.1   Writing plain English

Write plain English versions of the following. The first three are very similar to the instructions found on the packages of medication bought over the counter in chemist shops. The last three are very similar to passages in health promotion leaflets.

1. *Wheezoff* paediatric syrup is specially formulated for children. It is indicated for the relief of cough and its congestive symptoms and for the treatment of hay fever and other allergic conditions affecting the upper respiratory tract. Contraindications, warnings, etc. Hypersensitivity to any of the active constituents. If symptoms persist consult your doctor.

2. *Notwinge* cream – directions for use. Apply a sufficient quantity of balm to the part affected. Massage lightly until penetration is complete.

3. The baby lies curled up in what is called the fetal position. It lies in a bag of water and the membranes which make up this fluid-filled balloon are enclosed in the womb.

4. Vitamin B1, also called thiamin, is required for the functioning of the nervous system, digestion and metabolism. Insufficient vitamin B1 can cause anorexia and fatigue.

---

give a rough measure of readability for adult readers based on the principle that the combination of long sentences and long words is harder to comprehend. But note that many other factors that affect readability are not taken into account, such as how the text is laid out, the use of illustrations and the size of print.

NONSEXIST WRITING

The importance of material being nonracist and nonsexist has already been discussed, but using language in a nonsexist way presents particular challenges. One is the use of 'man' as a generic term for a person. For example, people talk about manning an exhibition stand when it is just as likely to be staffed by a woman. Many job titles end with 'man' and date from the time when only men performed these duties, for example postman.

Another problem is the generic use of the male pronoun. For example, 'Each doctor presented a case from his own practice', assumes that all the doctors are men. Although it may seem clumsy to

say 'he' or 'she', it can sometimes usefully emphasis that both sexes are involved. An alternative which has been used in this book is to turn the singular into a plural and use the words 'they' or 'their': changing 'A health promoter must be a fluent communicator. He must also be a good listener.' To 'Health promoters must be fluent communicators. They must also be good listeners.'

It may be possible to rephrase a passage to eliminate the pronouns altogether. So, instead of 'Information given to a social work agency is confidential in the same way as communications between a doctor and his patients', say '... in the same way as communications between doctors and patients'.

Another way is to use 'you' instead of 'he', 'she' or a noun that implies male or female. For example, in a leaflet on parenting, you could change 'A mother often finds difficulty in persuading her 2-year old to eat' to 'You may find difficulty in persuading your 2-year-old to eat' or 'Parents may find difficulty ...' This avoids the implication that only mothers (not fathers) have a parenting role.

Or avoid 'he' by finding another noun. Thus, in 'You may find it difficult to persuade your 2-year-old to eat. He may prefer throwing his food around instead' you could say '... A child at this age may prefer throwing food around instead.'

It is also important to avoid sexism when speaking as well as writing. So, for instance, a health promoter who refers to the women who attend a smoking cessation programme as 'the ladies' could affront the women in the group. It is far better to refer to the women who attend as 'patients' or 'clients'.

For further discussion of language barriers, see the section on overcoming language barriers in Chapter 10.

PRESENTING STATISTICAL INFORMATION

Numbers may be meaningless to lay people unless they are carefully presented in a visual way, such as in Figs 11.1 and 11.2. A wide range of computer software programmes facilitates the production of information in ways that are visually arresting and easy to understand. NHS organisations and local authorities are likely to have the equipment and expertise to support this production and there are Internet sites which also contain statistics reproduced visually. See, for example, the NHS Information Centre (http://www.ic.nhs.uk).

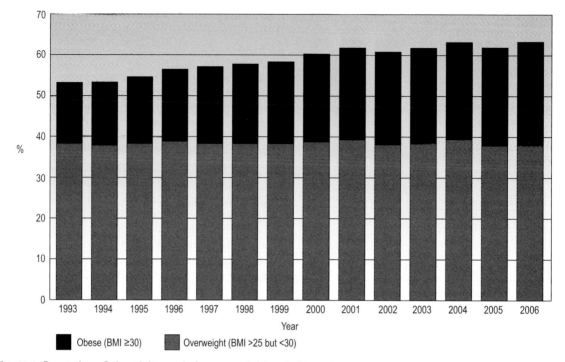

Fig. 11.1 Proportion of the adult population overweight and obese. *(Source: General Household Survey, Office of National Statistics (reproduced in Black 2008: 40)).*

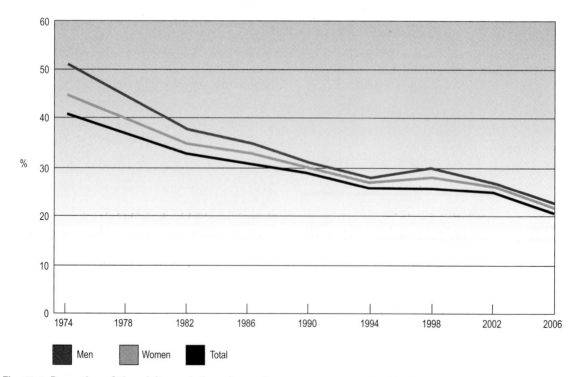

Fig. 11.2 Proportion of the adult population who smoke. *(Source: Health Survey for England (reproduced in Black 2008: 38)).*

USING MASS MEDIA IN HEALTH PROMOTION

The mass media are channels of communication to large numbers of people and include television, radio, the Internet, magazines and newspapers, books, displays and exhibitions. Leaflets and posters are also mass media when they are used on a stand-alone basis, as opposed to use as a learning aid in face-to-face communication with an individual or a group. However, usually when people talk about the media they are referring to television, radio, newspapers and magazines.

Health promoters are most likely to become involved with mass media when undertaking health promotion programmes or campaigns with the public, or when a public health issue becomes a news item. Probably most involvement will be with local newspapers and local radio or television. However, it is useful to put this into a wider context, and to appreciate the range of ways in which health issues and messages are portrayed via mass media.

MASS MEDIA AS TOOLS FOR HEALTH PROMOTION

Health messages and information are sent through the mass media in a number of different ways:

- Planned, deliberate health promotion, from posters and leaflets, displays and exhibitions on health themes, such as all of the mass media resources available for *Change4life* campaign, a society-wide movement that aims to prevent people from becoming overweight by encouraging them to eat a healthy diet and take more exercise (Department of Health (DoH) 2009a), to advertisements and campaigns on television, such as the *Worried* campaign based on teenagers' worries about their parents smoking (DoH 2009b) and in newspapers (see, for example, Martinson & Hindman 2005).
- Health promotion by advertisers and manufacturers of healthy products and services: for example the *Safety In The Sun* leaflet produced by Boots the Chemist helped convey the SunSmart message by providing information for customers (Cancer Research UK 2005).
- Books, television, newspapers and magazine articles about health issues which follow new research disseminated in academic conferences or journals or government publications. The

problem here is that the media may distort the evidence with attention-grabbing headlines which can give out unhealthy messages, such as the example in Box 11.1.

- Discussion of health issues as a byproduct of news items ('Rock star dies from drugs overdose') or entertainment programmes, notably soap operas/serial dramas where a character has a health problem, such as being abused as a child or suffering from cancer.
- Health (or anti-health) messages conveyed covertly or incidentally, such as well-known personalities or fictional characters refusing cigarettes or, conversely, smoking. The portrayal of alcohol on television, for example, conveys a norm of heavy drinking and associates consumption of alcohol with benefits rather than costs (Matthews 2007).
- Planned promotion of anti-health messages such as advertisements for alcohol (see Anderson 2009).
- Sponsorship of health promoting events and services by organisations or commercial companies, such as sponsorship of sporting events by alcohol companies (see, for example Swanton 2009) or health promotion events by commercial companies (see DoH 2000 for guidance on commercial sponsorship). By associating with a health promoting event or service, the sponsor's product or service is brought to the public eye with an implied stamp of approval and a sense that it is somehow associated with health.

USING MASS MEDIA FOR EFFECTIVE HEALTH PROMOTION

The fact that the message is sent via a medium, such as television, makes it difficult to obtain immediate feedback and modify the message to respond to the needs and characteristics of the audience. There can be some two-way communication through audience phone-ins, but mostly it is one way, which has implications. For example, it is not possible for the sender to repeat, clarify or amplify the message, so in general it is best to use mass media for conveying simple, rather than complex, messages.

Many research studies have shown that the direct persuasive power of mass media is very limited and will not result in long-term changes in health behaviour (Tones & Tilford 2001). Many health campaigns in the media are driven by the

---

BOX 11.1   New health research reported in the media can mislead with attention-grabbing headlines

Low or moderate dietary energy restriction for long-term weight loss: what works best?

Theoretical calculations suggest that small daily reductions in energy intake can cumulatively lead to substantial weight loss, but experimental data to support these calculations are lacking. A 1-year randomized controlled pilot study was conducted of low (10%) or moderate (30%) energy restriction (ER) with diets differing in glycemic load in 38 overweight adults. Food was provided for 6 months and self-selected for 6 additional months. Measurements included body weight, resting metabolic rate, adherence to the ER prescription. The 10% ER group consumed significantly less energy than prescribed over 12 months, while the 30% ER group consumed significantly more. Changes in body weight, satiety and other variables were not significantly different between groups. However, during self-selected eating (6–12 months) variability in % weight change was significantly greater in the 10% ER group and poorer weight outcome on 10% ER was predicted by higher baseline BMI and greater disinhibition. Weight loss at 12

months was not significantly different between groups prescribed 10 or 30% ER, supporting the efficacy of low ER recommendations. However, long-term weight change was more variable on 10% ER and weight change in this group was predicted by body size and eating behaviour. These preliminary results indicate beneficial effects of low-level ER for some but not all individuals in a weight control program, and suggest testable approaches for optimising dieting success based on individualizing prescribed level of ER.

(Adjusted from the abstract of an article by Das et al (2009). Please refer to the article for full details.)

When the research described above was published the *Sunday Times* ran an article with the following misleading title:

Can crash diets be good for you? New research shows that crash diets can be a safe and effective way of keeping the pounds off.

(Goodman 2009.)

---

need to do something, and to be seen to be doing it. So it is important for you to know what success you can realistically expect when you use mass media in your health promotion work. The research evidence tells us how mass media can be used effectively, and what it cannot be expected to achieve, as follows.

Mass media *can* be an effective health promotion tool if it fulfils the following criteria:

1. The information portrayed is:
   - perceived as relevant
   - supported by other approaches such as one-to-one advice
   - new and presented in an appropriate context.
2. The aim should be to:
   - raise awareness of health and health issues (for example, in order to trigger action to raise awareness about the impact of smoking on family members)
   - deliver a simple message (for example, to make quitting easier by providing details of a national helpline for people who want to stop smoking)
   - change behaviour (for example, to reinforce motivation and make quitting easier by phoning for a leaflet or other support).

3. The use of mass media is part of an overall strategy that includes face-to-face discussion, personal help and attention to social and environmental factors that help or hinder change. For example, mass media campaigns are just one strand in a long-term programme to combat smoking (DoH 2008).

What mass media *cannot* be expected to do is:

1. Convey complex information.
2. Teach skills.
3. Shift people's attitudes or beliefs.
4. Change behaviour unless it is a simple action, easy to do, and people are already motivated to change.

See Naidoo & Wills (2009) for a more detailed analysis of the mass media and health promotion and Wammes et al (2007) for research into the effectiveness of a mass media campaign aimed at weight gain prevention.

CREATING OPPORTUNITIES

You may be motivated to use the mass media, but you may have misgivings and feel the need for further training. For example, you may feel apprehensive of interviews with reporters from the local news media because of concerns about being misquoted or that the media might sensationalise the issue or that you will not perform effectively.

What can be done to overcome these concerns? Some NHS organisations and local authorities now have guidelines for dealing with the media (for example, Fay 2002, Jones & Hutchings 2003) and some professional bodies offer advice to their members in terms of media involvement (British Medical Association 2004) and some employ communications specialists, and their help can be enlisted (see Thake & Glendinning 2009 for an example of a media release from NHS Cambridgeshire).

Contact local journalists to establish a mutually beneficial relationship. You can give exposure to health topics and they want items for their reading, listening or viewing public. Get to know how they work and their special areas of interest. Also, remember that it is in both your interests to have good skills in communicating via the mass media, so ask for help with training needs. Short courses on using the media may also be available.

Keep a record of what you find out about local media, and update it regularly. Include information on names and special interests of journalists and the copy dates (deadline for submitting written information) for each of the media in your area. The daily newspapers should be able to respond immediately to a press release; radio often needs a few days to prepare coverage; television may need longer advance notice to allow time for booking a film crew.

WORKING WITH RADIO AND TELEVISION

Using radio or television effectively requires research, preparation and skill. The following checklists are prepared to help you get your health promotion story to the right person and have the best chance of getting coverage. You need to monitor your local radio and television to see which programmes might be interested in your kind of news.

Basic information

- What hours do they broadcast?
- What region do they cover?
- Who are the listeners? Does the profile alter according to the time of day?

The programmes

- What is covered on the news items?
- How many minutes of current affairs and local interest items?
- Are interviews used, or straight reporting?
- What are the different kinds of programmes, and what is the proportion of time they occupy (news, current affairs, weekly events, phone-ins, music)?
- Which programmes use guests or experts?
- Is there any local programme that regularly covers health issues?
- Is there a round-up of events in the week ahead? What is the deadline for information?
- How much detail do they give? What sorts of events are covered?

Interviews

- Which programmes use interviews?
- How many minutes?
- What is the tone (bland, chatty, aggressive)?
- How long is the average answer before the next question? Time it!
- Are they on location or in the studio?
- Are they recorded or live?
- Who are the presenters or interviewers on the programmes who might be interested in health? What is their style?

Finding out about a specific programme

- What programme is it? What sort of approach does the programme have? How long is it? When is it transmitted? What kind of audience does it have?
- Why is your topic of interest *now*? Is there some local or national controversy or news item that sparked off interest? If so, do you know all about it?
- How are you going to be presented: an information spot, an interview or a discussion panel?
- If you are going to be interviewed, who will do it? Will it be in the studio, on location or a telephone interview?
- If you are going to take part in a discussion, who else will be taking part?
- Will it be broadcast live or recorded first?

- How much time are you likely to have on the programme?
- When and where is the broadcast or recording to take place?

Preparing the message

- Do your homework. You may know a lot or a little about the subject, but in either case you need to identify exactly what it is you want to get across, and to have this very clearly in your mind *before* you go on air.
- Be positive. Emphasis the good news, *not* a series of don'ts. Tell people what they *can* do and emphasis the benefits.
- You should have two or three key points to put across, and *no more*. You can expand on these and describe them in different ways but do not overload your audience with too much detail or too many points. They will not remember the additional information, and may even forget the key points.
- Use anecdotes and analogies to illustrate what you mean; simple messages do not have to be bald and boring. Tell stories (short ones) and use real-life experiences. Put complex points over with everyday analogies.
- Avoid technical terms (unless these are essential, in which case use them and explain them) and jargon, but do not be patronising. It helps to pitch the level right if you imagine that you are talking to an intelligent 14–15-year-old whom you have never met.

Presenting your message

- If you are nervous, regard it as positive; it means that you will be keyed up to do your best. Remember that the interviewer is there to help you tell your story and to put you at ease.
- Perform with liveliness and conviction. Be alert and (if you are on television) look alert at all times. Always assume that the camera is on you even when you are not talking. Make sure you look convincing and involved.
- Speak with your normal voice; if you have a regional accent this will make you more interesting to listen to. Speak clearly and distinctly, and (especially on radio) vary the pitch and speed.

- Make sure you say what *you* want to say. You do not have to follow the line of the interviewer's questions if, for good reason, you do not wish to. Provided you stick to the broad framework of agreed subjects, you have every right to steer the interview or discussion in such a way that you get over what you want to say. Regard the questions as springboards from which to make your points. For example, if you do not like a question you can say:
  'I can't really answer that question without explaining first that ...'
  'The real problem behind all this is ...'
  'We don't know the answer to that at the moment, but what we do know is ...'
- When the interview is over, remain still, quiet and alert until you are *told* it is over.
- On television, wear what makes you feel comfortable and confident. Avoid wearing blue or bright red, predominant stripes, small patterns or flashing jewelry. As the camera will be on your face for most of the time, pay special attention to what you wear in the neckline area.

Practise your media skills by undertaking Exercise 11.2.

WORKING WITH THE LOCAL PRESS

Local community newspapers are an excellent medium for health promotion and journalists will be interested in newsworthy health issues. This is a checklist of what to look for when researching a newspaper.

Basic information

- Is it published daily or weekly?
- What are the copy deadlines?
- What locality does it cover?
- How many readers, and who are they?

The copy

- What is the style (bright, sober, campaigning)?
- What is the average length of articles (often different for news, business, features)?
- What percentage of articles have photos?
- How many photographs per page?
- How are photographs used generally?
- How are quotes used?

EXERCISE 11.2   Being an effective health promoter on television and radio

1. Prepare your message

Select a health promotion topic that you are familiar with, such as healthy eating, sensible drinking, breastfeeding, keeping fit, avoiding home accidents.

Identify *three* key points you would want to put across in a 5-minute radio or television interview. Be clear in your mind:

- What the three key points are.
- How you will explain them in an interesting way, what illustrations, analogies or anecdotes you could use.
- How you will develop your point further if you have time.

2. Practise your presentation

Get a colleague to act as your interviewer, and record your interview on an audio or a videotape. Ask a third person to be an observer. Play the tape back and assess your performance.

- Did you sound/look lively, alert and convincing?
- Was your voice clearly understandable? What did it sound like for speed and pitch?
- Did you get your key points across? Did you do so in an interesting way?
- Were you able to deal with difficult questions?

The subjects

- What sorts of stories are used (local, controversial, educational) and how are they treated?
- What is the ratio of coverage for news, features, business, diary, advertisements?
- How long and how full is the section publicising events ahead?
- Are there special sections or supplements on health, education, women? How long and on what day?
- Are there regular columnists? What are their special interests?

The language

- What is the average length of sentences?
- What is the average length of paragraphs?
- What kind of language is used (multisyllabic, slang, turgid, lively, short and simple)?

Your special interests

- Anything in the papers that may be of special use to you or to your organisation?

Gradually build up expertise, with a fact sheet on each newspaper. This will be indispensable for targeting your press releases.

How to write a press release

To write a press or news release you need to consider the following:

Headline. Create a catchy headline that is short and simple using less than 10 words. It should convey the key point made in the opening paragraph in a light-hearted manner that catches imagination and attention.

Collate and organise your facts. A simple rule is to find answers to questions pertaining to the five Ws: Who, What, When, Where, Why and then How. Identify your story's angle. A good story angle must have the following attributes. It must be the most important fact in your story, it must be timely, it must be unique, newsworthy or contrary to trends. The story angle must be presented in the first paragraph. Make your points in order of importance. Use short sentences, brief paragraphs and easy language, with no abbreviations or jargon. Put the most important message down into a quote. Journalists use quotes from the newsmakers to add an authoritative voice to their reports. If the press release contains quotes that are important and relevant they have more chance of being replicated in full in the published article.

Keep to one page if possible. If longer, type 'More follows …' at the bottom right hand corner. Do not carry over paragraphs or sentences to the next page. Type 'ends' after the last line of the release. End the press release with brief background information on your organisation and who to contact for further information.

Be specific. Focus on people rather than making generalised statements or quoting dry statistics. For example, say: 'Last week three Bloggsville children were admitted to the Royal Infirmary after accidentally swallowing weed killer. This brings the number of children accidentally poisoned this year to over 100. Sister Florence Nightingale, in charge of the Accident and Emergency Department, said: "It is heartbreaking to see the needless distress this causes" …'

Timing is vital. Your press release may not be used if a) it comes out on a day when there is news overload, such as on the day of election of a new prime minister; b) the news is not topical or current. Alert newspapers a few days in advance so that they can send reporters to cover an interesting event. For example, contact on a Friday or Monday is usually best for a weekly paper published on the following Friday. If you want to launch a story at a particular time, use the embargo system. This means writing, for example, 'Not for use until Wednesday September 2nd 2010' or 'Embargoed 6 p.m. September 2nd 2010' across the top of the press release. If it is for immediate release, then state: FOR IMMEDIATE RELEASE.

Presentation. Use A4 paper, headed with a logo if possible. Colour catches the eye, so a coloured heading or coloured paper will make your release stand out. Journalists work at speed, so make their task easier by:

- Using only one side of the page, placing the text centrally on the page.
- Using a lay out with double spacing.
- Leaving at least a 1-inch (2–3-cm) margin on either side.
- Putting a release date or embargo date at the top.
- Giving names and telephone numbers of people in your organisation for further information (including an after-hours telephone number).
- Sending it to a named journalist if possible.
- Not underlining any words (because this gives printers instructions to use italics; use **bold** for emphasis instead).

Photographs. If you are sending a photo, a 7×5 or 10×8, generally black and white, is preferred, with a full label on the back giving names and details. Include the names of everyone on the photo the picture shows, for example, 'left to right June Bloggs, Director of Public Health, Sam Smith, Health Promotion Specialist …' and explain what they are doing 'presenting Healthy Eating awards at 3 p.m. on Tuesday March 10th at Bloggsville Town Hall'. Never write directly on the back of a photo, as this will destroy its quality. Photos should be eye-catching and clear.

Communication. Send a copy of the press release to everyone who will be affected, including your organisation's communication or press officer, and to everyone mentioned or otherwise involved in the story.

BOX 11.2   Press release

Kofftown Primary Care Trust
PRESS RELEASE 1st September 2010
SMOKERS HOTLINE LAUNCHED

Kofftown's Smokers Hotline got off to a flying start this week, when Jo Goodheart, a health promotion specialist at Kofftown PCT, launched the service.

The hotline has been set up as part of Kofftown's Heart Week (1st–10th September), to help people who want to stop smoking. Anyone ringing 1234 567 890 will be sent a free pack of useful ideas to help them give up, including tips from ex-smokers and information about local stop-smoking groups.

'I smoked myself when I was younger and I remember what a struggle I had to stop. Many of my clients also find it incredibly difficult', said Joe Goodheart. 'That's why I'm delighted to launch this scheme. The pack has lots of useful information to help people over the difficulties.'

Smokers have a two to three times greater risk of having a heart attack than nonsmokers. At least 80% of heart attacks in men under 45 are thought to be due to cigarette smoking. Stopping smoking could lead to 150 fewer deaths each year of men and women under 65 in Kofftown.

For further information, please contact:

Jo Goodheart, Senior Health Promotion Officer, PCT, People's Lane, Kofftown KT1 2YZ

Telephone 1234 246 802 (day) or 1234 135 790 (evenings)

The above is based on ideas from *Pressbox: press release writing* (http://www.pressbox.co.uk). There are many websites with excellent ideas for writing press releases for the media. These can be found by simply using Google and the search term *press release*. See also the example of a press release in Box 11.2.

Writing letters to the editor

Another way of using the local paper as a medium for health promotion is by writing letters to the editor. This can keep an issue in the public eye for some time, and provides good opportunities for

---

EXERCISE 11.3   Writing for the local paper

1. Write a press release about a public health issue you are currently concerned about or working on, such as healthy school meals, binge drinking, drug taking by young people in local clubs, lack of play facilities for young children or poor public transport.
2. Write a letter to the editor supporting a current health promotion campaign or drawing attention to a specific need for health promotion.

---

public debate of controversial issues. Letters to the editor should be to the point, short (some newspapers restrict length) and be on one topic only.

Practise writing a press release and a letter to the editor by undertaking Exercise 11.3.

USING THE INTERNET FOR HEALTH PROMOTION

The Internet has revolutionised the way health promoters and the general public gain access to health information. Because of the massive growth of Web-based health information, the global nature of the Internet and the absence of real protection from harm for citizens who use the Internet for health purposes, quality is regarded as a problem (Risk & Dzenowagis 2001). Health promoters can use *He@lth Information on the Internet*, a journal which offers a guide to the most useful health websites and offers invaluable tips on how to find the information you and your clients need.

The Internet can be used to:

- support evidence-based health promotion practice
- disseminate resources and information to other health promoters
- provide information and support to the public.

See the section on evidence-based health promotion in Chapter 7.

SUPPORTING EVIDENCE–BASED HEALTH PROMOTION

The Internet provides the means of acquiring research evidence on the effectiveness of health promotion. There are a number of key websites which provide easy access to the best available information on what works to improve health and reduce inequalities, including effectiveness reviews that can be downloaded. These websites include the National Institute for Health and Clinical Excellence (NICE) (http://www.nice.org.uk). The Cochrane Centre (http://www.cochrane.co.uk) produces and disseminates systematic reviews and promotes the search for evidence in the form of clinical trials and other studies of interventions. The Cochrane Collaboration is named after the British epidemiologist Archie Cochrane.

Those health promoters working in a health setting can access Health Information Resources, formerly National Electronic Library for Health, which aims to provide accredited reference material for evidence-based practice. Other electronic databases that can be accessed include CINAHL and Medline.

DISSEMINATING RESOURCES AND INFORMATION TO OTHER HEALTH PROMOTERS

Organisations in which health promoters are located will generally have their own websites, and use them to disseminate reports of local projects and locally produced health promotion resources. Leaflets and resource packs are often available in PDF format so that visitors to the website can download the materials for their own use.

The Department of Health website (http://www.dh.gov.uk) (and the Irish, Scottish and Welsh equivalent) is an excellent resource for health promoters and contains significant amounts of policy and campaign/programme information and resources.

PROVIDING INFORMATION AND SUPPORT TO THE PUBLIC

A key objective of health policy (see, for example, DoH 2004) is to provide fast, convenient access for the public to accredited multimedia advice on lifestyle and health. One result of this has been the establishment of NHS Direct online (http://www.nhsdirect.nhs.uk) which aims to provide expert health advice and information.

Many health websites are read-only and are used to publish information for the user, a one-way process. But some also allow the user to interact. There are sites that offer interactive health guides such as the Department of Health site designed to support people in safe drinking (http://www.drinking.nhs.uk) by providing a unit calculator, drink diary, advise on how to cut down and other valuable materials. The Department of Health also uses YouTube (http://www.youtube.com).

These examples of e-health can be useful tools for health promotion. There is a growing body of debate about the effectiveness of computer-generated interventions (see Korp 2006, for example), and the volume of websites and blogs will present serious issues about the quality and accuracy of health advice.

ASSESSING THE QUALITY OF INFORMATION ON THE INTERNET

It is important that health promoters evaluate the quality of any website they use and/or advise their clients to use before trusting the information it provides (see Lewis 2006 for an interesting debate on the use of the Internet by the lay public). The following guidelines adjusted from LEARN NC (http://www.learnnc.org) may be useful in assessing the quality of a website:

1. **Who has written the information?** Who is the author? Is it an organisation or an individual person? Is there a way to contact them?
2. **Are the aims of the site clear?** What are the aims of the site? What is it for? Who is it for?
3. **Does the site achieve its aims?** Does the site do what it says it will?
4. **Is the site relevant to me?** List five things you want to find out from the site.
5. **Can the information be checked?** Is the author qualified to write the site? Has anyone else said the same things anywhere else? Is there any

way of checking this out? If the information is new, is there any proof?
6. **When was the site produced and last updated?** Is it up to date? Can you check to see if the information is up to date, and not just the site?
7. **Is the information biased in any way?** Has the site got a particular reason for wanting you to think in a particular way? Is it a balanced view ?
8. **Does the site tell you about choices open to you?** Does the site give you advice? Does it tell you about other ideas?

PRACTICE POINTS

- Communication tools for health promoters are wide ranging and need to be selected carefully and used effectively, with an assessment made of the advantages, uses and limitations of each kind of resource.
- Consider factors such as site, colour, language and style when creating displays.
- Written materials should be nonsexist, nonracist, in plain English and accessible to everyone, for example, ethnic minority languages, large type or alternative formats such as audiotape instead of written materials.
- Present statistical information with appropriate use of graphics to ensure clarity.
- You can use mass media successfully to raise awareness of health issues and deliver simple messages. You are unlikely to be successful if you try to use mass media to convey complex information or skills, or to shift attitudes, beliefs or lifestyle.
- Work effectively with local media by researching potential opportunities and carefully preparing presentations and press releases.

References

Anderson P 2009 Is it time to ban alcohol advertising? Clinical Medicine 9(2): 121–124.

Black C 2008 Working for a healthier tomorrow. London, The Stationery Office.

British Medical Association 2004 Focus on: dealing with the media. http://www.gp-training.net/training/docs/media.doc.

Cancer Research UK 2005 Schools fail to protect pupils from the sun.

Tuesday 19 July. http://info.cancerresearchuk.org/news/archive/pressreleases/2005/july/77637.

Das SK, Saltzman E, Gilhooly CH et al 2009 Low or moderate dietary energy restriction for long-term weight loss: what works best? Obesity 17(11): 2019–2024.

Department of Health 2000 Commercial sponsorship: ethical standards for the NHS. London, The Stationery Office.

Department of Health 2004 Choosing health: making healthy choices easier. London, The Stationery Office.

Department of Health 2008 Tobacco media/education campaigns. http://www.dh.gov.uk/en/Publichealth/Healthimprovement/Tobacco/Tobaccogeneralinformation/DH_4126098.

Department of Health 2009a Change4Life – eat well, move more, live longer. http://www.dh.gov.uk/en/News/Currentcampaigns/Change4Life/index.htm.

Department of Health 2009b Worried. http://www.dh.gov.uk/en/News/Currentcampaigns/DH_081137.

Fay S 2002 West Hertfordshire Hospital NHS Trust guideline for all members of staff in dealing with the media. Hertfordshire, West Hertfordshire NHS Trust.

Goodman J 2009 Can crash diets be good for you? New research shows that crash diets can be a safe and effective way of keeping the pounds off. Sunday Times, 7 June. http://www.timesonline.co.uk/tol/life_and_style/health/article6415198.ece.

Jones L, Hutchings K 2003 Homerton University Hospital NHS Trust. Trust media policy: guidelines for dealing with the media. Homerton, Homerton University Hospital NHS Trust.

Korp P 2006 Health on the Internet: implications for health promotion. Health Education Research 21(1): 78–86.

Lewis T 2006 Seeking health information on the Internet: lifestyle choice or bad attack of cyberchondria? Media, Culture & Society 28(4): 521–539.

Martinson BE, Hindman DB 2005 Building a health promotion agenda in local newspapers. Health Education Research 20(1): 51–60.

Matthews C 2007 Do soap shows encourage teenage drinking? The Food Magazine. http://www.foodmagazine.org.uk/press/soap_shows_and_drinking/.

Naidoo J, Wills J 2009 Using media in health promotion. In: Naidoo J, Wills J Foundations for health promotion, 3rd edn. Edinburgh, Baillière Tindall/Elsevier.

Risk A, Dzenowagis J 2001 Review of Internet health information quality initiatives. Geneva, WHO.

Robinson M 2002 Communication and health in a multi-ethnic society. Bristol, Polity Press.

Swanton W 2009 Incident makes you question sponsorship by alcohol companies. Sydney Morning Herald, June 6. http://www.smh.com.au/news/sport/cricket/incident-makes-you-question-sponsorship-by-alcohol-companies/2009/06/05/1243708626655.html.

Thake L, Glendinning R 2009 Media release: NHS Cambridgeshire and 200 GPs & surgery staff get together to help the people of Cambridgeshire lead a healthier lifestyle. http://www.cambridgeshirepct.nhs.uk/documents/News/2009/NHS_Cambs_3308_NHS_Cambridgeshire_Host_Major_Event.pdf?preventCache=09%2F01%2F2009+10%3A52.

Tones K, Tilford S 2001 The mass media in health promotion. In: Tones K, Tilford S (eds) Health education: effectiveness, efficiency and equity, 3rd edn. Cheltenham, Nelson Thornes.

Wammes B, Oenema A, Brug J 2007 The evaluation of a mass media campaign aimed at weight gain prevention among young Dutch adults. Obesity 15: 2780–2789.

Websites

http://www.cochrane.co.uk
http://www.dh.gov.uk
http://www.drinking.nhs.uk
http://www.ic.nhs.uk
http://www.learnnc.org/lp/external/QUICK
http://www.nhsdirect.nhs.uk
http://www.nice.org.uk
http://www.pressbox.co.uk/contpr2.htm
http://www.youtube.com/user/departmentofhealth

Chapter 12

Educating for health

SUMMARY

The first section of this chapter involves a discussion on the principles of learning. An exercise is used to analyse the qualities and abilities of an effective health educator, and some principles of facilitating health learning are outlined. Subsequent sections contain guidelines on giving talks, strategies for patient education and teaching practical skills for health. A role-play exercise is used to focus on skills of effective patient health education.

This chapter is about the skills and methods of educating for health, when the aims are primarily concerned with enabling people to acquire health knowledge and skills. Examples are: giving a talk on a health topic to a large community group; teaching an adult education class in food safety or a school class in sexual health; running cardiac rehabilitation sessions for patients recovering after heart attacks; giving information to a patient on a one-to-one basis about diagnosis, treatment and self-care; or teaching a small group of colleagues about the techniques and procedures used in a smoking cessation programme.

PRINCIPLES OF LEARNING FOR HEALTH

Some aspects of education, teaching and learning are relevant for health promoters.

Other relevant Chapters are 10, 11, 13 and 14.

BOX 12.1   Principles of learning as applied to health education

- Learning for health is most effective when the learner identifies their own learning needs and sets their own goals.
- The health educator's role is to enable or facilitate learning rather than to direct it. Health educators who adopt this approach often refer to themselves as facilitators.
- Learners are generally most ready to learn things that they can apply immediately to existing health problems or to their own situation.
- Learners bring with them life experience, which should be seen as a resource and to which new learning should be related.
- Learners can help each other, because of their experiences, and should be encouraged to do so.
- Learning is best when active (not passive), by doing and experiencing, for which learners need a safe environment where they feel accepted.
- Learners should be encouraged to carry out continuous evaluation of their own learning. Health educators should use this evaluation to fit the learning process to the learners' needs.

Health promoters generally have credibility because of their training and expert knowledge which is likely to be valued and respected by clients, but expertise alone does not make a good health educator. In order to get results in the form of measurable learning achievements, such as greater retention and application of health information and skills, health educators need to understand some principles of learning, such as the importance of participative learning. The basic principles of learning as applied to health are summarised in Box 12.1. For more details on adult learning see Rogers (2001); for an example of how the principles of learning can be applied in practice see Suter & Suter (2008); for a broader perspective on teaching and learning in nursing health promoting practice see Bastable (2002); and for health settings generally see Bastable (2004).

FACILITATING HEALTH LEARNING

Exercise 12.1 will help you to identify factors that have helped and hindered your learning, and to assess your own qualities and abilities. The following recommendations apply to health education with individuals or groups.

EXERCISE 12.1   What helps and hinders learning?

Think of two occasions when you have been a learner, such as when you were a health promotion student in class, or in the audience listening to a health talk, or when you were being taught on a one-to-one basis. These learning occasions need not have been connected with work, for example listening to an art lecture or taking a driving lesson. One should be when you felt, overall, that the session was *good* and the other when it was *bad*. The aim of the exercise is to identify the factors that made them good or bad for you.

In each of your two situations in turn, identify factors that helped you to learn, and factors that hindered your learning. Think of these factors in three categories:
1. Those to do with the *environment* (e.g. too hot? noisy? hard chairs? a spacious, comfortable room?)
2. Those to do with the *qualities of the teacher* (e.g. sense of humour? appeared bored? contagious enthusiasm? seemed unfriendly?)
3. Those to do with the *presentation* (e.g. talked too long? used relevant illustrations? involved audience?

muddled? used words you didn't understand? used audiovisual aids effectively?)
Enter these factors on the chart:

	Environment	Teacher	Presentation
Factors that helped			
Factors that hindered			

If you are working in a group, compare your chart with those of other people.
- What have you learnt about the importance of the environment?
- What qualities of a good health educator do you think you already possess?
- What helpful points about presentation do you think you already use, or will use, in your own work?
- What points about your own qualities or presentation would you like to improve?

PLAN YOUR SESSION

However skilled and knowledgeable you are about the health topic, it is vital to put thought and time into preparation. You need to think through what you aim to achieve, how you are going to introduce and develop your session and how you will involve your audience. Preparation is especially important when facilitating health learning is new to you, but even the most experienced and self-confident health educator needs to spend some time in preparation. Active participation is a more complex process and will require greater attention to planning.

WORK FROM THE KNOWN TO THE UNKNOWN

Time is wasted in teaching people something they already know so the starting point is finding out what your clients know. If you cannot do this in advance, spend some time at the beginning of the session asking a few questions. If you have a mixed audience with varying degrees of knowledge, it may be best to acknowledge that some people know more than others, and you will have to make a decision about the level at which to pitch your information: 'Some of you will probably know this, but I'll talk about it briefly because it will be new to others …'.

Your aim is to impart new health information, or new skills, onto what is already known.

AIM FOR MAXIMUM INVOLVEMENT

People learn best if they are actively participating in the learning process, not just passive listeners (see Jenson & Simovska 2005 for an interesting discussion of two models of participation).

First, where appropriate, involve your clients in deciding the aim and content of the session. If you are running a course, such as a series of antenatal classes or one on food hygiene, you might begin by explaining your aims, asking for comments and suggestions, and then going on to discuss the content. This will help to increase motivation by stimulating clients to think about their own needs and to take some responsibility for their own learning. The goals and content of a one-to-one session can be established by mutual agreement at the outset. As a general rule, it is worth considering how much room for negotiation there is in your health education role, and spending time to find out what people really want. Ask yourself 'Is what I cover what *I want to teach* or what *my clients want to learn*?'

Second, keep your clients involved as much as possible during sessions. This is a challenge if you are giving a talk or a lecture to a large audience, but there are possibilities, such as asking people to respond to a question, such as 'I'd like you to put your hand up if you made a new year resolution to take more exercise this year'. Or ask them to respond to a series of statements: for example, as an introduction to a talk on nutrition, ask the audience to stand up, then ask them to sit down if they: usually eat white bread … add sugar to tea and coffee … regularly eat fried food … add salt at the table … Most of them will be sitting down by now but will feel alert and involved. Another way of keeping an audience involved is to give them time to talk. This can be done by having question-and-answer sessions, or by allowing short breaks when they can talk about something in groups of two or three for a few minutes. In a talk on passive smoking, for example, you could give your audience a couple of minutes to tell their neighbours how they are affected by other people's smoke.

You can also keep people involved with eye contact. Make sure that you look round at everybody, not just the people immediately in front of you.

VARY YOUR LEARNING METHODS

It is natural to consider health educating from the health educator's point of view but it may be more helpful to look at it from the learner's point of view. For example, talking for half an hour demands concentrated effort and total involvement on your part; but all your audience is doing is listening, which involves only one of their senses and is highly unlikely to hold their full attention.

Variety can be brought into health teaching in many ways, including strategies that can be used with individuals, groups, large audiences, children or adults; see Table 12.1 for ideas.

DEVISE HEALTH EDUCATION ACTIVITIES

Listening is passive; activities are the means by which you help learners to think through what is being said and act on it, in their own way. It is not sufficient to ask a group 'What do you think?' at the end of a talk or after viewing a DVD; planned activities are necessary to help people to explore and

Table 12.1   Learning methods involving clients

CLIENT INVOLVEMENT	MATERIALS AND METHODS
Listen	Lectures, audiotapes
Read	Books, booklets, leaflets, handouts, posters, whiteboard, flip-chart, PowerPoint slides
Look	Photographs, drawings, paintings, posters, charts, material from media (such as advertisements)
Look and listen	DVDs, PowerPoint, demonstrations
Listen and talk	Question-and-answer sessions, discussions, informal conversations, debates, brainstorming
Read, listen and talk	Case studies, discussions based on study questions or handouts
Read, listen, talk and actively participate	Drama, role-play, games, simulations, quizzes, practising skills
Read and actively participate	Programmed learning, computer-assisted learning
Make and use	Models, charts, drawings
Use	Equipment
Action research	Gathering information, opinions, interviews and surveys
Projects	Making health education materials – DVDs, leaflets, etc.
Visits	To health service premises, fire station, sewage works, playgroups, voluntary organisations
Write	Articles, letters to the press, stories, poems

For discussion of some of these methods, see Chapters 13 and 14; for discussion on the use of audiovisual aids, see Chapter 11.

Table 12.2   Common types of learning activities

TYPE OF ACTIVITY	EXAMPLE
Guidelines for discussions with particular people about particular topics	Guidelines on 'what to do if you think your child is offered drugs' for discussion at a parent–teacher meeting
Analysing and discussing diary records	Ask people to keep a diary or write down what they ate or the alcohol units they consumed in the last 24 hours. Ask them to talk about what they are pleased about and not pleased about
Sentence completion	Ask people to complete a sentence such as 'I feel really stressed when ...'
Using checklists	Have a list of 'ways to make small changes to my lifestyle' such as taking the stairs and not the lift, walking (or cycling to work), joining an exercise class, and discuss how many you use
Identifying your own thoughts/feelings/ behaviour in particular situations	Ask people to think about and discuss what they feel when visitors to their home ask if they can smoke, and how they respond
Generate lists	Ask a group to make a list of all the ways they could deal with an obese client who will not comply with advice on healthy eating
Answer sheets	A quiz with yes/no or multiple answers on 'How much do you know about sensible drinking?'
Drawing charts or bubble diagrams	Draw a stick-person picture of yourself in a supermarket in the middle of a page. Draw bubble thoughts about all the things that influence what food you buy
Writing instructions	Ask a group learning about food hygiene to write down instructions for someone else on how to store food safely in a fridge
Practical skills development	Practise bathing a baby using a doll or a real baby.

apply ideas, feelings, attitudes and behaviour. It is more effective to have a mix of activities that are specifically tailored for a particular group of learners, so where possible develop the skill of devising your own activities rather than relying on learning aids made for general audiences. There is an almost infinite range of possibilities. Some of the more common types of activity are set out in Table 12.2.

There are also ideas in some of the exercises used throughout this book.

ENSURE RELEVANCE

You should ensure that, as far as possible, what you say is relevant to the needs, interests and circumstances of the clients. For example, recommendations about health-promoting activities that cost money may not be useful to an audience which has no money for extras. A discussion on childhood vaccination may be irrelevant to a pregnant woman whose overwhelming concern is the birth itself; she may not relate to an issue that will not meet her immediate needs.

You will help your clients to see the relevance of your subject if you use concrete examples, practical problems and case studies to explain and illustrate your points. It may be more difficult for your clients to relate to abstract generalisations, quotations of statistics or epidemiological evidence. For example say 'one person in ten' instead of 'X million people in this country', tell the story of a home accident rather than describe a list of risk factors, and describe 'increasing the risk' by saying 'It's like driving a car with faulty brakes, there's no guarantee that you will have an accident, but your chances of having one are greater'.

IDENTIFY REALISTIC GOALS AND OBJECTIVES

In Chapter 5 there was a discussion on the importance of clearly identifying health promotion aims and objectives, but it is worth emphasising again that it is essential to be clear about what you are trying to do (raise awareness of a health issue? give people more health knowledge?) and what you want your clients to know, feel and/or do at the end of your session. As mentioned above, your clients should be involved in these decisions.

See Chapter 5, section on setting aims and objectives.

Three or four key points are all that clients can be expected to assimilate from a session. Including more than that does not mean that they learn more; it usually means that they forget more. For example, if you are asked to give a talk on a huge theme, such as food for health, avoiding accidents, first aid or pollution, you will need to select what you feel to be the few points most relevant for your audience, and avoid the temptation to include everything.

USE LEARNING CONTRACTS

In some educational settings the learner is told what objectives or targets to work towards. This can conflict with some people's psychological need to be self-directing and may induce resistance, apathy or

withdrawal. Learning contracts are an agreement, decided together, about what is to be learnt. By participating in the process of diagnosing needs, formulating goals, choosing methods and evaluating progress, learners can develop a sense of ownership of the plan, and feel more committed and empowered.

The stages of developing a learning contract are described below.

Step 1: Diagnose health learning needs with the learners

First, decide the competencies required to carry out actions, behaviour or roles. A competency can be thought of as the ability to do something, and it is a combination of knowledge, understanding, skills, attitudes and values.

For instance, the ability to ride a bicycle from home to school involves knowledge of how a bicycle works and of the route from home to the school; understanding of the risks inherent in riding a bicycle; skills in mounting, pedalling, steering and stopping. It is useful to analyse competencies in this way, even if it is crude and subjective, because it gives the learners a clearer sense of direction.

Next, assess the gap between where learners are now and where they should be in regard to each health-related competency. Learners may wish to draw on the observations of friends, family or experts to make this assessment. Each learner will then have an idea of the competencies needed and a map of their health learning needs.

Step 2: Specify the learning objectives of each learner

Translate the learning needs identified in step 1 into objectives that describe what each learner wants to *learn*. All learners should state their learning objectives in terms most meaningful to them. For example, in order to ride a bicycle from home to school, learners may decide that they need knowledge of how to work the bicycle gears and improved skills of steering and stopping safely.

Step 3: Specify learning methods

Review the learning objectives of the learner or (if you are working with a group of learners) all the members of the learning group, perhaps through listing them on a flip-chart and identifying shared objectives and areas of difference. Now think about how you could go about accomplishing these objectives. Specify the methods you would use. In the bicycle example, you could specify that practical demonstration followed by supervised practice in a traffic-free area would be the way to learn. Ask learners to suggest the methods they prefer.

Step 4: Evaluate learning

Now describe what evidence you will need to show that these objectives have been achieved. For example, knowledge can be tested through quizzes; understanding can be tested through solving problems; skills can be tested through demonstrations of performance; attitudes can be tested through role-play and simulation exercises; values can be tested through line debates and value-clarification exercises.

> See also Chapter 5, section on planning evaluation methods.

An example of a learning contract for a group is provided in Box 12.2. Individuals in a group can have their own personal version of the learning contract.

> See Chapter 14, section on strategies for increasing self-awareness, clarifying values and changing attitudes.

ORGANISE YOUR MATERIAL

Whether you are talking to a group or an individual, it helps if you organise your material into a logical framework, and tell your client(s) what this is, both at the beginning and during your teaching session. For example, with an individual client in a smoking cessation course, say:

> 'We are going to:
> * Look at your smoking behaviour and the reasons why you smoke.
> * Identify the barriers to you giving up smoking.
> * Measure where you are in terms of your motivation to stop smoking.
>
> First, let us discuss your smoking behaviour and what prompts this behaviour.
>
> Second, what do you think will prevent you from stopping …
>
> Finally, let us see where you stand in terms of you wanting to stop smoking …'

The same principle applies if you are talking to a group. You tell them what you are going to tell them; tell them; then tell them what you have told them! This helps both you and the audience to know where you are and where you are going. Recapping where you are at intervals is helpful: 'That's all I've got to say on the benefits of yoga; now, to move on to how you can get started …',

---

BOX 12.2   Learning contract for Mary's young parents' group

Group members said they wanted to know more about how to cook cheap, interesting, healthy meals for their families, as a change from the usual ready prepared foods such as frozen fish fingers, cans of beans, frozen chips. Mary and group members worked out the following learning contract.

Learning objectives	Learning methods	Evaluation of achievement of objectives
Know what to eat to be healthy	Keep food diaries for 2 days. Mary to produce guidelines and members discuss how far their food matches up to guidelines	Be able to say what sort of food each member should aim to eat more or less of
Know where to buy healthy cheap food	Group members share experience of where they buy food, its price and quality	Two weeks later, members identify changes in where they buy food, and whether it is better quality and value for money
Be able to cook healthy meals that their families enjoy eating	Mary and group members bring recipes, choose some to try out and cook together	Have cooked new healthy meals at home

or 'Now I'd like to move on to my third and final point, which you may remember I said was about ...'

EVALUATION, FEEDBACK AND ASSESSMENT

It is important to get feedback, so that you can assess how much your client is learning and improve your own performance in the future.

See Chapter 5, section on planning evaluation methods, and Chapter 10, section on asking questions and getting feedback.

Assessing your own performance

You need to ask yourself what went well, what didn't, why and how things could be improved next time. You may find it helpful to use a simple form to record your thoughts. This is especially useful if your session is part of a course with a team of people involved. An example is given in Box 12.3, a form used by a group facilitator to record issues after a group session on healthy eating and cooking.

BOX 12.3	Nutrition and cooking project monitoring form

Session no:
Date:
Time:
Facilitator:
Number of attendees:
Number in crèche:
Activity:
Positive outcomes:
Negative outcomes:
Feedback/comments from participants:
Crèche issues:
Issues needing further action:
Action plan:
Completed by:

(Hartcliffe Health and Environment Action Group and health visitors from Hartcliffe and Withywood, Bristol. Reproduced with permission.)

Getting feedback

You could include oral feedback as part of your session. For example, at the end ask people to do a round of sentence completion:

'The thing I liked best about today's session was ...'

'The most important thing I am taking from this session is ...'

'The thing I liked least about today's session was ...'

However, people may find this intimidating, and might not feel comfortable with expressing what they feel. You may wish to use a written evaluation form; see the two examples in Boxes 12.4 and 12.5.

Assessing the health learning outcomes

Assessing learning outcomes is an important aspect of evaluation in health education. It is the process of measuring the extent and quality of your clients' learning: judging how successful they have been in progressing towards goals which they set themselves. It may be carried out very informally through getting apparently casual feedback from clients about how they have applied the learning to real-life situations, or it may involve setting tests in formal situations. Here are two examples of ways in which health promoters assess how well they are doing:

1. Sandra teaches yoga. She does not feel it appropriate to assess her students formally, so she uses the British Wheel of Yoga standards to check on their performance and give them feedback.

2. Marleen teaches cookery and healthy eating to adults with learning difficulties. She keeps records of their progress in relation to their

---

BOX 12.4	Evaluation form A

Title of session:
Date:
   Please help me to get the session right for you by completing the following sentences about how you feel. Thank you.
It helps me when ....
It is difficult for me when ....
I would like more of ....
I would like less of ....

BOX 12.5   Evaluation form B

Title of session:
Date:

   We would like your views to help us assess this session and make plans for similar sessions in the future. All your comments will be valued and used, and treated confidentially.

	Yes	No	Partly
1. Overall, have you found this session beneficial? (please tick)	☐	☐	☐

	Yes	No	Partly
2. Did the session match up to your expectations?	☐	☐	☐

3. What did you expect to gain from the session?
   Please comment:

4. Which parts of the session have you found most beneficial?

5. Which parts of the session have you found least beneficial?

6. How do you think the session could be improved?

7. Do you have any other comments you would like to make?

   Please write your name here (or leave blank if you prefer to remain anonymous).

   Thank you very much for filling this in.

---

previous level of competence in choosing healthy menus and cooking healthy meals.

Monitoring students' progress by keeping records of achievements can be valuable for helping them to see what they have achieved. If your health education is geared towards people learning to change behaviour, it can help to keep diary-type records of what they ate or drank, or their physical activity levels. If they are learning practical creative skills, photographic records can help. For example, on a course designed to help people cook and eat healthier food for their families, you could give them a single-use camera to make a pictorial record of the dishes they cooked and their family enjoying the meals.

GUIDELINES FOR GIVING TALKS

Giving a formal talk is often part of a health promoter's work. There are considerable disadvan-

tages in this method: a talk is largely a one-way communication process with little opportunity to assess how much people are learning or understanding, and with only a small proportion of it likely to be remembered at the end (and still less a few days later).

Despite these limitations, talks and lectures can be valuable for several reasons. A talk can be used to introduce a health topic by giving a broad overview of it, and this may lead people to take further action. For example, an introductory talk on first aid may lead people to enrol for a first aid course. A talk may also be an important source of health information and awaken a critical attitude in the audience, for example by drawing their attention to issues such as traffic pollution or misleading information on food labels. Giving talks is also a relatively economical way to use a health promoter's time, since large numbers of people can be addressed at one time. In order to ensure success, the following points need to be addressed.

CHECK THE FACILITIES

If possible, visit the place where you are going to give your talk and check the seating, lighting and audiovisual equipment, including electric power points and extension leads. On the day of the talk, arrive early so that you can arrange chairs, open windows and check that the equipment is working. Get your audiovisual equipment ready for use. If you need blackout, check that you can turn the lights on and off quickly so that you do not lose rapport with the audience while they are left in the dark.

MAKE A PLAN

It can be useful to make an outline plan of your whole session, indicating the sections, times and any audiovisual aids you are using. This is particularly useful if you are sharing a session with a colleague, so that you are both clear what you are doing. See the example in Box 12.6 and either use this as a skeleton overall plan to guide you when you make detailed notes to speak from (see section below) or it might be enough to enable you to speak from the plan itself.

MAKING AND USING NOTES

It is generally best to give a talk from notes. The more experienced you are the fewer notes you are

---

BOX 12.6   Plan for giving a talk

TALK ON 'SENSE IN THE SUN – PREVENTING SKIN CANCER'
Bloggshire Secondary School Parent–Teachers Meeting
21.10.2010: an hour at the end of the business meeting, 8.00–8.45 p.m.
SNS (school nurse) and JAS (deputy head)
AIM: to give parents basic information on risks and prevention of skin cancer

Time	Section	Content	Audiovisual aids PowerPoint (PP)	Who
8.00	Intros	Intro JAS & SNS Why we are now concerned about skin cancer – rising incidence?	PP graph showing rise in skin cancer in UK	JAS
8.05	What is skin cancer?	Different types of skin cancer. How you spot it? Who is most at risk (fair skin, sunburn, etc.)?	PP key points	SNS
8.15	Prevention	Key message: respect the sun – avoid exposure at hottest times, use good sunscreen, cover up with sun hats and light clothing. Be a mole-watcher	Examples of sun hats, light clothing (big, long-sleeved, cotton shirts, etc.). Examples of sunscreen creams	SNS
8.25	What the school can do?	Encourage the use of cover-up and sunscreen creams in outdoor PE. Include topic in health education and science teaching	Main points on PP	JAS
8.30	Summary	Aim for school and parents to work together. Main points to remember: Care in the sun, Cover up, use sunscreen Creams	PP: 3 Cs to remember: Care in the sun, Cover up, Creams. Leaflets to take away	SNS
8.35	Any questions?			SNS

---

likely to need, unless your talk is full of technical detail or likely to be taken down and quoted verbatim (for example, by the press). However, very few people can give a successful talk with no notes at all, and beginners may find it helpful to write out a talk in full before they transfer the main points to notes.

If you are writing out your talk in full to begin with, it is useful to know that a 50-minute lecture consists of about 5000 words, allowing for pauses and an estimated speed of delivery of about 110 words per minute. You can then try transferring the key points as notes to cards or paper.

Never give a talk by writing it out in full and then reading it. Unless you are an exceptional orator it will sound flat and stilted. Furthermore, you will find it difficult to look at your audience, because you will need to keep your eyes on the notes, and if you look up you are likely to lose your place.

PREPARE YOUR INTRODUCTION

Secure the attention of your audience with your opening words. Some ways of doing this are:

● State a surprising fact or an unusual quote.
● Ask a question that has no easy answer.
● Use a visual image to trigger interest.
● Get the audience to do something active (some suggestions are discussed in the earlier section on aiming for maximum involvement).
● Tell a joke, if you have the confidence to do it successfully.

Establish eye contact with your audience and, if necessary, ask them whether they can see and hear you.

State your aim and theme at the beginning of your talk. It should be a brief statement, not a complex summary of the whole talk. For example, say 'I'm going to talk about the benefits of incorporating more physical activity into your life and ways of making small changes to ensure you are getting sufficient exercise', but do not go into detail at this point; save that for the main part of the talk.

By the time you have finished the introduction, you should have:

- established your aim and theme with the audience
- obtained their interest and commitment
- ensured that they can hear and see you clearly.

PREPARE THE KEY POINTS

Identify the three or four main points you wish to make, and prepare your talk around each point in turn. Illustrate and support your points with evidence from your experience or from research, with examples, audiovisual materials, and so on.

See Chapter 11, on using and producing audiovisual materials, including leaflets, handouts and DVDs.

PLAN A CONCLUSION

You need to plan how you will end your talk in order to avoid rambling on or trailing off. Some ways of ending are:

- A very brief recapitulation (not a boring repetition) of what you've said, such as 'We've now covered the basics of exercising and lifestyle change'.
- A statement of what you hope the audience will do with the information you have given them, such as 'I hope that you can confidently make changes to your lifestyle to include more exercise'.
- A suggestion for further action: 'If you'd like to find out more about exercise and health please come to see me afterwards or contact me at … – giving e-mail/telephone and/or office address'.
- A question – 'What small lifestyle changes can you make to include more physical activity into your life?'
- Thanking the audience for their attention and/or participation.

ASK FOR QUESTIONS

If possible, include a question-and-answer session in your talk. It gives you feedback, and gives the audience a chance to participate.

When you ask for questions, allow people time to think; do not assume that there are to be no questions just because one is not instantly forthcoming. When a question is asked, it is often helpful to repeat it or summarise. This gives you a little time to consider the question, and ensures that everyone else in the audience has heard it. Never ignore or refuse to answer a question. If you don't know the answer, admit this and ask whether anyone else in the audience does. In any case, this helps to involve the audience; you could also ask for comments on answers: 'Does anyone else have suggestions for the person who asked that question?'

WORK ON YOUR PRESENTATION

Important points about presentation include pace and timing, which can mean consciously having to slow down your rate of speaking; the nervous beginner can speak too quickly. Other factors are looking at the audience and using notes appropriately.

Thorough preparation will help you to feel confident, but however nervous or inexperienced you may feel, do not apologise for being there. For example, if you have been asked to give a talk about your work, *do not say* 'I'm going to talk about the work of health visitors, but I'm afraid I've only been qualified for a year so there's a lot I don't know yet'. Instead, present yourself positively 'I'm going to talk about the work of health visitors. I've been qualified for a year now, and I'd like to share my experience of the work with you'.

The way to improve presentation is practise. Practise giving your talk out loud, or to friends or colleagues. Ask a trusted colleague to sit in when you give a talk, and to give you feedback afterwards. It is also helpful to have your talk recorded so that you can assess your own strengths and weaknesses.

PLAN FOR CONTINGENCIES

A major fear when giving a talk is that you might lose your place or your train of thought. If this is a possibility, it is better to think beforehand about what you will do if it should happen. It is best to acknowledge that you have a problem rather than leave an embarrassing silence. For example, say 'Sorry, I've lost my place'. Remember that an audience is likely to be friendly rather than hostile. So let them help by asking for time: 'Excuse me for a moment while I look through my notes'.

See also section on dealing with difficulties in Chapter 13.

Another fear is that audiovisual equipment may not work. You cannot insure against this, so it is best to have a contingency plan ready. For example, 'As we can't see the sequence on PowerPoint as I'd hoped, I'll write the stages up on the flip-chart and talk through them instead', or you may wish to ensure you have a back-up, such as overhead projector slides of the PowerPoint presentation.

IMPROVING PATIENT EDUCATION

Evidence suggests that patients want health information but some have difficulty in understanding and remembering what they have been told by their doctor, nurse or other health worker (see, for example, the research of Posma et al 2009 on older patients and the difficulties they have in processing and remembering information). Patients also often feel dissatisfied with the communications aspect of their encounters with health professionals, and are reluctant to ask for more information (see Jangland et al 2009 for reasons for this and recommendations

for improvement). Not surprisingly, a large proportion of patients do not comply with the advice and treatment prescribed for them (see, for example, Duke 2009).

There may be complex reasons for these apparent failures, but some of the cause will be the way in which information, advice and instructions are given to patients. Often the circumstances are less than ideal, because patients are distressed or feeling unwell, and there may be little time in a busy surgery, health centre, outpatient clinic or hospital ward. This is all the more reason to ensure that the best possible use is made of the time and opportunities for patient education.

All the basic communication skills discussed in Chapter 10, and the principles of helping people to learn outlined in this chapter, are important. There is also now a growing body of evidence in the field of patient education and information. See Cochrane website for various studies (http://www.cochrane.org). Some particular principles that have been found helpful in patient education are set out in Box 12.7. See also Pestonjee (2000) and Osborne (2004).

BOX 12.7   Some principles of patient education

- Say important things first: patients are more likely to remember what was said at the beginning of a session, so give the most important advice and instruction first whenever possible.
- Stress and repeat the key points: patients are more likely to remember what they consider to be important, so make sure they realise what the important points are. For example, say:
  - 'The most important thing for you to remember today is …'
  - 'The one thing it's really essential to do is …'

Repetition of key points also helps people to remember them.

- Give specific, precise advice: sometimes it is appropriate to give general guidance, but specific, precise advice is more likely to be remembered than vague guidance. For example, say:
  - 'I advise you to lose 5 pounds in the next month' rather than 'I advise you to lose weight'.
  - 'Try to take 30 minutes exercise every day' rather than 'Take more exercise'.
- Structure information into categories: this means telling the patient headings and then categorising

your material under these headings as you present it.

See 'Organise Your Material' above.

- Avoid jargon and long words and sentences: if you need to use medical terms or jargon, make sure the patient understands what they mean. Never use a long word when a short one will do. Use short sentences.
- Use visual aids, leaflets, handouts and written instructions.

See Chapter 11 on using communication tools.

- Avoid saying too much at once: three or four key points are all that you can expect someone to remember from one session.

See 'Ensure Relevance' above.

- Ensure advice is relevant and realistic in the patient's circumstances.
- Get feedback from patients to ensure that they understand.

See the section on asking questions and getting feedback in Chapter 10.

EXERCISE 12.2   Skills of patient education

Work in groups of three, taking each role in turn.

The **first person** takes the role of the health promoter. She selects the topic to be taught, drawing on her own experience, and tells the patient their medical history before role-play starts.

The **second person** plays the patient. This patient should have one of the following sets of characteristics:

■ Intelligent, but with very limited understanding of spoken English, no ability to read or write English and no one available to translate.

■ Extremely worried, tense and anxious about their medical condition and prognosis.

■ Has some learning difficulty, finds great difficulty in understanding and remembering instructions although they try hard to be cooperative.

The **third person** takes the role of the observer, using the observer's checklist below.

Role-play the scene in which the health promoter is teaching the patient for 10 minutes. The observer keeps time. Then give constructive feedback as follows:

■ First, the health promoter assesses themself, saying what they felt they did well, and identifying points they feel they need to work on in the future.

■ Second, the patient describes how it felt to be the patient, identifying what the health promoter did or said which made them feel at ease/put down/anxious/reassured/more confused, and so on.

■ Finally, the observer gives feedback using the checklist as a guide.

Communication checklist

1. Nonverbal aspects of communication, e.g. tone of voice, posture, gestures, facial expression and use of touch.
2. Sequence and structure of key points, e.g. important things first, logical sequence, information in categories.
3. Choice of language, e.g. appropriately simple and short, use of jargon/idioms, medical terms.
4. Two-way communication, e.g. encourage patient to talk and express feelings, get feedback about how much is understood, open/closed/biased/multiple questions.
5. Amount of information, e.g. too much or too little.
6. Clarity of objective(s).
7. Use of repetition.
8. Use of emphasis to stress important points.
9. Any assumptions made but not checked, e.g. about previous knowledge, facilities for carrying out instructions, willingness to comply.
10. Anything else?

Exercise 12.2 is designed to help you practise the skills of patient education and supplements the basic communication skills outlined in Chapter 10. Another useful way of learning to improve communication skills is to record and then analyse an interview with a patient.

TEACHING PRACTICAL SKILLS FOR HEALTH

Health promoters are often called upon to teach practical skills, such as relaxation or keep-fit exercises, how to bath a baby or change a nappy, and how to give an injection or test urine.

Teaching a skill is not just about giving the client information and teaching new practical skills. It is also necessary to pay attention to what clients *feel*. If people are afraid to do something because they are worried about looking foolish or doing it incorrectly, they are unlikely to succeed: encouragement

and step-by-step progress are needed. Confidence building is as important a part of the health educator's role as developing practical skills.

In order to develop clients' ability to perform a skilled task, a three-stage approach is most effective:

Stage 1. Demonstrate.
Stage 2. Rehearse.
Stage 3. Practise.

Clients will be watching and listening in stage 1, but they become actively involved in *doing* in stages 2 and 3.

It may be useful to begin by using a dummy, for example when teaching safe lifting techniques, or to use an orange instead of a person when teaching injection techniques. As skills develop, the techniques can be tried in real-life situations (lifting people, for example) and perhaps under more difficult circumstances.

Individual learners need to progress at their own pace and build up confidence at each stage. For this reason teaching practical skills needs time and patience, but it is worth the investment to get the right skills programme from the beginning. People who have lost confidence in their ability to do something are sometimes more difficult to help than a new learner.

PRACTICE POINTS

- To be successful in health education with clients you need to understand principles of learning and factors that help and hinder the learning process. You may find it helpful to use informal learning contracts.
- Giving talks on health topics requires detailed planning, preparation and practise.
- You can help patients to understand and remember more if you take account of some key principles of patient education.
- Use a three-stage approach of demonstration, rehearsal and practice when you are teaching practical health-related skills.

References

Bastable SB 2002 Nurse as educator: principles of teaching and learning for nursing practice. Sudbury, Jones and Bartlett.

Bastable SB 2004 Essentials of patient education. Sudbury, Jones and Bartlett.

Duke S-AS, Colagiuri S, Colagiuri R 2009 Individual patient education for people with type 2 diabetes mellitus. Cochrane Database of Systematic Reviews 2009, Issue 1. Art. No.: CD005268. DOI: 10.1002/14651858.CD005268.pub2.

Jangland E, Gunningberg L, Carlsson M 2009 Patients' and relatives' complaints about encounters and communication in health care: evidence for quality improvement. Patient Education and Counselling 75(2): 199–204.

Jenson BB, Simovska V 2005 Involving students in learning and health promotion processes – clarifying why? what? and how? Promotion & Education 12(3–4): 150–156.

Osborne H 2004 Health literacy for A–Z: practical ways to communicate your health message. Sudbury, Jones and Bartlett.

Pestonjee SF 2000 Nurses' handbook of patient education. Springhouse, Springhouse Corporation.

Posma ER, van Weert JCM, Jansen J, Bensing JM 2009 Older patients' information and support needs surrounding treatment: an evaluation through the eyes of patients, relatives and professionals. BMC Nursing. http://www.biomedcentral.com/1472-6955/8/1.

Rogers J 2001 Adults learning, 4th edn. Buckingham, Open University Press.

Suter PM, Suter WN 2008 Timeless principles of learning: a solid foundation for enhancing chronic disease self-management. Home Healthcare Nurse 26(2): 82–88.

Website

http://www.cochrane.org

Chapter 13

Working with groups

CHAPTER CONTENTS

SUMMARY

This chapter is about working with clients in groups and begins by discussing the range of groups in health promotion, potential benefits of group work and when it is appropriate to use it as an approach. Group leadership styles and responsibilities and individual group behaviour are considered. The last part of the chapter focuses on the competencies needed for working successfully with people in groups, including the practicalities and skills of setting up a group, getting groups established, discussion skills and dealing with difficulties. Exercises focus on identifying the benefits of joining a group, looking at your leadership style and planning a group meeting.

Health promoters work with many different kinds of groups in a variety of settings. Working with groups of colleagues is considered in Chapter 9; in this chapter, the focus is on the health promoter's work with groups of clients, but many of the skills discussed in Chapter 9 (such as coordination, team-work and working effectively in meetings and committees) may also apply when working with clients.

See Chapter 9.

Group work encourages clients to be active participants in their own health issues and with their communities. Many of the groups with which health promoters are involved will already exist, where members have come together for a common purpose and health issues form part, or the whole, of the agenda. The role of the health promoter may vary widely, from leading a one-off session to facilitating the development of a new group, or leading a group with a defined lifespan. Whatever the role, competencies in group work are needed. Leading therapeutic groups are excluded from the discussions in this chapter. Therapy requires in-depth professional training in a range of possible approaches, outside the scope of this book, but see Hogg & Scott Tindale (2002) Buckroyd & Rother (2007) and Bertram (2008) for discussion on therapeutic groups.

TYPES OF GROUPS

Groups are formed for a variety of purposes and are not simply a random collection of individuals. Members generally have a sense of shared identity, common objectives, defined membership criteria and their own particular ways of working. The term *group work* can be applied to a range of activities such as group therapy, social action or self-help. Groups in the context of health promotion are usually formed for one or more of the following purposes.

For raising awareness. To increase members' interest in, and awareness of, health issues through group discussion. This may be a group already in existence, such as a women's group, which may agree to discuss a health issue.

For mutual support. To support members in difficult decision making, to help each other to cope with shared health problems/disabilities, or to change a health-damaging behaviour. Examples are self-help groups such as patients' associations and Alcoholics Anonymous.

For social action. To use collective power to campaign for social change, for example tackling a local problem of drug misuse, housing standards or community facilities.

For education. To impart skills, offer information and sometimes to prepare members for specific life events, for example becoming a parent.

For group counselling. To help members to find solutions through exploring a shared problem with a counsellor, for example a group of menopausal women.

Being clear about the purpose of a group is important. Confusion can result if the tasks of a group are changed, especially if this means that individual members have to adopt different roles. For example, an individual will have difficulty if she attends a group to obtain support, and finds the task has changed to campaigning. A new group is required for the new task.

The type of task will determine the most effective size for the group; for example, educational groups may be larger than support groups.

Different kinds of groups may also require the health promoter to take on different roles, and use different skills. Leading or facilitating groups requires special skills and methods; later in this chapter group leadership and the skills you need to be effective as a group leader are discussed.

POTENTIAL BENEFITS OF GROUP WORK

It is important that a group leader or facilitator considers the benefits for the individual client of using a group as a medium for support (Stock Whitaker 2001). The *process* of being part of a group is often as important as the intended outcome of the group; for example, a young parent may gain friends and social skills by being part of a parenting group as well as learning parenting skills.

In addition to thinking of potential benefits for the group as a whole, the group facilitator needs to think about which benefits are relevant to individual group members. Different group members may benefit in different ways. Exercise 13.1 is designed to help you think about what joining a group could mean to a client.

WHEN TO USE GROUP WORK

Health promoters may be unsure about when it is appropriate to use a group work approach to health promotion. Group work is appropriate when your plans fulfill the following criteria:

See also Chapter 5, section on deciding the best way of achieving your aims.

- You have looked critically at what other health promotion opportunities exist, and you have concluded that group work is needed to meet the particular needs of specific groups of people.
- You have evidence that group work is effective for this particular client group.
- You are going to be working with a defined group of people over a period of time, which will allow the group to build up trust and be able to help each other, for example a group of teenage mothers, a self-help group of patients

---

EXERCISE 13.1   How can joining a group promote health?

Think of a group that you have:
- set up in the past, or
- intend to establish in the future, or
- belonged to yourself.

Consider the list of potential benefits below. Which ones could apply to members of your group?

Trying out new behaviours that are better for the group members or other people they have contact with.

Gaining new health knowledge, becoming better informed.

Learning new ways of doing things and acquiring new skills for health.

Finding better ways of coping with everyday life.

Feeling less isolated, reducing the sense of being alone with an illness or problem or that nobody else understands.

Developing more confidence, with group members having a more positive view of themselves.

Group members recognising that they can make changes, they can see new possibilities.

Revising previously held assumptions group members had about themselves and/or others; they think differently about themselves and others.

Developing an understanding, or a fuller and more accurate understanding, of how past experiences have, until now, influenced group members.

Feeling able to work with other people to take action about a health issue group members feel strongly about.

Can you think of any other benefits?

(This exercise is adjusted from Stock Whitaker 2001.)

---

who are recovering after heart attacks, or people who have been diagnosed as HIV positive.
- You have access to a comfortable, private and relaxed environment in which to run the group, for example a community centre.
- You have access to support and supervision in order to provide you with assistance when you need it and help you to develop your group work.

In some circumstances group work may be particularly helpful. Examples are:

- You are planning to work with people who are already in a close small group, and possibly already used to group work, for example a group of young people who are in a residential drug rehabilitation setting.
- You are establishing a connection with a number of people who have a common interest, and wish to develop an equal and respectful partnership with them, for example a group of people with mental health problems who have recently moved into a group home.
- You want to work with a particular ethnic minority community but you do not come from that group yourself and are faced with issues of differences in culture and language. In this case, it could be helpful to run a group to look at health issues in partnership with a link worker or health advocate who can offer culturally sensitive help and skills in translation and interpretation.

There are times when it may not be advisable to embark on group work, or to continue to run an existing group. These may include situations when:

- You have not consulted with prospective clients to establish their needs.
- Group members are from such a diverse range of backgrounds that they have little in common and feel uncomfortable with one another.
- The cultural or psychosocial background of the group will make it difficult for them to adapt to group work.
- The group will meet only once or twice, which means that people will not have long enough to get to know and trust one another.
- The membership of a group is not stable and people are constantly leaving or joining.
- Your aim is solely to transmit information, so that a talk with questions and answers would be better.
- The aim of the group is to encourage a change towards a healthier lifestyle but the people concerned do not have the opportunity to make changes because of lack of money, skills, support or facilities.
- You do not have suitable accommodation for meetings; for example, you only have available a large, tiered lecture theatre.
- You do not yet have the competencies to facilitate group work, or access to the necessary training and support.

GROUP LEADERSHIP

Two aspects of group leadership are useful to consider. One is your leadership style and the other is your responsibilities as a group leader.

LEADERSHIP STYLE

It is important that all the members of the group are agreed on who is the leader, and support the leader in this role. The leadership style needs to be compatible with the group members, especially if the group has to work together to complete complex tasks. For example, a group of highly motivated and trained professionals will work best with a leader who encourages participation and shared decision making. It is essential for leaders to be aware of which style members prefer, and to develop the ability to adjust their style if the situation demands it.

A key dimension of leadership style is where the leader stands on a continuum from authoritarian to participative.

authoritarian _____ *participative*

An **authoritarian** style is directive, with the group leader acting as a source of expertise. If you adopt this approach, you rely on your status, credibility and expertise to ensure acceptance of your views and leadership role.

The *strength* of this style is that children and vulnerable people (such as those who are sick or distressed) may feel secure, reassured and protected from harm.

The *weaknesses* of this style are that clients may become fearful, anxious and reluctant to take independent action; it does not develop their ability to take responsibility for their own decisions and actions. Furthermore, clients may respond by rebelling and rejecting your guidance.

A **participative** style involves shifting power from the group leader so that it is shared between the leader and the group members. This means using all the skills and knowledge of the group members as well as the leader, who is more likely to choose the title of facilitator. As a facilitator, you will need to show warmth and empathy, encourage group members to express their feelings and provide counsel and encouragement. You will need to be tolerant of different viewpoints, showing fairness and impartiality. You will need skills and

ability to confront difficult issues and resolve conflict using a problem-solving approach.

See Chapter 9, section on understanding conflict and Exercise 9.3 on identifying your conflict resolution style.

The *strength* of this style is that clients learn to trust their own judgements and at the same time to appreciate other people's rights and opinions.

The *weaknesses* of this style may be that strong feelings are uncovered and distress experienced by the client and yourself, which might be difficult to manage. Also, clients who are used to being told what to do may feel confused and dissatisfied because they are not receiving advice and direction. They will need to have the approach explained to them and be given suitable learning experiences to show them that it works.

Group leaders can operate somewhere between the two extremes, providing some authoritative leadership while also encouraging a degree of participation. Successful group leadership depends on a variety of factors such as:

- The leader's preferred style of operating and personality. For example, if you have been used to being perceived as the expert, with the authority of professional knowledge that you want to pass on, you will probably feel (and look) uncomfortable if you try to switch to a facilitator style without sufficient training, and this may produce tension in the group.
- The group members' preferred style of leadership in the specific circumstances of the group. For example, if group members are low in confidence, they may need you to be more authoritarian to start with, so that they feel secure. You can then gradually encourage participation and adopt a more facilitative style as members learn to trust you and each other, and feel confident enough to join in.
- The group's objectives and tasks. For example, a group that has the objective of learning new skills (such as an exercise class) will need a more authoritarian leader who will tell them how to do the exercises properly, whereas a group of parents in a support group that aims to help them recover from the death of a child will need a facilitator to help members to express and work through their grief.
- The wider environment, such as the culture of the group members, and of the organisations they belong to. For example, the cultural norm

of some ethnic minorities may be passive, and they may not only lack confidence about active participation in groups but may also perceive it as inappropriate.

You need to consider these factors and how they might be modified in order that the group achieves its purpose. The easiest thing to modify in the short term should be your own style, but in the long term it may also be possible to make other changes, for example to develop the group members' confidence so that they are willing to take on more responsibility and participation.

See Chapter 3, section on analysing your aims and values: five approaches.

The participative style fits best with the self-empowering client-centred approach to health promotion. However, some health promoters will have been trained in an authoritarian style and will have modelled themselves on this experience. If this is true in your case, you will need to learn how to work in a participative style in order to become more effective in empowering your clients.

Finally, a participative style must be distinguished from a permissive style. A permissive style lets clients come to their own conclusions and aims to avoid conflict and keep everyone happy. Helping the clients to enjoy the experience is more important to the leader than achieving the goals of the group. Difficulties and conflict are not confronted and the clients may feel neither nurtured nor secure. Group leaders may need to build up their own assertiveness skills in order to avoid an overly permissive approach. Undertake Exercise 13.2 to determine your leadership style.

LEADERSHIP RESPONSIBILITIES

The responsibilities of group leaders will depend on the role they take; for example, whether they are responsible for the practical organisation such as booking a venue. But whatever the role, a leader's responsibilities may include:

- Helping members to identify and clarify their interests and needs, and what they would like to gain from the group in the short and long term.
- Helping to develop a relaxed atmosphere in which members feel able to be open and trusting with each other, and able to participate freely.
- Offering expertise to the group on the understanding that members are free to accept or reject the offer.
- Accepting and valuing all contributions from group members.

But it is not only the group leader who has responsibilities: group members have them too. They may include:

EXERCISE 13.2   Looking at your leadership style

The following questions aim to help you to examine your own leadership style. Put a tick in the appropriate box.

	Never	Sometimes	Usually	Always
1. Do your clients say what they feel?	☐	☐	☐	☐
2. Do clients finish what they are saying before you respond?	☐	☐	☐	☐
3. Do you think you are able to see things from your clients' point of view?	☐	☐	☐	☐
4. Do clients disagree with you?	☐	☐	☐	☐
5. Do you explore with your clients the consequences of alternative actions?	☐	☐	☐	☐
6. Do you help clients to discuss painful memories or sensitive issues?	☐	☐	☐	☐
7. Do you share all the information at your disposal?	☐	☐	☐	☐
8. Do you help clients to discover their own strengths?	☐	☐	☐	☐
9. Do you respect your clients' right to reject your advice?	☐	☐	☐	☐

What leadership style – authoritarian, participative or permissive – do you think you usually use?
What influences led you to develop this style?
Can you identify any advantages in using alternative leadership styles in your work?
Can you identify any aspects of your leadership style that you would like to change?

- Participating in clarifying the aims of the group.
- Choosing whether and how much to participate.
- Identifying personal goals and concerns.
- Deciding which challenges and risks they are prepared to take. For example, how much are they prepared to expose their own weaknesses and vulnerability to other people in the group?

GROUP BEHAVIOUR

Health promoters will be able to work with a group more effectively if they are aware of the group dynamics and the ways in which people are likely to behave when they come together in groups. There are three aspects of group behaviour that you may find particularly useful: the pattern of behaviour that usually develops in a group's life, the different roles group members may perform and the concept of hidden agendas.

GROUP DEVELOPMENT

Groups tend to show a particular pattern of behaviour as they mature and develop. An early and much quoted study characterised a group developmental process in to four stages (Tuckman 1965):

1. Forming. The group is forming. People meet each other, and get to know one another, with individuals establishing their own identity and role within the group. The group's purpose and way of working are established.

2. Storming. Most groups go through a conflict stage when the leadership and ways in which the group is working are challenged. For example, people may question how things are being done and what the leader's role is, and may get into heated discussions with each other. This can be a difficult period for both leader and members, but it is a vital stage in the group's maturing process, rather like the period of rebelling and questioning during adolescence. Successful handling of this period leads to the development of open communication, trust and shared responsibility for achieving the purposes of the group.

See Chapter 9, section on understanding conflict.

3. Norming. At this stage the group settles down, with the norms and accepted practices of the group established.

1. Performing. The group is fully effective at this stage and is able to concentrate on its tasks.

When the developmental process fails in some way, attempts to sabotage the group may occur. It is thus worth investing time and effort to help new groups to develop successfully.

Many groups have a limited life, meeting for a set number of sessions or until a particular task has been completed. At the end of a group's life, it may be helpful to have a final session, which could give group members an opportunity to express their appreciation and perhaps arrange a follow-up or reunion.

GROUP MEMBERS' ROLES

An early study established the characteristics of members of teams identifying that a mix of nine roles is needed for full effectiveness (Belbin 1981) These roles are also relevant to a group's effectiveness and are outlined in Box 13.1.

At different times, each group member may play a variety of these roles, and most people have personal characteristics which might result in more affinity with a particular role. If one or more of these roles is lacking, a member or leader can help

---

BOX 13.1   Roles needed for effective groups and teams

The Coordinator – clarifies goals, promotes decision making, delegates well to enable the group to work effectively.

The Shaper – is action oriented and encourages the group to get on with its tasks.

The Plant – is the creative source of ideas and proposals.

The Monitor/Evaluator – is good at analysing and criticising.

The Resource Investigator – has a good network of contacts and liaises with other people and agencies.

The Company Worker – is good at organising and administration.

The Team Worker – supports the members of the group and is a good listener.

The Specialist – provides specialist knowledge and skills.

The Finisher – contributes foresight and perseverance to ensure that the group completes its tasks.

to make a group more successful by consciously adopting a new role, or encouraging other team members to adjust their roles.

HIDDEN AGENDAS

People will have their own individual reasons for joining a group, which may be in addition to, or instead of, the reason expected. For example, a woman may attend a women's health group because she is lonely and sees the group as a way of meeting people; she has not joined because she is particularly interested in health issues. Or a group member may seek a prominent position in a group, such as being the Chair or Secretary, to fulfill their need to feel valued and useful; they may or may not also be committed to the work itself and the aims of the group. In these examples, fulfilling these personal objectives are hidden agendas.

Most people bring their own hidden agendas to groups, in addition to the agreed group objectives; these commonly include meeting the need for social contact, or making a particular alliance. Members will work together best when there is communication about individual objectives or agendas and agreement about shared objectives. Otherwise members may promote their own interests at the expense of the group. You will be more effective as a group leader if you are aware of the hidden agendas in the group and can find ways of dealing with them.

SETTING UP A GROUP

Planning and preparation are essential for successful group work. The sections below take you step by step through the thinking and planning you need to do when setting up a group.

Why are you proposing to run the group?

- Are you reacting to a demand from clients, other professionals, a community or your own observations?
- Are you trying to develop your health promotion role and see this group as a way of progressing?
- Are you aiming to provide advice and support, to supply information or to help people to change health-related behaviour?

- Are you aiming to satisfy your own needs or your clients' needs? (Your reasons can include both, but it is helpful to distinguish between them.)

Who will the members be?

- Will the members be referred (from their GP, for example), will they be coerced into joining or will membership be entirely voluntary?
- Have you given everyone an equal opportunity to join (such as ensuring facilities for wheelchairs, disabled toilets, signing for those hard of hearing, hearing loops, translation into appropriate minority languages)? Have you made provision for people to let you know of any special needs?
- How will you identify the potential members of your group – from individuals requesting a group, from local or national registers, from people with shared characteristics (such as age, sex, lifestyle, culture, job, health concern), or by other means?
- How will you recruit your members? Do you need to advertise?
- How many members do you aim to have? What is the ideal number, bearing in mind the purpose of the group and any constraints imposed by your location?

What are the group's aims and objectives?

- Are these within the realistic abilities of yourself and the members?
- Can all the potential membership understand them?
- Are you clear about your own objectives in setting up the group, and whether these are different from the members' objectives?
- Are all members clear about their individual objectives, i.e. the specific outcomes they hope to achieve through attending the group?

Where will the group meet?

- Is the location appropriate? For example, a health centre or hospital could appear clinical and cold and remind people of illness. Neutral territory, such as a room in a community centre, or someone's house, may be more relaxing and inviting.

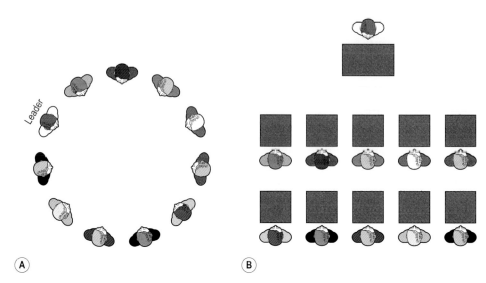

Fig. 13.1 (A) Seating in a circle – best for group work; **(B)** traditional seating in rows – not suitable for group work.

- What is the seating like? If you are aiming for participative group work, seating people in a circle is best (see Fig. 13.1), with physical barriers to communication such as tables or desks removed. Can you put chairs in a circle, where all group members can see each other?
- What are the facilities like? Is there enough space for the activities you plan? Is the floor covering suitable for the purpose? Is the temperature suitable and adjustable if necessary? Are the facilities adequate for the purpose (for example, access for pushchairs, toilets, catering facilities, washing/shower rooms, crèche)? Are there facilities for people with special needs (for example, wide access for wheelchairs, disabled toilets, hearing loops, signs in minority languages)?
- Is access good? Is the venue accessible by local transport? Do you have transport for members who cannot manage on public transport? Are parking arrangements satisfactory?
- What are the security arrangements? Where the fire extinguishers and what is the fire drill? In case of an emergency, who do you contact? Do you need insurance cover?

What resources do you need?

- Do you need any special equipment, for example audiovisual equipment? Are you

familiar with the equipment and confident you can operate it? Does the equipment have to be booked in advance? If so, are you familiar with the booking system?
- Do you need any additional resources such as DVDs, leaflets, posters, books, outside speakers? If so, have you made all the necessary arrangements in advance?
- Do you need to pay for anything? If so, have you identified a source of funding (for example, a charge to the group members or a sponsor)?

When will the group meet?

- Is the time you have chosen the best one for the clients, or have you chosen it to suit yourself?
- Does the length of meetings suit members and take into account their other commitments?
- Have you consulted potential members about timing and tried to satisfy the majority?

How will the group be run?

- Will it be a self-help group and directed by the members, or led by a health professional?
- To what extent will the structure be flexible and the content negotiable?
- Will the group be open (anyone can join at any time) or will there be restrictions on admitting new members once the group has started?

How will the group be evaluated?

- At the end of each meeting? At the end of the group? Or both?

  See also Chapter 12, section on evaluation, feedback and assessment.

- Verbally, or in writing, or both? How will you ask questions in order to obtain accurate feedback from members (for example, by providing opportunities for anonymous feedback)?
- How will you know that the group, individual and your own objectives have been achieved?
- Were there any unplanned outcomes of the group? Were these desirable or undesirable? What caused them?
- What have you learned? What would you do differently next time?

(See Doel 2006 for more details in setting up a group and group work in general.)

GETTING GROUPS GOING

Some people may feel nervous about going to a group meeting for the first time, especially if they are unlikely to know other members. The initial task for the group leader is to help people to feel at ease.

  See also Chapter 5 on the basic planning and evaluation process.

BEFORE THE FIRST MEETING

If you know in advance who is coming to a group meeting, it may be helpful and welcoming to confirm by letter or telephone that you are expecting them, and the time and place. If anyone has let you know they have special needs, contact them in advance to discuss their needs and let them know what facilities will be available.

ON ARRIVAL

It helps if clients can be greeted personally, introduced to other people or given something to do: 'There are some books and leaflets on the table if you'd like to look at them until everyone has arrived'. Ensure that anyone with special needs has appropriate facilities and assistance.

GETTING TO KNOW EACH OTHER

Knowing each person's name and something about them is the first step towards constructive group work because it helps them to feel valued as a member of the group, and is the beginning of openness and trust between members.

There are many ways of going about this, some of which are as follows.

Introduction in pairs

Ask each person to sit next to someone they have not met before. One person in each pair then interviews their partner. After a few minutes (the leader keeps the time) the partners swap roles. Then, in turn, each member of the group introduces their partner by name and says something about them. You may like to remind people that no one has to answer any questions if they do not wish to.

The leader could also suggest appropriate questions. For example, in groups for prospective parents the leader could suggest that partners find out if this is the first baby, where the mother goes for antenatal check-ups or where she is booked to have her baby.

Name games

Group members sit in a circle and you, the leader, take an object, such as a pen, and hand it to the person on your left, saying 'My name is A and this is a pen'. You ask the person who now holds the pen to say 'My name is B and A says that this is a pen'. B then passes the pen to the person on his left, who says 'My name is C and B says that A says that this is a pen'. This continues until the pen gets back to the beginning. If group members forget someone's name the rest of the group can prompt them. This helps to establish a cooperative and supportive atmosphere as well as helping people to learn each other's names. Any tension and embarrassment is relieved by laughing and tension is effectively broken.

At subsequent group meetings, it is often helpful to do a quick round of names at the beginning, for example 'Who would like to have a shot at naming every member of the group?' or 'I'm going to try to see if I can remember everyone's name'.

You might like to set the tone by suggesting how people are addressed, by first names or more formally. The important thing is to encourage people to use whatever feels comfortable: 'My name is Ann Jones, and I'm happy for you to call me Ann'.

Sharing initial feelings and expectations

People may be helped to relax if they know that others also feel nervous or shy. So ask 'What did you feel about coming here today? Did anyone feel nervous? Did anyone almost *not* come?' This can open the way for people to express their anxieties. You can also encourage them to say why they have come to the meeting and what they expect to gain from it. It might help to ask members to complete a checklist, ticking statements that are true for them. Such statements could include:

- I'm worried I won't have anything to say.
- I'm afraid I'll talk too much.
- I'm worried I'll make a fool of myself.
- I'll be too embarrassed to join in.
- I'm afraid I might get upset.
- I'm concerned I may be bored.
- I want to meet other people in the same situation.
- I enjoy talking to others.
- I enjoy a good debate.
- I want to get out of the house.
- I want to go somewhere different.
- I enjoy listening to other people.

People can then compare their list with that of one or two other people, and then it may be helpful to share what has been discovered with the whole group.

SETTING GROUND RULES

People joining a group will have different expectations and assumptions about how the group will run. Problems can arise if these are not brought out in the open and clarified at the beginning. For example, people may assume that what they say in a group will be treated confidentially, and then be upset if they find that another member did not realise this and had discussed the issue elsewhere; or some members might expect the group leader to take all the responsibility for organising the group, and may feel let down if they later discover that the leader expects them to do some of the work.

To prevent these difficulties, it is often helpful to establish a set of ground rules. Early on in the group's life, members need the opportunity to explore their expectations, and reach agreement about issues such as the following:

- How members are expected to behave in the group.
- Are any rules and sanctions to be set, for example about nonattendance at group meetings or whether members can join in if they arrive late?
- What is confidential to the group?
- Can new members join at any time, or is the group closed to new membership?
- How will the leader and the members exercise control in the group?
- Who has responsibility for the practical aspects of running the group, such as bringing refreshments along or booking the room?

For example, in a self-help group, mutual rights and responsibilities will be agreed on the basis of equality of leader and clients, but in reality the power balance will not be completely equal and a contract will help with power sharing. In a counselling group the power of the counsellor is much greater than that of the clients and the leader has a duty to respect the members and to promote their autonomy.

DISCUSSION SKILLS

A discussion may not happen just by putting a group of people together and saying 'Let's discuss …'. Discussion needs planning and preparation, and there are many ways of triggering it off and providing structures that will help everyone to participate.

TRIGGER MATERIALS

Discussion can be triggered by providing a focus, preferably a controversial one. This can simply be a question 'What do you think about the call to ban child-in-car smoking?', but it might also be a leaflet, a poster, a health promotion campaign film or an item in a newspaper or magazine ('What do you think the makers of this alcoholic drink are trying to convey in this advertisement?'). Choose something that people are likely to have strong views about.

Some health promotion campaign films are specially made as trigger materials, presenting situations for people to talk about. Helpful notes for group leaders often accompany such campaign films.

BRAINSTORMS/THINK SESSIONS

Brainstorming is a useful way to open up a subject and collect everyone's ideas. Ask an open question to which there is no single right answer, such as 'Why do some young people binge drink?' or 'What do you feel you need to know before your baby is born?' Accept every suggestion, without comment or criticism, and write them down in a list on a flip-chart or blackboard. Ask the group not to start discussing the ideas until everybody has finished. You can make your own suggestions and write them down along with others.

In this way all members' contributions are equally valued and everyone has a chance to participate. Encourage shy members by asking 'Anything else?' and allowing silent pauses while people think.

Then you can set the group to work by asking them to put the ideas into categories, and to identify the key features of each category. For example, people might categorise reasons for binge drinking into a *constructive* category: 'It helps me to socialise' or 'It helps me to relax, to feel good', and an *escape* category: 'I can forget my problems' or 'It stops me from feeling upset'.

ROUNDS

A round is a way of giving everyone an equal chance to participate. You invite each group member in turn round the circle to make a brief statement. You might like to start the round yourself or to join in when your turn comes in the circle. For example, ask everyone to make a brief statement about one of the following:

'My first feelings when I knew I was pregnant were …'
'What I think about jogging is …'
'The main reason why I can't lose weight is …'
'The thing that has helped me most in my efforts to give up smoking is …'

There are four essential rules for successful rounds, which must be explained and gently enforced if necessary. These are:

- No interruptions until each person has finished his statement.

- No comments on anybody's contribution until the full round is completed (no discussions, interpretation, not even 'I think that too' remarks).
- Anyone can choose not to participate. Give permission, clearly and emphatically, that anyone who does not want to make a statement can just say pass. This is very important for reinforcing the principle of voluntary participation.
- It does not matter if two or more people in the round say the same thing. People should stick to saying what they had intended even if someone else has said it already; they do not have to think of something different.

Rounds are also useful ways of beginning and ending sessions. For example:

'One thing I've put into practice since last week is …'
'The main thing I've got from today's session is …'
'One thing I'm going to find out by next time we meet is …'

It is also a useful way of getting feedback. For example:

'One thing I really liked about today's session was …'
'One thing I didn't like about today's session was …'
'One thing I wish we'd done is …'

BUZZ GROUPS

Buzz groups are small groups of two to six people who discuss questions or topics for short periods, usually about 10 minutes. It is especially useful for large groups to be divided up in this way, as it gives everyone more chance to talk. Form the groups first of all, then say what you would like each one to do, such as 'Make a list of the times when you want a cigarette' or 'Talk about the things you find helpful when you feel stressed', and how long they have in which to do it. If you want people to share ideas with the rest of the group as a whole afterwards, it may be helpful to provide large sheets of paper and felt-tip pens, so that feedback posters can be put up for everyone to see and discuss.

SAFE REVELATIONS

Sometimes people may hesitate or refuse to say what they really feel for fear of looking silly, being embarrassed or getting upset. One way of overcoming this is to give everyone a piece of paper and ask them to write down, for example, what their biggest worries are, or what they really want to know. All the papers are then folded and put in a receptacle, such as a waste-paper basket or a shopping bag. Each person in turn picks out one piece of paper and reads aloud what is written on it. Tell people not to say if they happen to pick out their own piece of paper, and that, of course, nobody needs to identify themselves as the author of any of the statements.

The aim is to find out the concerns of the group members in the security of anonymity. Make sure that everyone listens and does not comment until all the papers have been read out. Then you can discuss what was discovered.

DEALING WITH DIFFICULTIES

Acknowledge the potential difficulties of running a group and work out strategies for coping should the problem actually arise. Some common problems and possible strategies for coping are as follows.

SILENCE

Silence can be useful; it can be time that group members need to think. Silence often does not feel as threatening to group members as it may do to the facilitator; however, you may find it helpful to:

- Run a group with a partner, so that you can help each other out if either of you gets stuck.
- Ensure thorough preparation, so that you have planned activities and questions. Write down a plan and a list of questions to ask (such as at the end of showing a DVD).
- Have an additional activity ready to use if the reason for the discussion closing down is that what you have planned does not seem to be working.

DISASTERS

Unexpected disasters include such things as arriving late, or finding that too few or too many people have turned up. There is no blueprint strategy to cope with the unexpected, but it will help if you acknowledge what has happened and share it with your group: 'I'm delighted that so many of you have come along, but I wasn't expecting such numbers, so we may be a bit crowded this week'. Also share your plans for dealing with the disaster ('I'm going to try to get a bigger room next time' ... 'I'm going to start 10 minutes late'). Sharing the problem and enlisting cooperation can have the positive benefit of encouraging mutual support; *not* sharing it can leave your group feeling angry.

DISTRACTIONS

Distractions can take many forms: noises outside the room (such as road works), noises inside the room (such as crying babies, coughing), people coming in late or leaving early, or interruptions. Distractions can also be caused by group members themselves, for example by someone becoming very angry or upset.

As a rule, there are three choices for you as group leader:

- **Ignore them.** This is seldom a good idea, as it leaves people wondering whether you are going to do anything, and this in itself is a distraction.
- **Acknowledge and accept them.** This is generally best with things you cannot change 'I know the traffic is really noisy, but there's nothing we can do about it, so I think we'll just have to put up with it this time and I will find a different room/venue for future meetings'.
- **Do something about them.** It is preferable to involve the group in the decision: 'As so many of you found it difficult to get here by 2 o'clock, shall we start at 2.15 next week?' or 'Do you think it would be helpful if you took it in turns to look after the babies in the next room?'

If someone is showing emotion, such as crying, acknowledge it: 'I can see that you're upset', and offer reassurance that it is OK to show emotion: 'There's no need to be embarrassed ... we don't mind if you cry ...', and offer the opportunity to talk about it: 'Would you like to tell us what is upsetting you?' or to take some time away from the group, accompanied by you or someone else: 'Shall we go outside for a few minutes?' Do not put any pressure on people in distress. Help them to do what they want to do, whether it is cry, talk, keep silent, stay, leave or be by themselves. But *do not* ignore a show of emotion; ignoring it will only cause tension and embarrassment.

DIFFICULT BEHAVIOUR

How group members behave can pose difficulties for the leader. There are two broad categories of difficult behaviour: nonparticipation and talking too much. The latter category takes many forms: the person who dominates and always responds with the answers and prevents other people contributing, people who launch into long stories, people who interrupt, people who talk off the point, people who always disagree and people who always crack jokes. Note that people often change their behaviour as they get to know others and feel more comfortable in a group, but here are some points about dealing with people who talk too much, and about encouraging quiet members to engage.

- Think about why dominant people are behaving like this. Are they nervous, threatened or worried? Are they desperately in need of attention? If you can deal with the underlying cause, the situation is likely to improve.
- Get people to work in pairs or small groups, which can help quiet members to join in and give others a break from the constant talker.
- Use structures in your discussion such as rounds, or make a point of asking for other people's opinions: 'Would someone else like to say what he thinks?' or 'Would you like to give us your opinion, Ann?'

- Finally, it may be necessary to confront a person who talks too much, but not in front of the rest of the group. For example, you could say: 'I've noticed that you contribute a great deal to the group discussions. That makes me concerned about whether other people are getting enough chance to talk. I'd like to suggest that you keep your comments to just a couple of sentences. Would you feel OK about doing that?'

Exercise 13.3 offers you the opportunity to apply all the points above when planning a group meeting. Case study 13.1 is an example of good practice in the use of group work.

PRACTICE POINTS

- In health promotion, groups are useful for raising awareness of health issues, mutual support, social action, education and group counselling.
- Group work covers a wide range of activities and has a number of potential benefits for individual group members.
- Group work is not always the most appropriate health promotion method to use; you need to be sure that it is right for your particular clients and circumstances.
- You need to develop skills of group leadership, appreciate the range of leadership styles and understand the roles and responsibilities of both

---

EXERCISE 13.3   Planning a group meeting

1. Identify a health promotion opportunity that you have encountered or are likely to encounter, where informal group work would be appropriate

For example, this could be a group of food handlers, a pre-retirement group, an antenatal group, a group of patients in hospital recovering from a heart attack, a stop-smoking group or a group for healthy eating and weight control.

   Assume that your group consists of about 12 people who do not know each other, and that this is the first of several meetings.

What do you think would be the best place and time to meet, and the best physical features of the meeting room?

What are your aims for the first meeting?

What are your objectives for your group members for the first meeting?

Complete the following:

At the end of the first meeting, each group member will:

1...............
2...............
3...............
etc. ....

2. Make a plan for what you will do

- As people start to arrive.
- To get people to become acquainted with each other.
- In the main part of the group meeting.
- To round off the meeting at the end.
- To evaluate whether you have achieved the objectives you set.

CASE STUDY 13.1 GOOD PRACTICE IN GROUP WORK

The Family Links Nurturing Programme is a support programme which works with parents and has been developed in all the schools in South Southall, London. It complements the existing parental support provided by schools and helps to build capacity for further outreach work with families. The programme consists of 10 weekly group work support sessions at the schools which focus on parents sharing techniques with one another in order to build better relationships with their children and improve their confidence in parenting. The group work programme is based around four main ideas: building self awareness and self esteem, developing appropriate expectations, empathy and positive discipline. The support groups are designed to promote emotional health in adults and children, enable families to improve their relationships and empower parents to fulfill their potential in all aspects of their lives.

The programme benefits both adults and children by:
- promoting emotional literacy and emotional health
- raising self-esteem

- developing communication and social skills
- teaching positive ways to resolve conflict
- providing effective strategies to encourage cooperative, responsible behaviour and managing challenging behaviour in children
- offering insights into the influence of feelings on behaviour
- encouraging adults to take time to look after themselves.

The nurturing group supports positive behaviour in children and explores the emotional needs behind their behaviour. Overall, the programme is founded in the knowledge that empathic relationships in childhood have an important effect on the developing brain, on the way we learn to manage emotions and sensitively relate to others. These are both key factors in the way we behave and an important contributor to lifelong health and wellbeing.

(Case study produced by Natalie Shepping, South Southall Extended Schools Coordinator, London.)

leaders and members and the way in which groups develop over time.
- Thorough planning and preparation are essential for successful group work, which includes having a clear rationale and aims, and paying attention to recruitment, venue, facilities, resources, timing and evaluation.

- If you facilitate groups, you will find it helpful to develop a range of skills and strategies for getting groups going, encouraging discussion, and dealing with difficulties.

References

Belbin RM 1981 Management teams: why they succeed or fail. Oxford, Butterworth-Heinemann.

Bertram L 2008 Supporting postnatal women into motherhood: a guide to therapeutic groupwork for health professionals. Oxford, Radcliffe.

Buckroyd J, Rother S 2007 Therapeutic groups for obese women: a group leader's handbook. Chichester, Wiley Blackwell.

Doel M 2006 Using groupwork. Oxford, Routledge.

Hogg MA, Scott Tindale R (eds) 2002 Blackwell handbook of social psychology: group process. Oxford, Blackwell: Chapter 26.

Stock Whitaker D 2001 Using groups to help people, 2nd edn. Hove, Brunner-Routledge.

Tuckman BW 1965 Developmental sequence in small groups. Psychological Bulletin 63: 384–399.

Chapter 14

Enabling healthier living

CHAPTER CONTENTS

SUMMARY

This chapter considers the approaches used to support people in making changes to their health-related behaviour. In the first section there is an overview of two behaviour change models. This is followed by a section on working with a client's motivation and how to work towards client self-empowerment, strategies for increasing self-awareness, clarifying values and changing attitudes. Strategies for decision making and for changing behaviour follow. The chapter ends with principles for using behaviour change approaches effectively and summarises key points. It includes exercises, examples and a case study.

This chapter focuses on the competencies you need when you are enabling people to make changes to their health-related behaviour and lifestyles. Health behaviour may have developed without conscious decision making and in response to individual and group circumstances and external events. Active control of behaviour is different because it involves committing time and effort (yours and your client's) to understanding the factors that influence health choices and behaviour, and to taking considered decisions and actions.

However, it has to be accepted that people may prefer to carry on with behaviour that seems unhealthy to you. To a client, it may not seem unhealthy as the benefits outweigh the risks. Respect for people's values, opinions and their right to choose are fundamental to establishing relationships between health promoters and their clients.

See Chapter 10, section on exploring relationships with clients.

On the other hand, you also have to consider that a person's right to individual freedom of choice has to be balanced against the effect of that choice on other people; for example, a parent choosing to smoke could affect their children's health by subjecting them to passive, secondary smoking.

Furthermore, choosing a healthy behaviour does not automatically lead to practising it. Changes such as taking more exercise, practising relaxation, wearing ear protectors in noisy surroundings, eating healthier foods and stopping smoking can require self-discipline and overcoming barriers which make these changes stressful. Social or economic circumstances can be a significant obstacle to people carrying out new health behaviours, even if they would like to (Parliamentary Office of Science and Technology 2007).

However, despite these limitations, it can be very rewarding to enable people to look at their motivations, beliefs, values and attitudes, and to make and carry out decisions that will lead to improved health and wellbeing (Box 14.1).

MODELS OF BEHAVIOUR CHANGE

Health-related behaviour change is a very complex process involving a web of psychological, social and environmental factors. Using behaviour change models will help you to clarify your thinking and make your practice more effective. Models are simplified ways of describing reality and provide frameworks and routes to help you know where to start and what to do. Two models that can be used by health promoters are the Health Action Model and the Stages of Change Model.

THE HEALTH ACTION MODEL

The Health Action Model (HAM) was devised by Tones (1987, and Tones & Tilford 2001) and emphasises the important influence of self-esteem on behaviour. It assumes that someone with high self-esteem and a positive self-concept is likely to be more motivated towards ways of healthier living and that people with low self-esteem may feel that they have limited control over their behaviour and that they are victims of bad luck or fate. Many health promoters, particularly those working in the field of drugs, have used this model, through

---

> **BOX 14.1   Counselling about a health choice**
>
> A health visitor has the task of helping parents to decide what to do about having their baby vaccinated. The stages could be:
>
> **Stages 1 and 2. Identify and explore the need**
>
> For example, are the parents worried about having the child vaccinated at all, or is it just the whooping cough vaccination which is worrying? Is it *when* to have the child vaccinated, or *if?*
>
> **Stage 3. Help the client to set goals and establish options**
>
> For example, the parents may identify the goal of the child having the best possible chance of staying healthy.
>   The options might be: no vaccinations at all, some vaccinations or all the vaccinations.
>
> **Stage 4. Help the client to decide which option to choose**
>
> - Weigh up the pros and cons. The health visitor provides unbiased information on the risks from catching each disease compared with the risks of having the vaccinations.
> - Consider the likely consequences of pursuing each alternative: for the child in terms of health risk, for the parents, in terms of anxiety, guilt and responsibility, for other people in terms of spreading the diseases.
>
> **Stage 5. Help the client to develop an action plan**
>
> For example, the parents may decide to go ahead with the vaccination programme, but also to join a parents group, in order to get support from other parents facing the same anxieties and decisions. The health visitor suggests to the parents that they keep a record of the vaccinations for future reference, and provides them with a record card for their child. They set a date for the first vaccination.

---

concentrating on boosting people's self-esteem and their skills in resisting peer group pressure. According to this model, learning life skills such as how to be assertive may be essential before someone is ready to change their lifestyle.

The HAM identifies a variety of psychological, social and environmental influences which research and practice have shown to be important determinants of a number of health choices. The model offers an explanation about how these influences

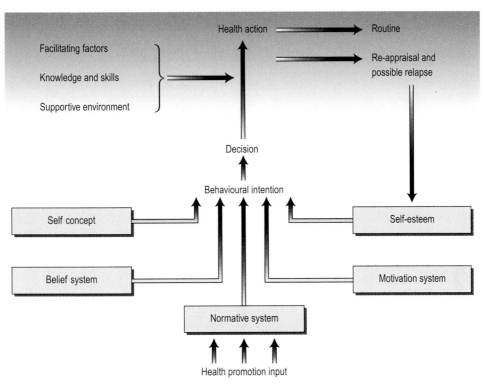

Fig. 14.1 The Health Action Model. *(Source: Tones 1995. Reproduced with permission from the Health Education Authority).*

work. It suggests that health decisions and actions are influenced by our beliefs, our values, our motivation, our expectations of how other people will react to our actions and our self-concept and self-esteem (see Fig. 14.1).

The HAM is concerned with empowerment, with increasing the control people have over their lives. It suggests that health promotion should not just focus on the provision of information and the pros and cons of particular behaviours. More important than this are interventions that enable people to value themselves, and to acquire the skills to assert themselves. Equally important is the provision of environmental circumstances that facilitate healthy choices, rather than acting as barriers. And at a broader level, national and local policy needs to address the broader determinants of health, such as poverty and deprivation.

TRANSTHEORETICAL MODEL (TTM) AND STAGES OF CHANGE

One way of supporting people in making health-related decisions and changing their behaviour is to

consider all the stages in the process, and how people move from one stage to another. The Trans-theoretical Model (TTM) developed by Prochaska & DiClemente (1982) is rooted in extensive research and integrates a range of psychological theories. The TTM has evolved over time and now contains five core constructs: stages of change, processes of change, decisional balance, self-efficacy and temptation (Prochaska & Velicer 1997) which provides a valuable conceptual framework for how people naturally change their behaviour. However, there is controversy and debate about whether this can consistently be translated into an intervention programme (see, for example, Aveyard et al 2009 and Prochaska 2009). Studies based on this model, such as Aveyard et al (2006) found no evidence that the smoking cessation intervention based on the model was more effective than a control intervention that was not tailored for stages of change. Armatage (2009) offers a useful critique of the model and an assessment of three studies that deemed to have successfully utilised the processes of change to reduce alcohol consumption, encourage smoking cessation and increase physical activity. It is important before using the approach to be abreast of the controversy and the systematic reviews on it's effectiveness. A useful summary with a full set of up-to-date references is presented on Wikepedia (http://en.wikipedia.org).

The stages of change component of the TTM identifies a number of stages that a person can go through during the process of behaviour change. It takes a holistic approach, integrating factors such as the role of personal responsibility and choices, and the impact of social and environmental forces that set very real limits on the individual potential for change. It provides a framework for a wide range of potential interventions by health promoters, as well as describing the process individuals go through when acting as their own agents of change; for example, when someone stops smoking without any professional support. The main stages identified in the model are set out in Fig. 14.2 (see also Prochaska 2005).

The key to the model is to regard the cycle in the centre as a series of stages that people go through

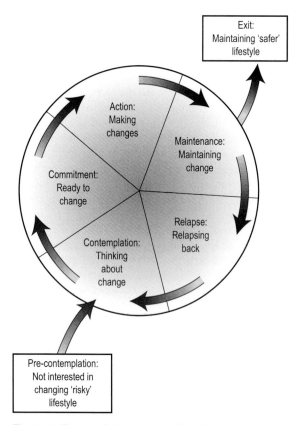

Fig. 14.2 Stages of changing health behaviour. *(Adapted from Prochaska & DiClemente (1984) and Neesham (1993)).*

in the process of changing health behaviour, such as stopping smoking, taking more exercise regularly or adopting healthier eating. A crucial point is that the cycle can be thought of as a revolving door, because people usually go round more than once before emerging to a permanently changed state. It is also important to recognise that some people may never get as far as entering the revolving door.

Pre-contemplation stage. The stage that precedes entry into the change cycle is referred to as pre-contemplation. At this stage a person has no awareness of a need for change, or does not accept it, and has no motivation to change habits or lifestyle.

Contemplation stage. This stage is the way into the revolving door cycle of stages of change. People enter this stage when they have enough motivation to contemplate seriously changing their habits; the entry stage is therefore called contemplation.

Commitment stage. If people continue to progress round the cycle, they enter the commitment stage, in which they make a serious decision to change the particular habit concerned, such as stopping smoking or taking more exercise.

Action stage. They next enter the action stage as they actively begin to change the habit.

Maintenance stage. At this stage people struggle to maintain the change and may experiment with a variety of coping strategies.

Relapse stage. Although individuals experience the satisfaction of a changed lifestyle for varying amounts of time, most of them cannot exit from the revolving door the first time around. Typically, they relapse; for example, they start smoking again. Of great importance, however, is that they do not stop there, but move back into the contemplation stage, engaging in the cycle all over again. Prochaska et al (1992) found that, on average, successful former smokers take three revolutions of change before they find the way to become fully free of the habit, and exit from the revolving door.

Exit stage. This is the stage in which people are settled into a changed behaviour, such as stopping smoking permanently.

By identifying where clients are in the stages of change, health promoters can tailor their interventions to the particular stage. For example, behaviour change strategies are appropriate for someone in the action or maintenance stages; education and awareness raising are appropriate for someone in the pre-contemplation stage; working for client self-empowerment is appropriate for someone in the contemplation stage; strategies to help people to make decisions are useful for those in the commitment stage.

The model can be useful in primary healthcare settings, because clients' needs can be assessed and appropriate advice or information given, within the constraints of a short consultation.

WORKING WITH A CLIENT'S MOTIVATION

Motivation is a state that changes frequently depending on lots of different factors. If people are struggling to maintain their new behaviour, what gets them through this difficult time without relapsing? It is thought that both the *importance* of the new behaviour (in terms of the expectation of costs and benefits) and the *confidence* of the person being able to maintain the new behaviour are essential to prevent relapse. The following suggestions can help you explore the importance of the new behaviour with clients, and to build their confidence.

Ideas for exploring importance

- What are the positive aspects of the current behaviour?
- What are the negative aspects of the current behaviour?
- Summarise and ask 'And is there anything else?'
- Where does that leave you now?

Ideas for building confidence

- Get the client to identify as many solutions as possible which will help to prevent relapse.
- Ask 'What have you learned from previous attempts to change about what works (or doesn't work) for you?'
- Ask 'Are there methods that you know have worked for other people?'
- Aim to help the client develop a clear plan but explain that it can be reviewed at any time.

It is essential to listen actively to the client when exploring readiness to change. Confidence can be divided into *self-efficacy* and *self-esteem*. Self-efficacy is concerned with a person's confidence in being able to make a specific change in behaviour; self-esteem is a more general sense of wellbeing that a person has about themselves. Self-efficacy can vary in different situations, and you can help your clients look at different approaches for improving self-efficacy in situations where they feel less confident.

This section is partly based on Rollnick et al (1999). See also Botelho (2004) and Rollnick et al (2007) for more on motivational practice.

DANGEROUS ASSUMPTIONS ABOUT MOTIVATION

Health promoters can become very focused on health issues, and may forget that there are other motives for change and that health might not be one of them. The list below illustrates some of the other assumptions that are easy to make when counselling clients.

- This person ought to change.
- This person wants to change.
- It is the right time for this person to change.
- If this person decides not to change, this intervention has failed.
- A tough approach is always best.
- For this person, health is a prime motivator.
- I'm the expert. This person must follow my advice.

WORKING FOR CLIENT SELF-EMPOWERMENT

Making health choices and carrying them out can bring benefits. These are not only the benefits that go with a healthier lifestyle, such as improved health and wellbeing, but also increased self-esteem from the feeling of taking active control over a part of life, such as being in control of the smoking habit rather than cigarettes being in control. In other words, making a positive choice about health can be a self-empowering process.

There are a number of different ways of working towards self-empowerment. Using the Stages of Change is empowering, because people can follow their own progress. It may encourage them to try to get to the next stage of the cycle, and not to see change as all-or-nothing. Also, the recognition that relapse can be part of the process of changing behaviour is important (see Marlatt & Donovan 2007). Behaviour change messages can be tailored to individual need, for example through providing clients with access to specially designed computer programs (Walters et al 2006). Other methods include group work and experiential learning, individual counselling and therapy, and advocacy, all of which are considered in the following sections, except therapy, which is beyond the scope of this book. Unless you are a mental health specialist, most people you work with probably do not need in-depth therapy.

The process of empowerment involves helping clients to become more self-aware, and have greater insight into, and understanding of, themselves, their attitudes, values, motivations and feelings

STRATEGIES FOR INCREASING SELF-AWARENESS, CLARIFYING VALUES AND CHANGING ATTITUDES

Many of the strategies that are useful for increasing self-awareness, clarifying values, developing belief systems and changing attitudes for the contemplation stage of change are designed for group work. However, some of them can be adapted for health promoters to use in one-to-one situations.

See Chapter 13, Working with groups.

All these strategies use the principle of experiential learning, which emphasises the importance of personal experience as a source of learning. Experiential learning has evolved from two sources. One is from the theories of the American philosopher Dewey (1938). Another is from humanistic psychology. Humanistic psychology sees people as free decision makers actively controlling their own destinies. Humanistic psychology has had a huge influence on healthcare, education and health promotion both in the UK and worldwide. The literature is vast. One classic text is Rogers (1967). Experiential learning is active learning undertaken through exercises and other activities designed, for example, to increase self-awareness or aid decision making.

See Chapter 12 on helping people to learn.

DECIDING WHAT TO CHANGE

Some clients could benefit from making several lifestyle changes to improve their health, and it can be tempting to try to address all of them at the same time. But people are often at different stages of readiness to change on different issues. For example,

a person considering making improvements to his diet might be ready to make one change (such as eating more fruit and vegetables) but not ready to make others, such as changing to lower fat milk; an overweight person may be ready to take more exercise but not to change his eating habits. By writing down all the areas or issues that could be changed and asking 'Are there any of these you think you could discuss changing?', you can get agreement to discuss one particular topic (Rollnick et al 1999).

RANKING OR CATEGORISING

Ranking is a way of analysing an issue in order to distinguish the relative importance of different aspects. It is therefore useful for clarifying values. For example, in Exercise 1.1 in Chapter 1, readers are asked to rank aspects of being healthy. Health is a value and that exercise is designed to help readers to clarify which aspects of health they value most.

See Chapter 1, section on what does being healthy mean to you?

Another approach to increasing self-awareness and values clarification is to generate a list of items, and then code them into different categories. Exercise 14.1 illustrates this approach; it is designed to raise awareness of the link between enjoyment and health.

USING POLARISED VIEWS

This is a way of getting people to clarify their views about a particular issue. Views about the issue are polarized and phrased to reflect extremely different views. For example, if the issue was 'Is jogging good for you?', polarised views could be summed up as 'Jogging kills people and only very fit athletes should do it' or 'Jogging is very beneficial to health and all people would be fitter if they took it up'. Examples of polarised views can be described by the group leader or taken from writings that express opposite views.

The group leader may ask people to work in pairs, with each individual acting as if he fully adopted one of the points of view for the duration of the exercise, whatever his personal opinions. First, each person writes down all the arguments he can think of that support his position, without discussing it with his partner at this stage. After a few

---

EXERCISE 14.1   Enjoyment and health

Quickly list as many things as you can think of that you enjoy doing. Write them down the left-hand side of a piece of paper. On the right-hand side, code each item according to the following categories.

£ – any items that involve spending money.

A – any items that you do alone.

P – any items you do with other people.

R – any items that involve some kind of risk.

F – any items that help to keep you fit.

C – any items that involve creativity.

D – any items that involve consumption of drugs (including alcohol and tobacco).

H+ – any items that positively affect your health.

H– – any items that negatively affect your health.

Items may be coded in more than one category. For example, if one of the things you enjoy is going out to the pub for a drink, this may be coded £, P and D, as well as H+ and/or H–.

What have you learned about enjoyment and health through doing this exercise?

---

minutes, the partners are asked to start arguing the case, usually for about 15 minutes. The leader then lists the points in favour of each view by asking each pair in turn to contribute one point, until all the points have been collected. She then asks the group to comment on what they have learnt. In this way, members of the group can consider a whole range of arguments, which helps them to understand other people's points of view, tolerate differences of opinion, clarify their own views and perhaps see the issue in a new light.

> Another example of a values clarification exercise using the polarised arguments approach is Exercise 3.1 in Chapter 3.

USING A VALUES CONTINUUM

This is an extension of the polarised argument technique. It helps people to understand the spread of opinion on a particular issue and to clarify where they stand.

The leader describes two extremes of opinion and asks the group to imagine that these can be represented by two points, A and B, joined by a straight line. With a small group this line can be across a room; with a large group it could be drawn

on the blackboard. The group members are then asked to mark or place themselves at a point along the line that best reflects their own view. For instance, in the jogging example discussed above, pro-joggers place themselves at one end, with the most extreme at the farthest point, people with moderate views stand around the middle, and the most ardent anti-joggers stand at the other end. The leader asks each person to state his views briefly as he takes up his position. Other people are asked not to interrupt or comment until everyone has taken up a position, or has passed if they choose not to participate.

This technique can encourage a more detailed discussion of the range of possible options than the polarised argument technique. On the other hand, if everyone seems moderate, a better discussion may be stimulated by the polarised argument technique.

> The values continuum technique is used in the last task of Exercise 3.1 in Chapter 3.

USING ROLE-PLAY

Role play generally means taking on the role of another person in a specified situation, and acting out what that other person might do and say in that situation. This helps people to understand what it feels like to be in another person's shoes. For example, health promoters role-playing non-English-speaking patients visiting a clinic may be helped to understand how those patients feel, especially if the role-play is given added authenticity by using a foreign language that the health promoters do not speak.

It is also possible to role-play oneself in a new situation. This is a useful way of practising a new skill or rehearsing for a future event. For example, patients can role-play a consultation with a doctor in order to practise the skills of presenting their health problems to doctors.

> For an example of a role-play exercise, see Exercise 12.2 in Chapter 12.

USING STRUCTURED ACTIVITIES

Structured activities, usually for a group of people but sometimes for one or two people only, can be used to meet a variety of aims. One is to help people to get to know each other – icebreakers; other activities are devised to help people trust each other, communicate more openly or to increase self-awareness.

See Chapter 13, section on getting groups going, for icebreaker ideas.

For example, activities can be used to help people to identify irrational beliefs. Irrational beliefs are misconceptions that hinder people from achieving their goals. For a detailed overview of irrational beliefs see David et al (2009). There are three major irrational beliefs:

1. I must win everybody's approval otherwise I am worthless.
2. Other people must treat me exactly how I want them to, and if they don't they must be blamed and punished.
3. Life must give me everything I want and nothing I don't want.

These beliefs lead to self-defeating thinking, which in turn can affect health. It can lead to health-related behaviour with destructive consequences, such as emotional disorders, heavy drinking and physical ailments. The quiz in Exercise 14.2 aims to help you identify your own irrational beliefs.

STRATEGIES FOR DECISION MAKING

As a health promoter, you may be involved in counselling with the aim of enabling people to make a choice, such as which treatment to have, whether to have a blood test for HIV, or how to select healthy foods in particular circumstances.

See Chapter 10 on Fundamentals of communication.

Basic skills of counselling to help people make decisions at the commitment stage of change are those discussed in Chapter 10: understanding non-verbal communication, listening, helping people to talk, asking questions and obtaining feedback. For those of you who require a level of counselling skill but are not trained counsellors or therapists, see Mcleod (2007) for an introduction to counselling techniques across all disciplines.

There are at least five stages involved (adapted from Burnard 1985 and Inskipp 1993). These stages may seem familiar to you because counselling involves a framework of planning and evaluating similar to the one we used in Chapter 5.

See Chapter 5, Planning and evaluating health promotion.

EXERCISE 14.2   Beliefs quiz

Look at the following statements and put a tick in the appropriate column:

	Agree	Disagree
1. I believe in the saying, 'A leopard cannot change his spots'.		
2. I believe that 'wait and see' is a good philosophy for life.		
3. I want everyone to like me.		
4. I usually put off important decisions.		

Now identify your rational beliefs and your irrational beliefs (misconceptions):

Q1. If you agreed with this statement you may believe that the past has a lot to do with determining the present and that people are largely unchangeable. 'I'm made that way'. The idea that you are no good at playing sports, for example, can be used to avoid trying out new behaviour and learning the skills necessary to participate in a sport. The truth is that people who take risks, experiment and work on things generally find that they can become reasonably competent at most of the things they attempt; not necessarily perfect, but good enough.

Q2. If you agreed with this statement you may believe that human happiness can be achieved by hoping for the best and waiting to see what happens. This belief could result in you becoming merely a spectator in life, watching television every night and somnolent on a sun-lounger for the whole of your holidays. Getting more actively involved could be more satisfying and actually provide you with more energy. If you feel too exhausted, now may be the time to take a close look at how you are managing your life and make some changes.

Q3. If you agree with this statement you may believe you are only as good as other people think you are. Because of this you may feel worthless if, despite your efforts, people don't seem to like you. Having the approval of others is pleasant, but in order to run our own lives we shall almost certainly have to do some things some people do not like. Work on giving yourself the approval you deserve.

Q4. If you agreed with this statement you may believe that life's problems will go away if you avoid them. Don't waste your time hoping that things will work out; make them.

Stage 1: Identify the need and create the climate

Rogers (1983), an early pioneer of counselling, identified the qualities necessary for a counsellor to establish a climate in which a client can open up. These are warmth, openness, genuineness, empathy and unconditional positive regard. Unconditional positive regard is the quality of totally respecting the worth and dignity of a person, irrespective of whether you like the person or agree with his views or behaviour.

The practical aspects of creating the climate include ensuring that you will not be interrupted and cannot be overheard, that you have sufficient time and that you are comfortably seated in chairs of the same height, with the counsellor adopting an open posture and making direct eye contact when appropriate.

Stage 2: Explore the needs and the concerns

Through giving full attention and actively listening, by encouraging the client to talk and by asking questions, the counsellor begins to establish trust and to enable the client to move from superficial issues to deeper needs and concerns.

Stage 3: Help the client to set goals and identify options

Having gained a new perspective on the issues and concerns, it becomes possible for the client to identify goals and ways these might be achieved. The counsellor could help the client to identify themes or to get a clearer vision of the future by asking key questions, such as:

'How would you feel if …?'
'If things were exactly how you wanted them to be, how would they be different from now …?'
'Have you ever felt like that on other occasions …?'

The counsellor may also provide the client with information in order to establish options:

'If you do X, what's likely to happen is …'
'If you do Y, the chances are that …'
'You might find it helpful to consider that …' and so on.

Stage 4: Help the client to decide which option to choose

The important thing about this stage is that the choice must be the client's, not the counsellor's. Making decisions – that is, choosing between alternative options – is a highly complex process. It involves:

● Weighing up the pros and cons of the alternative options.
● Considering the likely consequences of pursuing each alternative.
● Deciding which is the best alternative.
● Having the confidence to pursue the best alternative.

If the client is reluctant to commit to a decision, then both parties need to consider whether it is worth undertaking further work at stages 2 and 3.

If the client chooses an alternative that the counsellor feels may not work, they should nevertheless back the client's choice and help them to develop an action plan, knowing that if it doesn't work, there is still the possibility for exploring other options.

Stage 5: Help the client to develop an action plan

Having made a decision, the client now needs to think about turning that decision into action. They may need to identify coping strategies and sources of support. Once an action plan has been agreed, the final details are to set a review date and to clarify how progress will be monitored.

See next section on strategies for changing behaviour.

STRATEGIES FOR CHANGING BEHAVIOUR

Having made a choice, people may need considerable help to carry their decision through into the action stage of change. A number of techniques developed from behavioural psychology are useful, and the philosophy behind them, that people are responsible for their own behaviour and are capable of exercising control over it, is as important as the techniques themselves. For further reading on strategies for changing behaviour see Jenkins (2003) and Browing (2005).

A variety of material has been developed to help people to change different aspects of their behaviour. For example, the Department of Health *Change for Life* campaign (http://www.dh.gov.uk) has a range of interactive tools and information that clients would find useful in supporting their change efforts.

Some useful techniques are as follows.

SELF-MONITORING

Self-monitoring involves keeping a detailed and precise account, often in the form of a diary, of behaviour that is to be changed. Its aim is to help people to analyse their pattern of behaviour and become fully aware of what they are doing, which is a starting point for gaining control. Second, the diary provides a baseline against which progress can be checked.

Self-monitoring involves answering questions such as:

● How frequently does the problem occur?
● When the problem occurs, what else is happening, both externally (in the environment), and internally (in thoughts and feelings)?
● What event leads up to the problem?
● What happens afterwards: the consequences?

Box 14.2 is an example of a smoker's diary.

IDENTIFYING COSTS, BENEFITS AND REWARDS

The cost of changing behaviour can be considerable, involving deprivation of what might have become support mechanisms, such as cigarettes, and pleasures, such as eating and drinking, or there may be a heavy price to pay in terms of time, effort and perhaps money. So it is helpful to identify the benefits clearly, and set up a system of rewards to encourage perseverance.

Benefits may be long term, such as better health or increased life expectancy. They may be abstract: 'It will prove I've got will-power', or in other people's interests: 'For the family's sake'. These benefits may be important but it is also necessary to find immediate, short-term rewards that people genuinely enjoy, such as small treats.

SETTING TARGETS AND EVALUATING PROGRESS

Targets should be realistic rather than idealistic. Losing up to a kilo in weight a week is realistic for most people; losing 7 kilos in a month usually is not. People may have unrealistic hopes and expectations about what can be achieved, which lead to disappointment and a sense of failure when they don't meet the target.

BOX 14.2   A smoker's diary

Day........................ (Complete one of these charts every day.)
  Each time you smoke a cigarette, note down in the columns:
1. The time.
2. How urgent your craving for a cigarette is, on a scale of 1–10 (1, very little craving; 10, extremely high craving).
3. Where you smoke the cigarette.
4. Whether you are alone or who you are with.
5. Do you smoke it with drinks (coffee, tea, alcohol)?
6. Do you smoke it after a meal?
7. What else are you doing at the time (for example, chatting, reading the paper, working, talking on the phone)?
8. Why did you decide to smoke this cigarette?
9. What do you feel about it afterwards?

Time	Craving	Where	Who with	With drinks	After meal	Doing what	Why	Afterwards

In order to evaluate progress, it is necessary to keep a record of behaviour so that achievements can be seen clearly. Progress should be assessed once the new behaviour has been given a fair trial, perhaps for 2 or 3 weeks, although short-term reviews ('How have I done today?') can also be useful.

If the target is not being achieved, possible reasons must be looked for and changes made. For example:

- Is the target too difficult? Should it be lowered?
- Are the rewards too distant? Is there a more immediate reward that could be more encouraging?
- Is there an unforeseen crisis or illness? If so, encouragement to continue self-monitoring and to look on the setback as a learning experience may be needed.
- Are other people unhelpful? More strategies to cope with the negative influence of other people may be needed.
- Are there other problems which require support, such as learning to cope with anxiety or stress, lack of the resources required to fund changes?

DEVISING COPING STRATEGIES

Changing behaviour can mean coping with numerous difficulties, for at least a short period of time, until the new behaviour becomes a normal part of life. Someone who is stopping smoking has to cope with problems such as the craving they feel, the need to put something in their mouth, not knowing what to do with their hands, doing without their accustomed tension reliever in moments of stress and resisting the offer of a cigarette.

People adopt a wide variety of coping strategies, and it is often useful to get a group to share their ideas about what helps them to cope. The list of strategies here is certainly not exhaustive.

- Finding a substitute, such as substituting chewing gum for cigarettes or eating low-calorie instead of high-calorie foods.
- Changing some routines and habits that are closely associated with the unhealthy behaviour. Examples are drinking tea or fruit juice instead of coffee, because coffee is closely associated with cigarettes.
- Making it difficult to carry on with the unhealthy behaviour by, for example, not keeping alcohol in the home or restricting eating to meal times, not between meals.

What all these strategies have in common is that they require only a small step to achieve a large degree of help for self-control. Other strategies may be:

- Getting support from other people in the same situation, who might be from a weight control group, a smoking cessation clinic or a self-help group. Another helpful way of getting support is by linking with another person on the understanding that each may telephone or meet the other if they need help.
- Practising ways of responding to unhelpful social pressures, for example refusing the offer of a cigarette or a drink.
- Adopting a 1-day-at-a-time approach. The prospect of the whole of the rest of life without a cigarette may be overwhelming, but the prospect of 1 day without one is far more tolerable. Even shorter time spans may be helpful, such as putting off eating, drinking or smoking for just 15 minutes at a time.
- Learning relaxation techniques and other ways, such as exercise, of relieving stress. Simple relaxation routines that can be practised at any time and place can be helpful in coping with stressful moments when the habit would have been to reach for a drink or a cigarette.

USING STRATEGIES EFFECTIVELY

A number of different strategies have been covered that you can use when you are trying to help clients to increase their self-awareness, clarify their values and beliefs, change their attitudes and behaviour and maintain behaviour change; in other words to move them through the Stages of Change cycle. While it may be relatively easy to influence attitudes and behaviour in the short term, it can be difficult for people to sustain behaviour change over a longer period. In order to use these strategies with maximum effect there are a number of principles to bear in mind.

ADVOCACY AND WORKING IN PARTNERSHIP

Some people may need extra help to make health choices. Advocacy is generally taken to mean representing the interests of people who cannot speak up for themselves because of illness, disability or other disadvantage. In the context of health promotion, it is better seen as a variety of ways of empowering those people who are disempowered in our society. It is concerned with using every possible means to assist people to become independent and self-advocating.

There can be deep conflicts of loyalty for health promoters who take on an advocacy role. There may be a need to challenge employers, or those in authority, about services that fail to meet people's needs.

For example, if a patient complains to a community mental health nurse that his drugs are making him feel drowsy and generally unwell, but the doctor insists they should continue to take them, where should the nurse's loyalties lie: to the patient, to the doctor, to the health service (their employer) or to their professional body? How can the nurse most effectively act as an advocate in this situation?

Because of such conflicts of loyalties, many advocacy schemes use nonprofessional workers who come from a similar background to those they are empowering. For example, Maternity-Links schemes provide workers as advocates and interpreters for Asian mothers who do not speak English (http://www.bfwh.nhs.uk). The workers are Asian themselves but able to speak English as well as their own mother tongue, and the organisation may be run with health service funding but managed independently.

In order to reach and influence disadvantaged groups of people successfully, many projects involve professionals working in partnership with lay volunteers. For example, a community mothers' programme involved nonprofessional mothers as volunteers working with disadvantaged first time mothers to improve their parenting skills (Settles et al 2000).

MAKING HEALTHIER CHOICES EASY CHOICES

People make health choices in the context of their own environment, subject to all the pressures and influences that surround them. If this environment is conducive to a healthier lifestyle, clients have greater freedom to choose the healthier alternatives and change their behaviour. For example, the provision of cycleways makes it easier to take regular exercise by cycling to work; provision of litter bins, combined with frequent emptying, helps people to maintain a litter-free environment. National and local policies can create a climate where it is easier to adopt healthier behaviour.

> See Chapter 1, section on what affects health and Chapter 16, section on changing policy and practice.

Undertake Exercise 14.3 to apply some of these ideas to an example of a behaviour change scenario.

RELATING TO CLIENTS

> See Chapter 10, section on exploring relationships with clients.

Clients are more likely to change if the health promoter understands the client, sees things from their point of view and accepts them on their own terms. Achieving this relationship may be the most difficult part of helping people to change.

Sometimes it is difficult to start a discussion about changing behaviour, and establishing good rapport is essential for an honest discussion and openness for change. One way you can understand your client and also assess readiness to change is to ask the client to take you through a typical day with reference to a particular behaviour.

It is important to note that the attitude and behaviour of the health promoter may influence the outcome. For example, an obese health promoter may find it more difficult to encourage an obese client to adjust their dietary habits. The experiences of health promoters in trying to change their own behaviour, however, can be valuable in helping them to understand the difficulties that their clients experience. However, it is important to remember that everyone is different and that, although for some people making a particular change may be easy, for others a similar change may prove very difficult.

DEALING WITH RESISTANCE

It is sometimes difficult for health promoters to stop providing advice when they know that a particular behaviour, such as stopping smoking, can have huge benefits for the client. It is important to recognise when your clients are showing signs of resisting the suggestion to change. When you see this resistance, it is better to express empathy, emphasis-

---

EXERCISE 14.3   Changing behaviour in practice

Read the following example of behaviour change approach and answer the questions that follow:

Gemma is a single parent. She has a toddler who constantly wakes her at night. She has used various strategies, including trying to tire him out physically just before bed time, keeping him up later, leaving toys for him to play with in the night and playing with him herself in the night. She has started to buy vodka cocktails and cans of lager in the supermarket to drink in the evenings to help her relax and now finds that she needs another drink to help her get back to sleep after getting up in the night.

She phones her health visitor – Mary – for help. Mary goes to see her and asks her to describe a typical day (and night) in order to understand the situation better. She asks Gemma to describe the situations she struggled with, how she felt at the time and what she did. As Gemma's story unfolds Mary gains knowledge of Gemma's variation in mood states, existing coping strategies and support base.

Mary gets Gemma to reflect on her daily achievements and emphasises that it must be a struggle for her without much sleep. Gemma says she wants to do something to help her child sleep. Mary explores how confident Gemma feels in being able to make some changes. Mary also asks Gemma if she knows of anything that seems to help her child to relax, and using her suggestions they devise a suitable bed-time routine for Gemma to try out. Mary recognises that Gemma is concerned about her drinking and asks her for suggestions of what she could do about it. Gemma says she feels that her drinking is related to her stressful situation and that once her child sleeps better she will feel more in control.

Finally, Mary suggests that she should come back to see Gemma in 2 weeks' time to discuss whether the new routines are helping her child to sleep. Gemma agrees. Mary makes a note to ask Gemma about her drinking on the next visit.

- What strategies does Mary, the health visitor, use to help Gemma?
- What other strategies could Mary have used?
- What strategies might Mary want to use at the follow-up visit?

---

ing that it is the client's personal choice and that they have control over their lifestyle choices. Useful strategies for these clients at a later date are to reassess readiness to change, establish how important the behaviour change is to them and how confident they feel about making the change.

USING METHODS SENSITIVELY

People invest a great deal of emotion in their values and attitudes, which means that the exercises described here, especially those that are designed to encourage people to explore feelings, need to be handled with care and sensitivity. Special training in the use of experiential methods is recommended but, at the very least, health promoters should not attempt to use them unless they have experienced them first themselves. Some points to remember are as follows:

- Explain the activities carefully and thoroughly, and check to ensure that everybody understands what the exercise is for and what they are expected to do.

- Emphasise that participation is entirely voluntary.
- Allow plenty of time for discussion at the end. If people's opinions and cherished ideas have been challenged, they are likely to feel strongly about it. Increased self-awareness may be a very uncomfortable experience too. The group leader should ensure that people have time to express their feelings and get any support that they need before they leave the group.
- Ensure that there is an atmosphere of confidentiality and trust, so that people feel free to explore their views and feelings in safety.
- Save your own views to the end, after the group members have had a chance to think things through for themselves. Be open and honest about yourself and your beliefs, and nonjudgemental of values that might conflict with your own.

Finally, for detailed guides to changing health behaviour see Rutter & Quinne (2002) and Kerr et al (2005).

PRACTICE POINTS

■ For individuals to be ready to change a particular behaviour they need to feel confident in being able to adopt the new behaviour. The new behaviour also needs to be important to them and have clear benefits. You may need to help clients develop a number of competencies or life skills to do with social interaction, assertiveness and time management, and possibly specific skills (such as those needed to participate in a physical exercise programme).

■ In order to devise the appropriate strategy for each individual you need to start by exploring clients' health knowledge and beliefs related to the issue of concern, the stage of change they are at and what outcomes they desire. Asking the client to describe a typical day in relation to the behaviour is a useful approach.

■ You need to be aware that clients may be resistant to change. In these situations it is best to emphasise that it is the client's personal choice and that they are in control. At a later date you could go back to explore again the individual's confidence about changing and how important the change is to them.

■ You need to tailor an action plan to the specific needs of each client and provide positive consequences for the desired healthy behaviour (such as praise or rewards) in order to maintain behaviour change.

■ You can improve success by combining a number of strategies. For example, a patient who is being rehabilitated after a heart attack could have an interview with a hospital doctor, a home visit from a nurse to encourage support from family members, and small-group self-help sessions to help patients to manage their problems.

■ Records are important for follow-up. They are most effective if they are kept and owned by the individual concerned, for example in the form of a diary.

■ Providing a supportive environment can be the key to success, so that people find it easier to change to and maintain a healthier lifestyle.

References

Armitage CJ 2009 Is there utility in the transtheoretical model? British Journal of Health Psychology 2: 195–210.

Aveyard P, Lawrence T, Cheng KK et al 2006 A randomized controlled trial of smoking cessation for pregnant women to test the effect of a transtheoretical model-based intervention on movement in stage and interaction with baseline stage. British Journal of Health Psychology 2: 263–278.

Aveyard P, Massey L, Parsons A et al 2009 The effect of transtheoretical model based interventions on smoking cessation. Social Science and Medicine 68(3): 397–403.

Botelho R 2004 Motivational practice: promoting healthy habits and self-care of chronic diseases. Rochester, MHH.

Browning C 2005 Behavioural change: an evidence-based handbook for social and public health. London, Churchill Livingstone.

Burnard P 1985 Learning human skills: a guide for nurses. Oxford, Heinemann Nursing.

David D, Lynn S, Ellis A 2009 Rational and irrational beliefs: research, theory, and clinical practice. NY, Open University Press USA.

Dewey J 1938 Experience and education. New York, Collier Books.

Inskipp F 1993 Counselling: the trainer's handbook. Cambridge, National Extension College.

Jenkins CD 2003 Building better health: a handbook of behavioral change. Geneva, World Health Organization.

Kerr J, Weitkunat R, Moretti M 2005 ABC of behaviour change: a guide to successful disease prevention and health promotion. London, Churchill Livingstone.

Marlatt AG, Donovan DM (eds) 2007 Relapse prevention: maintenance strategies in the treatment of addictive behaviors. 2nd edn. NY, The Guilford Press.

Mcleod J 2007 Counselling skill. Maidenhead, Open University Press.

Neesham C 1993 A model for change. Healthlines, September: 15–17.

Parliamentary Office of Science and Technology 2007 POSTNOTE: health behaviours. May. No 283. London, Parliamentary Office of Science and Technology.

Prochaska JO 2005 Stages of change, readiness and motivation. In: Kerr J, Weitkunat R, Moretti M (eds) ABC of behaviour change: a guide to successful disease prevention and health promotion. London, Churchill Livingstone.

Prochaska JO 2009 Flaws in the theory or flaws in the study: a commentary on 'The effect of transtheoretical model based interventions on smoking cessation'. Social Science and

Medicine 68(3): 404–406; discussion 407–409.

Prochaska JO, DiClemente C 1982 Transtheoretical therapy: towards a more integrative model of change. Psychotherapy: Theory, Research and Practice. 19(3): 276–288.

Prochaska JO, DiClemente C 1984 The transtheoretical approach: crossing traditional boundaries of therapy. Harewood IL, Dow-Jones.

Prochaska JO, Velicer WF 1997 The transtheoretical model of health behavior change. American Journal of Health Promotion 12(1): 38–48.

Prochaska JO, DiClemente CC, Norcross JC 1992 In search of how people change. Applications to addictive behaviors. American Psychology 47(9): 1102–1114.

Rogers CR 1967 On becoming a person: a therapist's view of psychotherapy. London, Constable.

Rogers CR 1983 Freedom to learn for the eighties. Columbus OH, Charles E Merril.

Rollnick S, Mason P, Butler C 1999 Health behaviour change: a guide for practitioners. London, Churchill Livingstone.

Rollnick S, Miller WR, Butler CC 2007 Motivational interviewing in health care: helping patients change behavior. New York The Guilford Press.

Rutter DR, Quinne L 2002 Changing health behaviour: intervention and research with social cognition models. Buckingham, Open Univeristy Press.

Settles BH, Davies JE, Grasse-Bachman C et al 2000 Developing community and peer support for young parents: process and outcome evaluation inputs in prevention programs. Family Science Review 13(2): 182–196.

Tones BK 1987 Devising strategies for preventing drug misuse: the role of the Health Action Model. Health Education Research 2(4): 305–317.

Tones K 1995 Making a change for the better. Healthlines, November: 17

Tones K, Tilford S 2001 Health education: effectiveness, efficiency and equity, 3rd edn. Cheltenham, Nelson Thornes.

Walters ST, Wright JA, Shegog R 2006 A review of computer and Internet-based interventions for smoking behavior. Addictive Behaviors 31(2): 264–277.

Websites

http://www.bfwh.nhs.uk/departments/maternity/links.asp

http://www.dh.gov.uk/en/News/Currentcampaigns/Change4Life

http://en.wikipedia.org/wiki/Transtheoretical_Model

Chapter 15

Working with communities

SUMMARY

This chapter begins with a discussion of community-based work in health promotion and an overview of the range of activities it may include. Some key terms and principles are explained before an examination of three particular ways of working with communities: community participation, community development and community health projects. Each of these includes an exercise, and there is also a case study of a community development project. The chapter finishes with a consideration of the competencies health promoters need to work effectively with communities.

See Chapter 2, section on defining health promotion.

As discussed earlier, health promotion is the process of enabling people to increase control over, and improve, their health (World Health Organization 1986). The challenge this presents is considerable when working with people in the community who may be disadvantaged and discriminated against, and who may feel powerless to do anything about their health. This chapter is about working with communities in a way that enables them to take more control over their health.

See Chapter 7, section on local health strategies and initiatives, for information on government-funded initiatives focusing on disadvantaged communities.

COMMUNITY-BASED WORK IN HEALTH PROMOTION

Community-based work in health promotion involves working with groups of the public in a sustained way which will enable them to increase control over and improve their health. It may involve different kinds of activities, including:

- Community development work.
- Setting up a group and working with members on health issues (such as a group with learning difficulties addressing issues of sexual health).
- Working on projects or campaigns focusing on a particular community-identified health need (such as drug misuse).
- Outreach work, which means health promoters going out to meet people where they are, rather than expecting people to come to them (such as community work on sexual health, which might involve working with people in the sex industry on the streets or in clubs and massage parlours).
- Providing health information services (such as well-women information centres).
- Health-related work undertaken by organisations with wider remits (such as health courses for older people run by national older people's organisations).
- Advocacy projects (such as organisations undertaking interpreting and/or advocacy for Asian women).
- Self-help groups getting together for mutual support on health problems.

This list (adapted from London Community Health Resource and National Council for Voluntary Organisations 1987) begins to identify the activities that health promoters may engage with at a community level, but first the key terms and principles involved in community-based work need to be clarified.

KEY TERMS

Community

Traditionally a community is seen as a group of interacting people living in a common location. The word is often used to refer to a group that is organised around common values and social cohesion within a shared geographical location, generally in social units larger than a household. Essentially, a community is a network of people. The link between them may be:

- Where they live (such as a housing estate or neighbourhood).
- The work they do (such as the farming community or school community).
- The way they live (such as new-age travellers or homeless people).
- Common interests or shared values (such as a church community).
- Other factors they have in common (such as sexual preferences, so the gay community).

The people in the network come together on the basis of a shared experience or concern, and identify for themselves which communities they feel they belong to. Networks may be formal or informal and since the advent of the Internet, the concept of community no longer has geographical limitations, as people can now virtually gather in an online community and share common interests regardless of physical location (see http://en.wikipedia.org for a full discussion of the nature of community from a range of disciplinary perspectives).

Community work

This means working with community groups and organisations to overcome the community's problems. Community work aims to enhance the sense of solidarity and competence in the community. For example, a community development worker may take on a health promotion role by working with particular communities in order to collectively bring about social change and improve quality of life. This involves working with individuals, families or whole communities to empower them to:

- Identify their needs, opportunities, rights and responsibilities.
- Plan what they want to achieve, and take appropriate action.
- Develop activities and services to improve their lives.

(For more details see http://www.prospects.ac.uk.)

Community health work

This is community work with a focus on health concerns, but generally health is defined broadly to include social and economic aspects, so that community health work may encompass almost as broad a range of activities as community development work.

Community action

This means activity carried out by members of the community under their own control in order to improve their collective conditions. It may involve campaigning, negotiating with or challenging authorities and those with power.

Community participation

This is about involving the community in health work that is led by someone outside the community; for example a worker employed by a statutory agency. The degree of participation may vary.

Community development

This means working to stimulate and encourage communities to express their needs and to support them in their collective action. It is not about dealing with people's problems on a one-to-one basis; it aims to develop the potential of a community as a whole. A **community development approach to health** involves working with groups of people to identify their own health concerns, and to take appropriate action. **Community development health workers** are essentially facilitators, locally based, whose role is to help people in the community to acquire the skills, knowledge and confidence to act on health issues. They are usually community workers by background, rather than health professionals.

Community health projects

This is a loose term applied to programmes of work that are organised by agencies for the improvement of health in a community, or to local organisations aiming to improve health by supporting some combination of community activity, self-help, community action and/or community development. To read more on terms and projects linked to the community go to the Community Development Foundation (CDF) website (http://www.cdf.org.uk). The CDF is the leading source of community development expertise and delivery. As a public body and a charity it bridges government, communities and the voluntary sector, and has a range of information on the types of projects that lead to community cohesion, community engagement and community development.

Finally, it is worth mentioning that in the health service the word community is often used as an adjective to describe anything that is not based in hospital. Examples are **community care**, **community nurses** and **community services**.

PRINCIPLES OF COMMUNITY-BASED WORK

There are four key principles, as follows.

1. The centrality of the community

It is the community which defines its own needs. Community-based work is essentially a bottom-up process, rather than being top down expert led where those with power and authority make the decisions. Health promoters recognise and value the health experience and knowledge that exists in the community, and seek to use it for everyone's benefit. Both legislation and policy recognise the importance of community involvement in their own affairs (see Department for Communities and Local Government 2006).

2. The facilitator role of community health promoters

Community health promoters do not perceive themselves as experts in health, but as facilitators whose role it is to validate, encourage and empower people to define their own health needs and to meet them. They start where the community is, recognising and valuing people's own abilities and experiences. They involve people in community health work from the very beginning, encouraging and supporting them in working together. Knowledge and skills are shared and demystified. Community health promoters aim to complement as well as challenge statutory services by making people's access to statutory agencies easier, and making the agencies more accountable to the people they serve.

3. The importance of addressing inequalities

See Chapter 1, section on inequalities in health.

A central concern in community-based health promotion work is the need to challenge and change the many forms of disadvantage, oppression, discrimination and inequalities that people face, and which adversely affect their health.

Work therefore has focused particularly on the needs of disadvantaged groups. A central way of working is to bring people in such groups together for support and information sharing, and to enable them to bring about change through collective action. The work can be political, because it often involves working towards equality, social inclusion and social justice with people who experience powerlessness and inequality as part of their everyday lives.

4. A broad perspective on health

Health is perceived broadly and holistically as positive wellbeing including social, emotional, mental and societal aspects as well as physical. It is not seen merely as the absence of disease, and is not limited by medical or epidemiological views of what constitutes a health problem or issue. Health is seen to be affected by social, environmental, economic and political factors.

COMMUNITY PARTICIPATION

Participation is a word that is used widely to mean a range of activities, from those that are merely tokenistic to those which are firmly rooted in the concept of empowerment. Partnership, public participation and public decision making are all key issues in health services and local authorities. However, in reality some organisations may make decisions without having any wish to engage with the public (see Scriven 2007 for a detailed overview of collaboration and partnership working with communities).

COMMUNITY PARTICIPATION IN PLANNING

See also Chapter 6, section on public views.

The amount of community participation in planning health work organised by an agency (such as an NHS organisation or local authority) can vary along a spectrum of none to high, as shown in Table 15.1. In the health service, such participation can be called public involvement or service user involvement. (See Rosato et al 2008 for an interesting discussion on the value of community participation for health outcomes and Coulthard et al 2002 for an overview of people's perception of community participation.)

WAYS OF DEVELOPING COMMUNITY PARTICIPATION

Community participation can be encouraged and supported in many ways at different levels. If you work for a public sector agency such as a local

Table 15.1 Community participation in planning health promotion work	
No participation	The community is told nothing, and is not involved in any way
Very low participation	The community is informed. The agency makes a plan and announces it. The community is convened or notified in other ways in order to be informed; compliance is expected
Low participation	The community is offered 'token' consultation. The agency tries to promote a plan and seeks support or at least sufficient sanction so that the plan can go ahead. It is unwilling to modify the plan unless absolutely necessary
Moderate participation	The community advises through a consultation process. The agency presents a plan and invites questions, comments and recommendations. It is prepared to modify the plan
High participation	The community plans jointly. Representatives of the agency and the community sit down together from the beginning to devise a plan
Very high participation	The community has delegated authority. The agency identifies and presents an issue to the community, defines the limits and asks the community to make a series of decisions that can be embodied in a plan which it will accept
Highest participation	The community has control. The agency asks the community to identify the issue and make all the key decisions about goals and plans. It is willing to help the community at each step to accomplish its goals, even to the extent of delegating administrative control of the work.

The table is adapted from Brager & Sprecht (1973). See also Scriven (2007).

authority or the health service, the following suggestions may be useful (adjusted from Adams & Smithies 1990 and Labyrinth Consultancy 2000).

Be open about policies and plans. Publicise your policies, invite comments and recommendations on your plans, and involve representatives on planning and management groups. This is an intrinsic part of policy. See, for example, Department for Communities and Local Government (2009), the government response to the White Paper *Communities in Control: Real People, Real Power* (Department for Communities and Local Government 2008). This White Paper is about passing power to communities and giving real control and influence to more people.

Plan for the community's expressed needs. When planning health promotion services, help the community to express its own needs.

Decentralise planning. Set up planning and management of health promoting and allied services on a neighbourhood basis, encouraging and enabling the public's involvement.

Develop joint forums. Develop joint forums, such as patient participation groups in doctors' practices, where lay people and professionals can work together in partnerships. Mental health services often have joint forums to involve service users in service development.

Develop networks. Encourage individuals or groups to come together, thus increasing their collective knowledge and power to change things. Value interagency links and gain the support of workers from different organisations because competition and lack of understanding of each other's roles and cultures can hinder progress.

Use electronic networking. Electronic networks can provide community information and a means of communication within and between communities (see http://www.partnerships.org.uk). For example, rural communities with poor transport facilities can use electronic networks (e-mail and websites), which go some way towards addressing the problem of social exclusion caused by lack of information. Not only can groups and individuals find and supply information on the Internet, they can participate in democratic processes. For example, Communities UK uses Twitter (http://www.twitter.com) as does the National Council for Voluntary Organisations (NCVO). Many organisations also use YouTube (http://www.youtube.com). Another example is the use of virtual councillor's surgeries (for an example see http://www.stockton.gov.uk).

Provide support, advice and training for community groups. Provide opportunities for lay people to develop their knowledge, confidence and skills. CommunitiesUK have developed a guide for this purpose, *Community Power Pack: Real People, Real Power* (Communities and Local Government and Involve 2008), which is online (http://www.communities.gov.uk) or can be ordered free.

Provide information. Provide information about health issues, details of useful local and national organisations, leaflets, posters, books and websites.

Provide help with funding and resources. Help local groups to obtain funding from statutory agencies, and provide other sorts of practical help such as a place to meet or facilities to photocopy materials.

Provide help with evaluation. Being able to show real changes in community resources, services and health outcomes increases respect and confidence from communities, funders and agencies.

Support advocacy projects. Support projects that enable people who are otherwise excluded to have a voice, such as mental health advocacy schemes (see Foley & Platzer 2007).

Exercise 15.1 offers the opportunity for you to consider how you can encourage community participation in your work.

COMMUNITY DEVELOPMENT

However much you might seek people's participation, it may be that they feel so alienated, dissatisfied or overwhelmed with problems that they reject participation. In this situation, it is necessary to develop a climate and culture where participation can happen. You need to encourage, enable and support people, and community development is a way of doing this. Evidence suggests (although measurement is difficult) that encouraging autonomy, strengthening social networks and other aspects of social capital are prerequisites for good health (Morgan & Swann 2004).

Community development is much more than community participation. It means working with people to identify their own health concerns, and to support and facilitate them in their collective action. It means adhering firmly to the principles of community-based work outlined above, with the

---

EXERCISE 15.1   Developing community participation in your health promotion work

Consider the following list of ways in which you can encourage community participation in working for health.

- Be open about policies and plans.
- Plan for the community's expressed needs.
- De-centralise planning.
- Develop joint forums and networks.
- Offer support, advice and training for community groups.
- Provide information.
- Provide help with funding and resources.
- Provide help with evaluation.
- Support advocacy projects

(If you are not sure what is meant by these, look back at the explanations above.)

To what extent do you think these things are desirable?

To what extent do you do these things already?

From this list, can you identify ways in which you would like to increase community participation in your work?

Can you identify any other ways in which you would like to increase community participation in your work?

Given that there may be some obstacles to doing what you would ideally like to do, can you identify a practical way forward for acting on at least one of the things you would like to do?

Work individually, in pairs or small groups.

EXERCISE 15.2   Thinking about community development

Working individually, or in pairs or small groups, work through the following questionnaire. If you are working with other people, discuss the reasons for the answers you give. You do not have to reach a consensus. When you have listened to each other's views, you can agree to disagree.

Tick whether you think each of the following statements is true or false:

Community development is about:	True	False
1. Fostering a sense of community among people.	☐	☐
2. Helping people to see the root causes of their ill health.	☐	☐
3. Enabling a statutory authority to show it cares.	☐	☐
4. Getting involved in a political process.	☐	☐
5. Doing away with experts and professionals.	☐	☐
6. Confronting forms of discrimination such as racism and sexism.	☐	☐
7. Saving money on services by helping people to help themselves.	☐	☐
8. Promoting equal access to resources such as health services.	☐	☐
9. Enabling a community worker to become a leader/spokesperson for the community.	☐	☐
10. Helping people to develop confidence and become more articulate about their needs.	☐	☐
11. Campaigning for a better environment such as improved housing, transport and play facilities.	☐	☐
12. Controlling social unrest, by providing, for example, activities for bored young people.	☐	☐
13. Helping people from lower socioeconomic groups to change their attitudes and behaviour.	☐	☐
14. Recognising and valuing the skills, knowledge and expertise of individuals and groups in the community.	☐	☐
15. Beginning a process of redistributing wealth, power and resources.	☐	☐

Now add any other points you think community development is, or is not, about.

(Adapted from a questionnaire by Adams & Hawkins (undated and unpublished) and reproduced by kind permission).

---

community development worker having the role of a facilitator.

Exercise 15.2 is designed to help you to consider what community development work means in practice.

Case study 15.1 illustrates community development in practice, demonstrating how the community and the community's own expressed needs were central, the workers acted as facilitators, inequalities in health were addressed and a broad

CASE STUDY 15.1   BE WELL

Be WELL Community Health Project came into being as a result of the vision of a group of people working in the area who were concerned that local people should be involved in determining their own health needs and participating in defining what could contribute to their enhanced health, wellbeing and social functioning.

Be WELL operates from two refurbished former council houses and is often referred to by local people as *The Healing House.* The project is open to anyone living in Craigmillar (Scotland) or who is registered with a Craigmillar GP.

The project aims to provide a community health resource, operating on community development principles, where local people can meet to:
- Draw on the support and strengths of the community.
- Explore their health issues and concerns.
- Formulate a collective response to those concerns.
- Develop a creative and responsive range of services and activities which local people have identified as enhancing physical, emotional and social wellbeing.

Be WELL also aims to help improve the health of the community and address health inequalities both locally and in a wider context by:
- Working with a range of local, city-wide and national agencies in a collaborative, multiagency or partnership way as appropriate.

- Fostering and facilitating a two-way exchange between service planners and local people.

At Be WELL, a wide range of services is offered and a changing programme of activities which include:
- **Drop-in** – 3 days a week. One day includes activities such as crafts and storytelling. The drop-in is run by volunteers who provide tea and healthy snack lunches. Project users have the opportunity to enjoy a warm, welcoming and supportive environment.
- **Complementary therapies** – acupuncture, reflexology, therapeutic massage, craniosacral therapy and kinesiology.
- **Counselling service** – open-ended, person-centred counselling by trained volunteer counsellors.
- **Groups and short courses** – communications skills, confidence and assertiveness, relaxation, breastfeeding support, café and line dancing.
- **Men's group** – self-support group, offering a meeting place for men which they decide how to use.
- **Heart to heart group** – nonmedical source of support, information and encouragement to people suffering from, or recovering from, heart disease or surgery.
- **Free crèche.**
- **Annual stakeholders' away day.**

(Adjusted from http://www.lchpf.co.uk/bewell.htm. See website for full details and more case studies.)

perspective on health was taken. It also shows how local people were empowered to take action.

SOME IMPLICATIONS OF THE COMMUNITY DEVELOPMENT APPROACH

If you choose to adopt a community development approach, it is important to appreciate the implications and that areas of tension are likely to surface. These are identified below, as are suggestions for trying to prevent them.

1. Different priorities and agendas

Priorities chosen by communities may not be the same as those of local statutory agencies or the funding organisation. For example, health priorities for health promoters may be influenced by

government targets with lifestyle risk factors for major illnesses, and low uptake of health services dominating the agenda. Community priorities, on the other hand, may be about social conditions, such as poor housing and lack of good public transport. Conflicting agendas must be clearly understood and dealt with at the outset of any community development work.

2. Threat to local health workers

If local people gain confidence, become assertive and more articulate through the process of community development, they could voice concern and criticism about local health services. Furthermore, the prospect of members of the community taking an active role in policy making and planning may be alien to many managers in statutory agencies. A thorough educational grounding in the rationale and principles of community-based work is required, although setting this up and getting people to listen may in itself be a difficult task.

3. No instant results

It takes time to get to know a community and to build up trust with local people, and it may be years before there is any tangible outcome. A common problem is that projects with fixed-term funding for a year or two are often expected to achieve substantial outcomes in these short timescales, which is unrealistic. Secure long-term funding, with achievable objectives, is fundamental to success.

4. A token gesture or an easy option

Well-meaning authorities who prioritise inequalities in health may consider a community health project as a way of addressing the issue. The inequalities issue is complex, involving deeply rooted causes of poor health; a community health project can make a valuable contribution, but it can also divert attention from political solutions to the problems.

5. Evaluation conflicts

Outside agencies may expect to see results in terms of normative outcomes such as improved immunisation rates, a measurable change in community behaviour (less binge drinking, vandalism or crime, for example) or lower rates of hospital admission. However, the objectives of a community development project are rarely couched in such terms, and are more likely to be concerned with far less easily measured results such as increased public participation in health planning, or better communication between the community and statutory agencies. Open debate about the process, principles, aims and possible outcomes is essential (see Green & South 2006 for an excellent discussion of evaluating community-based projects and ASH Scotland 2003 for an example of evaluating a specific community project).

COMMUNITY HEALTH PROJECTS

A community health project aims to improve health usually by combining a number of approaches such as self help, community action and/or community development. Considerable insights can be gained from existing community health projects; some have been written up to include the processes, outcomes and lessons learnt. See, for example, the website of Lothian Community Health Projects Forum (http://www.lchpf.co.uk), which is where Case study 15.1 originated.

> See Chapter 5, Planning and evaluating health promotion.

It is important to adopt a systematic approach to planning a community health project. Fig. 15.1 summarises the planning and evaluation flowchart taken from Chapter 5, highlighting issues relevant to community health project work. This is not a comprehensive guide to setting up and running community health projects; it is intended to be complementary to the information in Chapter 5.

Stage 1. Identifying needs and priorities

At this stage, two particular issues are: how do you get to know the community and who do you consult?

Getting to know the community and its needs. Get all the relevant information you can about the health of the community. Search out data from local health services and the local authority.

Try contacting neighbourhood centres, community groups, voluntary organisations and tenants' associations. People who might be able to put you in touch with these include local workers in health and social services, local churches and schools, the local Council for Voluntary Service and the local Council for Racial Equality. Talk to members of the public, perhaps at local markets and festivals, or conduct a small survey. It might be necessary to hold public meetings to elicit full participation.

Talk to local professionals, but bear in mind that professional perceptions will often stem from a problem-centred view of a locality: for example, police may talk about crime, and social workers about the numbers of children on the at-risk register.

Local newspapers are a useful source of information about the needs, interests and activities of a locality, and may even have a library service to select material on a particular issue for you. Another approach is to walk, not drive, around the neighbourhood. Groups of young people on street

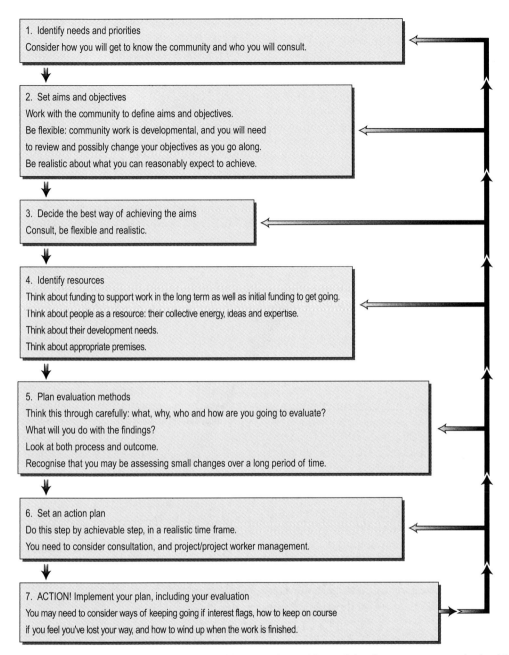

1. Identify needs and priorities
Consider how you will get to know the community and who you will consult.

2. Set aims and objectives
Work with the community to define aims and objectives.
Be flexible: community work is developmental, and you will need
to review and possibly change your objectives as you go along.
Be realistic about what you can reasonably expect to achieve.

3. Decide the best way of achieving the aims
Consult, be flexible and realistic.

4. Identify resources
Think about funding to support work in the long term as well as initial funding to get going.
Think about people as a resource: their collective energy, ideas and expertise.
Think about their development needs.
Think about appropriate premises.

5. Plan evaluation methods
Think this through carefully: what, why, who and how are you going to evaluate?
What will you do with the findings?
Look at both process and outcome.
Recognise that you may be assessing small changes over a long period of time.

6. Set an action plan
Do this step by achievable step, in a realistic time frame.
You need to consider consultation, and project/project worker management.

7. ACTION! Implement your plan, including your evaluation
You may need to consider ways of keeping going if interest flags, how to keep on course
if you feel you've lost your way, and how to wind up when the work is finished.

Fig. 15.1 Flowchart for planning and evaluating health promotion, with special reference to community health work.

corners, smells from fast-food shops and the range and price of goods in shop windows can reveal a lot about local lifestyle and socioeconomic conditions.

Consulting before setting up. Consult with local health and social service workers at a very early stage and also elicit community participation so that they have ownership of the project. Only do this if you are confident the project is likely to secure funding, as you could raise community members' expectations falsely and diminish their trust.

Stages 2 and 3. Setting aims and objectives, and deciding the best way of achieving them

Key issues here are about being flexible and realistic. It is important to have full participation from the people you have already made contact with, and the management group/steering group of the project (if there is one). These people are vital to setting realistic, achievable aims and objectives, and working out the best means of achieving them.

Flexibility is vital because community health work is essentially a developmental process, so you need to review and, if necessary, modify your objectives regularly. Objectives may change, and indeed should change, if new opportunities arise and/or previous objectives no longer seem achievable or compatible with changing needs.

Be realistic: this applies to identifying what you plan to achieve, and when. For example, if you are planning a community development approach, ensure that you have a realistic time scale; 3 years is suggested as a reasonable minimum.

Stage 4. Identifying resources

Funding. Funding can come from statutory organisations, such as the local authorities or the health service, sometimes in partnership. Projects may also be funded from the voluntary sector through funding from government grants and independent funds, such as the Big Lottery Fund (see http://www.biglotteryfund.org.uk for the full range of Reaching Communities funding, and also for case studies and evaluation reports). Uncertain funding arrangements can increase difficulties in planning and evaluating work and can divert efforts from project work to fundraising. It is important to think about long-term funding, otherwise there is a danger of work being dropped when funding runs out.

People. By bringing people with a common interest or experience together, you may find that the collective energy of the group generates ideas for future action. Your role may also begin to change, from being an initiator/facilitator to being a supporter.

It is also important to think about what training and development is needed, who will do it and how it will be funded. Not only project workers but also the project management committee (if there is one), local lay people and health professionals may need

help in understanding what this type of work is all about.

Premises. You need to consider what premises you need: rooms for large and small meetings, a room for a crèche, a place to keep and use equipment such as video equipment and photocopiers, a library/place where people can look up information and use computers with access to the Internet and e mail. Is there access for wheelchairs, push chairs and prams? Running water and toilets? Facilities for making refreshments or meals? Good access by public transport? Well-lit premises so that people feel safe going there after dark?

You also need to consider the nature of possible premises. If you are offered space in a clinic, for example, this may mean that people perceive the project to be part of the statutory health services.

Webpage. Many community health projects now have webpages (such as http://www.lchpf.co.uk), so it is important to consider who will fund and develop this resource.

Stage 5. Planning evaluation methods

It is vital that evaluation is planned at the outset, as this will avoid misunderstandings and false expectations. All parties (funders, managers, workers, participants) need to agree on key issues:

- Why are you undertaking an evaluation? Who and what is it for?
- What will you be evaluating?
- How will you do it? What methods will you use?
- Who will do it? Will you evaluate yourselves or will you use someone who is not involved in the work as an external evaluator?
- Who will be involved in the evaluation process? Will it involve the community, the workers, the funders, the steering group?
- What will you do with your evaluation findings? Will you publish a report? Who will be responsible for publication? Who will the evaluation report be distributed to? Who will own it? Will findings be widely disseminated, such as in journal articles?

(Based on ideas in DeGroot 1996.) Identify evaluation conflicts and ensure that your evaluation looks at process, impact and outcome, and identifies realistic ways of assessing what may be very small changes over long periods of time. It will probably not be possible to evaluate every element of a project so it may be necessary to prioritise which elements will be assessed.

It may be helpful to think in terms of charting changes as they occur, using a framework to record these systematically. An example of this approach is the outcome measures checklist used in a community health project described in Case study 15.2.

Stage 6. Setting an action plan

There are many things to consider here, but the main one is to identify what you plan to do, step by step.

You may need to build the following activities into an action plan:

Reviewing aims and priorities. It is necessary to review continuously the aims and priorities originally set down for the project, and compare them with those of the people who are now involved. You may need to modify the original aims, and regularly check that the agenda is meeting community needs.

Consulting and being accountable to the community. The community participation established at the outset needs to continue throughout. Once the project is established, you have a continuing responsibility to involve the community. This could be through meetings, newsletters, electronic networks and open days, for example.

Arranging a management committee or steering group. A management committee or steering group should provide a secure foundation for the project, taking responsibility for its continued development, its policies and management tasks such as fundraising and recruiting. It should also provide support for the project workers. Usually these are members of the group; they should not be expected to run the management committee themselves, but sometimes this is the case. This is not desirable because it leads to confusion about who is managing whom, and puts an unreasonable burden on the workers.

A management group could consist of both local workers, such as health visitors and social workers, and local people, perhaps representing the community groups involved in the project.

It may be helpful to get the members of a management committee/steering committee together for a day, to talk through the issues, clarify aims and foster a sense of teamwork.

Writing job descriptions. Paid project workers need clear job descriptions, specifying what is included. For example, does the job include fundraising, doing your own typing, servicing or even running the management committee meetings, keeping the accounts, evaluating, writing progress reports?

Ensuring support for the project workers. Recognise the value of networking as a means of informal training and support. Networking requires making time and other resources available to meet people doing similar work and to link with other community health projects in different parts of the country. This enables information and ideas to be shared and problems discussed. Access to e-mail and the Internet is essential. The need to ensure that project workers are not isolated is crucial.

Networking also means that more people will know about the project and you may get more support.

Formalising your project group. It may be helpful at some stage to look at the costs and benefits of formalising a project group that started off as a loose collection of interested people. The advantages of having a formal organisation are that it can apply for financial help and for recognition as a legitimate body; the disadvantages might be that control could be exercised from outside. The local Council for Voluntary Service can be extremely useful because it provides a helpful service for newly formed groups, and affiliation to the Council brings credibility in itself.

Dealing with opposition. The health issues the project is concerned with will probably have a local history, and be likely to have both won and lost support in the past. You need to identify opposition and plan a strategy for dealing with individuals or groups who may oppose the project.

Stage 7. Implementing your plan

As the project is implemented, it may run into difficulties because of a) flagging interest, b) lack of direction, and c) the project coming to an end.

Keeping going. Over time, the community may lose its enthusiasm. You may be able to provide additional impetus by being involved as a whole or part of your paid work. You need to be sensitive to the many ways in which a project can lose direction, and in such circumstances you may be able to help by:

● Discovering what similar activities are taking place elsewhere and circulating details.

CASE STUDY 15.2   A CHECKLIST FOR CHARTING CHANGES IN A COMMUNITY

A 3-year project ran on a housing estate where residents were identified as being at high risk for heart disease. Using a community development approach, a community health promoter worked with local residents on issues which residents identified as important. Over the life of the project, changes were noted, many of which became embedded as permanent features in the community. These changes were charted in a systematic way, using the following outcome measures checklist.

Type of change	Information recorded	Examples
Participation of target population in health-related action	Numbers and characteristics (age range, sex, etc.) of people who attend groups and community activities	Number and age range of young parents attending a new parent and toddler group
Perceived changes in knowledge, attitude and behaviour of target population	Changes in attitude towards participation in group and community activity; change in beliefs about ability to have control over one's own life and the power of group action; changes in the subjective experience of belonging to a community; changes in the capacity of local groups to identify problems and collaborate to solve these	Action group set up by local people to get better play facilities on the estate. Led to establishment of local playgroup run by local women. Many members stopped smoking
Changes in demand for health-related services	Changes in demand or requests for services or facilities	Groups requested talks from health visitors on health issues. Request for more accessible primary healthcare facilities on the estate
Changes in the availability of support, facilities and resources for people wanting to change lifestyle	Changes in group and community activities, informal social and support networks within the community	New groups to support young single parents. 'Get Cooking' group to help people learn to cook healthier food for their family. Exercise group for older people
Other physical changes to the environment	Any changes to the built or natural environment	Playground built. Traffic-calming schemes introduced
Changes in knowledge, attitudes, skills and practices of local health and allied workers	Changes in attitudes towards local residents to exercise choice and control over the services they receive, or changes in ways of working	Local health visitors use experienced local mothers to support young new parents
Changes in policy and procedures by local statutory and voluntary organisations	Changes that enable local people to have more say in decisions about local services	Consultation with local residents about location and design of new GP surgery on the estate
Dissemination of good practice	What information was sent out and why, talks, presentations, papers published and any evidence that good practice elsewhere has been affected	Article in community health journal. Community health projects featured in health authority public health report
Any other outcomes	Any other outcomes, expected or unexpected, which fall into the above categories	

(Based on Bruce et al 1996 and Ewles et al 1995, 1996.)

- Drawing the issue to the attention of relevant statutory agencies, and conveying the response to the group.
- Helping the group to produce its own health promotion materials such as posters, leaflets, Web site or video, and distributing them.
- Looking at other health promotion material on topics of interest.
- Encouraging members of the project to talk about their work to other people, such as groups of interested professionals and students.
- Sending memos or e-mails to everyone to remind them of meetings.
- Providing practical support such as photocopying or access to a computer.
- Introducing new members.

Working out what to do next. If you feel that you have lost direction, it can help to write down what information you have found, what contacts you have made, what needs and aims you have identified and what you have done so far. Then seek the views of your management/steering group (if there is one) or the impartial views of someone who has not been involved. Exercise 15.3 may help to provide a focus for working out what to do next.

EXERCISE 15.3 Planning community health promotion work

The following exercise may be useful when you are starting community health work or taking stock part way through a community health project.

Complete the following statements as fully as you can:

The key issue is ...
The people I need to consult/participate with are ...
The documents I need to read are ...
I can get to know more about the community by ...
The information that is likely to be available is ...
I intend to look for this information by ...
Work done on this issue elsewhere is ...
The people who are likely to be supportive are ...
The people I should avoid offending are ...
The period of time I can spend on this issue is ...
The amount of time I can give it during this period is ...
The person/people I will consult/participate with in order to work out what to do next are ...

Leavings and endings. There comes a point when your involvement has to stop, maybe because you change your job or the priorities of your work, or because the project work has been taken on by local people. Occasionally, you will need to recognise that you have done all you could do, and that there is now no potential in the project. Ending your involvement provides the opportunity for a final evaluation of what has been achieved and what your own contribution has been, and for making recommendations for future action.

DEVELOPING COMPETENCE IN COMMUNITY WORK

To be a successful community health worker, you need a range of competencies. You will also need to be committed to the principles and ideals of community-based work outlined earlier in this chapter: the centrality of the community, your own role as a facilitator rather than an expert, the importance of addressing inequalities and a broad perspective on health.

> See Chapter 1, section on inequalities in health and Chapter 3.

In order to adhere to these principles, you will need knowledge of key issues, such as the extent and cause of inequalities in health, the effects of racism, sexism and other forms of oppression on health, and awareness of the structures, policies and powers which influence the lives and health of communities. You will also need to be clear about your own particular political ideologies.

> See the section above on getting to know the community and its needs, Chapter 4, section on agents and agencies of health promotion and Exercise 4.1, and Chapter 6, section on finding and using information.

Other areas of knowledge include familiarity with local health resources: who and where to go to for information, advice and materials on health issues. Knowledge of local health services and social services is vital; so is understanding how local statutory and voluntary agencies work, and how to use the system effectively. An understanding of the community itself is of course vital.

A range of skills is required. It is important to have competencies in raising awareness of inequalities and discrimination, and being able to counter these by taking positive action when appropriate and working in an antidiscriminatory way.

See Chapters 5, 7, 8 for planning and managing; 10 for communication; 11 for using communication tools; 13 for working with groups.

Other skills link to working with people: being able to communicate well, facilitate groups and run effective meetings. You also need skills of planning and management, using and producing health promotion materials, and working for political change (Smithies 1987, North Cumbria Health Development Unit 2001).

PRACTICE POINTS

- Community-based health promotion involves working with communities (rather than individuals) over a period of time to enable them to increase control over, and improve, their health. It may involve community development work, specific community health projects and group work.

- A key principle is that community work is bottom up, not top down. This means that you respond to issues that the community identifies, rather than working on issues identified by people outside the community, such as health workers from statutory agencies.
- Community health workers take on the role of facilitators rather than health experts, to develop the community's abilities to both identify and meet health needs.
- Work is often focused on addressing inequalities and working with people who are disadvantaged.
- Health is interpreted holistically to encompass social, emotional and societal wellbeing.
- Community participation is fundamental to health planning and health promotion activity.
- You need particular skills and processes for successful community development work and community health projects. You need to be aware of the potential conflicts and difficulties inherent in this kind of work.

References

Adams L, Smithies J (eds) 1990 Community participation and health promotion. London, Health Education Authority.

ASH Scotland 2003 Evaluating community development work: briefing paper 3: the tobacco and inequalities project. Edinburgh, ASH Scotland.

Brager G, Specht H 1973 Community organizing. New York, Columbia University Press.

Bruce N, Springett J, Hotchkiss J, Scott-Samuel A 1996 Research and change in urban community health. Aldershot, Avebury.

Communities and Local Government and Involve 2008 Community power pack: real people, real power. http://www.communities. gov.uk/publications/communities/ communitypowerpack.

Coulthard M, Walker A, Morgan A 2002 People's perception of their neighbourhood and community involvement. London, The Stationery Office.

DeGroot R 1996 Much is written, but little is read. Community Health Action 1(41): 3.

Department for Communities and Local Government 2006 Strong and prosperous communities – the local government White Paper. London, The Stationery Office.

Department for Communities and Local Government 2008 Communities in control: real people, real power. London, The Stationery Office.

Department for Communities and Local Government 2009 Communities in control: real people, real power. Government response to the improving local accountability consultation. London, The Stationery Office.

Ewles L, Miles U, Velleman, G 1995 Promoting heart health on an urban housing estate. Community Health Action 1(35): 12–14.

Ewles L, Miles U, Velleman G 1996 Lessons learnt from a community heart disease prevention project.

Journal of the Institute of Health Education 34(1): 15–19.

Foley R, Platzer H 2007 Place and provision: mapping mental health advocacy services in London. Social Science and Medicine 64(3): 617–632.

Green J, South J 2006 Evaluation. Maidenhead, Open University Press.

Labyrinth Consultancy 2000 Community participation for health: a review of good practice in community participation health projects and initiatives. London, Health Education Authority.

London Community Health Resource and National Council for Voluntary Organisations 1987 Guide to community health projects. London, National Community Health Resource.

Morgan A, Swann C 2004 Social capital for health: issues of definition, measurement and links to health. London, Health Development Agency.

North Cumbria Health Development Unit 2001 Building healthy communities: a resource pack for multi-agency health improvement. Wokingham, North Cumbria Health Development Unit.

Rosato M, Laverack G, Grabman LH et al 2008 Community participation: lessons for maternal, newborn, and child health. Lancet 372: 962–971.

Scriven A 2007 Developing local alliance partnerships through community collaboration and participation. In: Handsley S, Lloyd CE, Douglas J et al (eds) Policy and practice in promoting public health. London, Sage.

Smithies J 1987 Training needs of community health workers. National Community Health Resource. Unpublished report on community health workers' training project.

World Health Organization 1986 The Ottawa charter for health promotion. Geneva, WHO.

Websites

http://www.biglotteryfund.org.uk/prog_reaching_communities.htm
http://www.communities.gov.uk/publications/communities/communitypowerpack
http://www.lchpf.co.uk/bewell.htm
http://www.lchpf.co.uk/changes.htm
http://www.partnerships.org.uk
http://www.prospects.ac.uk/p/types_of_job/community_development_worker_job_description.jsp
http://www.stockton.gov.uk/yourcouncil/egenda/cllrsvirtualwardsurg
http://twitter.com/CommunitiesUK
http://twitter.com/ncvo
http://www.youtube.com/NCVOonline
http://en.wikipedia.org/wiki/Community

Chapter 16

Influencing and implementing policy

SUMMARY

The focus of this chapter is on how health policy at local and national level is made, how it can be influenced and how health promoters can challenge health damaging policies. The characteristics of power and the politics of influence are discussed and illustrated with a case study. There are sections on developing and implementing policies, a case study on the politics of influence and an exercise on policy implementation. The chapter ends with a section on planning a policy campaign.

See Chapter 7, section on linking your work into broader health promotion plans and strategies, for information on national and local public health strategies and plans.

Health promoters have an important role in influencing and implementing policies that affect health. A policy is a broad statement of the principles of how to proceed in relation to a specific issue and can be at a number of levels, from international (see Duncan 2002 for a debate on the way EU health policy impacts on UK policy), to national, regional and organisational level.

In order to influence policy you need to understand how power is distributed and exercised between people at various levels and be able to use that knowledge to further your work and shape policy decisions. In other words, you need to be political.

Another relevant and important aspect of policy is managing change, discussed in Chapter 8.

Being a policy activist involves working with statutory, voluntary and commercial organisations to influence the development of health promoting policies. It also includes working for healthy public policies (see Scriven 2007 for a detailed overview of healthy public policies) and economic and regulatory changes that might require campaigning, lobbying and taking political action.

MAKING AND INFLUENCING LOCAL AND NATIONAL HEALTH POLICY

Working for policy change is an integral part of health promotion action, with health promoters able to press for the introduction of policies at both national and local levels and influence how they are implemented. The development of local health policies cannot be divorced from the central government's policies that shape the organisation and funding of health service, local authority and voluntary agency work at a local level. National policy is in turn influenced by consultation with and representations from health services, local authorities and voluntary agencies.

Other bodies such as national health promotion agencies and public health organisations such as the Royal Society for Public Health (http://www.rsph.org.uk) are also highly influential in the field of policy development. For an example of a national agency contribution to policy, see the report of the 20-year legacy of the Health Promotion Agency (HPA) of Northern Ireland (HPA 2009).

LOCAL HEALTH POLICY

At a local level, during the last decade healthy public policies and priorities have increasingly been jointly agreed by health, local authority and voluntary agencies. This has been made easier through national policy initiatives such as the implementation of local strategic partnerships (LSPs), where health and partner agencies are required to deliver joint plans for health and wellbeing. This means that policies have to be agreed by local authorities, primary care trusts (PCTs) and other relevant community organisations.

The structure of the NHS, including PCTs and strategic health authorities, is outlined in Chapter 4; see Figure 4.2.

Some health organisations and local authorities undertake health impact assessments (HIAs) or environmental impact assessments of their services and related policies. The Association of Health Observatories Health Impact Assessment gateway has many examples of HIAs at http://www.apho.org.uk (see, for example, Health Inequality Impact Assessment into the Leicester LIFT project). HIA involves examining the impact on health and/or the environment of all current and planned policies and activities. The purpose is to develop practical ways in which current health and environmental impact of services could be improved and to inform the development of a corporate approach to new health and environmental policies.

See Chapter 7, section on health impact assessment.

HEALTH POLICY IN THE NHS

The task of commissioning health services and programmes was undertaken by health authorities until 2002, when it passed to PCTs. *Commissioning* health services means deciding what health services, policies and programmes are needed to improve the health status of the local population and ensuring that they are provided.

PCTs provide opportunities for the public to comment on health service plans. There are representatives of the public on PCT management boards (usually called lay representatives) and PCTs generally consult the public on any significant proposals for policy change. Individuals, groups, professional associations and others are able to express their views on, for example, the balance of money spent on treatment and care compared with health promotion and disease prevention. Some PCT board members have responsibility for ensuring that the PCT properly addresses specific policy areas such as inequalities in health.

IMPLEMENTING NATIONAL HEALTH POLICIES AT LOCAL LEVEL

National strategies for health are outlined in detail in Chapter 7, and referred to in Chapters 1 and 4.

National strategies for health have been in place since the early 1990s with targets that set specific health outcomes. PCTs and partner agencies from the public, private and voluntary sectors translate these national targets into local ones, and may add other local targets. These targets, and the priorities and objectives they are derived from, are an important influence on policies and on health promotion programmes and activities.

For example, the *National Service Framework for Coronary Heart Disease* (Department of Health (DoH) 2000a), a policy document setting out the standards for services about prevention and treatment, has national targets for reduced death rates and changes in risk behaviour, such as smoking. These targets are translated into local targets that include health promotion programmes on smoking prevention, such as providing smoking cessation help as part of maternity services. In this way, national policies and strategies influence directly local interventions. For an assessment of the impact and progress toward implementing the *Coronary Heart Disease National Service Framework* in the 8 years since its publication, see DoH 2008.

See also Chapter 7, section on local health strategies and initiatives, for more on local plans and strategies.

LOCAL AUTHORITY CONTRIBUTION TO HEALTH POLICY

The local authority contribution to health policy is made at a strategic level through LSPs and the development of local area agreements (LAA). LAAs simplify some central funding, help join up public services more effectively and allow greater flexibility to develop policies to meet local health needs (for further details on LAAs, see http://www.communities.gov.uk).

LSPs bring together people from the public, private and voluntary sectors. They aim to avoid duplication and to rationalise partnerships and plans to make it easier to deliver policies around health improvement, education and crime. The Neighbourhood Renewal Strategy (Social Exclusion Unit 2001) is a catalyst for these partnerships and plans and has a direct impact on health gain (see Leathard 2003, for a critical overview of the link between NHS LSP and community strategies).

See also Chapter 7, section on local health strategies and initiatives, for more about local plans and strategies.

Another important way in which health services and local authorities can work together at local level is through cooperating in implementing international agreements such as the UN Agenda 21 and Millennium Development Goals (http://www.un.org). These are agreements forged by governments at international levels, which focus on ways of achieving sustainable development in relation to the environment and the wider determinants of health.

Local authorities have to work with a broad range of agencies and consult their communities about developments in relation to implementing international polices at a local level. Health promoters, in both their working role and their role as private citizens, can play their part.

THE VOICE OF THE CONSUMER IN THE NHS

In *The NHS Plan* (DoH 2000b) the government made a clear commitment to being responsive to the needs of all citizens by allowing their voices to be heard in relation to health-related public policies, planning and provision of services.

A number of steps have been taken to enable consumers to express their views. One example of this is the NHS Constitution for England (DoH 2009) which makes important pledges in relation to how people access NHS services, what commitment people can expect from the NHS and what their rights and responsibilities are in terms of influencing policy and service provision. A patient advice and liaison service (PALS) (http://www.pals.nhs.uk) was set up in every NHS trust for patients to get their concerns addressed. Other measures introduced to ensure that citizens and patients have more influence at all levels of the NHS include:

- Increased lay representation, such as on the National Leadership Network for Health and Social Care (http://www.nationalleadershipnetwork.org) and the Care Quality Commission (http://www.cqc.org.uk). See *Voices into Action* (Care Quality Commission 2009) for details of how lay voices are heard.
- A new Citizens' Council, to advise the National Institute for Health and Clinical Excellence (NICE). The Citizens Council brings the views of the public to NICE decision making about guidance on the promotion of good health and the prevention and treatment of illhealth. A group of people drawn from all walks of life, the Citizens Council tackles challenging questions about values, such as fairness and need (http://www.nice.org.uk).

While the means for lay involvement are in place, a recent review by the government select committee on health (House of Commons Health Committee 2009a,b) suggests that there is a risk the NHS may still not be engaging the public in a meaningful way.

CHALLENGING POLICY

As a heath promoter you may find you are expected to implement policies that you perceive as health damaging or contrary to health promotion principles. This can be difficult because such policies can emanate from national government or your employing organisation or even your direct manager. To challenge may create a conflict of loyalty between wanting to press for what you see as right and what is decreed to be right by your employing authority. To protest may be seen as too political. There is no easy answer to this issue, but there are some positive steps worth considering.

- **Use your vote**. At the next general or local election, look at the health implications in the policy manifestos. Raise questions about health policy with doorstep canvassers, at public meetings and by writing to candidates. All this can be done in your capacity as a private citizen rather than a health worker.
- **Use your professional association or trade union**. These groups can raise issues at a national and local level, and can be a powerful voice. You can play your part by joining and supporting their activities, and raising the issues you feel strongly about.
- **Use your representative**. There are many people whose job is to represent your interests. At European Union or national level, it is your Member of the European Parliament (MEP) or your MP. So if you want to raise an issue at these levels, lobby your MEP or MP: send letters, telephone, attend politicians' surgeries. At local level, do the same with your local councillor. You could also contact your professional association or union local branch representative.
- **Use your collective power**. If you are concerned about an issue at your place of work, it may help to find out if colleagues feel the same. If they do, join together so that you raise the issue collectively: this can give it more impact. Or at a national level, join with others

who share your concern to improve health and challenge health damaging policies. For example, members of the UK Public Health Association (UKPHA) aim to widen the focus of health policy in the UK towards creating a healthy environment, reducing inequalities and improving quality of life.

However, many areas of policy development are not controversial, and can be a positive and rewarding part of the day-to-day work of health promoters. The main thrust is likely to be in developing, changing and implementing local policies. To do this you need to understand the characteristics of power and influence and be competent at exerting influence when necessary.

CHARACTERISTICS OF POWER AND INFLUENCE

Power is the ability to influence others. There are four generally recognised types of power that are relevant to health promotion work:

1. **Position power** is the power vested in someone because of their position in an organisation. For example, a Director of Public Health has position power.
2. **Resource power** is the power to allocate, or limit, resources, including money and staff. It often goes hand-in-hand with position power. For example, a senior health service manager has both position power and the power to regulate the use of resources. You have a source of power if you have the authority to control the allocation of any resources. Every health promoter will have some power because people want the skills or services on offer.
3. **Expert power** is power related to expertise. Directors of Public Health have the expert power associated with their specialty.
4. **Personal power** is the power that comes from the personal attributes of a person, including strong personality, charisma and ability to inspire. It is closely related to leadership qualities and intelligence, initiative, self-confidence and the ability to rise above a situation and see it in perspective. However, effective leaders are not always charismatic, and what makes a leader effective in one situation may cause them to be less effective in changed circumstances. The classic example of this is Sir Winston Churchill. The attributes that

made him effective in wartime were not so appropriate in peacetime.

You may sometimes be in the position of wanting or needing to exert influence on people who have a stronger power base. For example, a health visitor may wish to influence a general practitioner to adopt a policy of supporting the running of ante-natal clinics in the local ethnic minority group's community centre, or a community worker may want to lobby local councillors about the need for more recreational facilities for young people on a housing estate. To do this requires skills in influencing and negotiation (see Cialdini 2007 and 2008 for overviews on the science and practice of influence and the power of persuasion).

Before attempting to influence someone who has position or resource power, first consider the basic questions in the planning process, such as: What are your aims? What resources do you need? Is the investment of your time in influencing others going to be worth it? Could the aim be achieved more easily another way?

> See Chapter 5, Planning and evaluating health promotion.

THE POLITICS OF INFLUENCE

There are four key elements of a strategy aiming to change policy:

1. planning
2. making allies
3. networking
4. making deals and negotiating.

Planning

Three particular aspects of planning are useful to consider: undertaking a force field analysis, identifying stakeholders and considering your timing.

Undertake a force field analysis. A force field analysis identifies the helping and hindering forces and helps to pinpoint how you can influence the process to make progress towards change. You identify how you can increase the power of the helping forces and decrease the power of the hindering forces.

> There is an example of a force field analysis at the end of Chapter 4, Exercise 4.2.

Identify the stakeholders. The stakeholders are those people with a vested interest in the issue, who wish to influence what is done and how it is done.

They are obviously powerful forces in the situation. It could be difficult to identify all the stakeholders, because some of them may not wish to be visible and try to work covertly through others.

Time your action. It is also important to consider when to introduce a proposal or when to delay. If people are already preoccupied with other major issues, it might not be the right time to make a new proposal. On the other hand, if a proposal will help other people to attain their own objectives, it will be a good time.

Making allies

Identify which of the stakeholders could be allies, and gain their trust and confidence in order to establish and maintain an alliance. It helps to pay attention to their concerns, values, beliefs and behaviour patterns, and to see what you need to do in order to form an effective working alliance.

For example, if you are concerned about the way in which people with disabilities are treated in an organisation, you might identify the person in charge of human resources as a key stakeholder. So find out if they are concerned about it and if they think it is important for the organisation. What kind of way do they work, are they likely to respond best to a lively discussion on the subject or to a well argued paper on the need for policy, backed up with facts and figures? Do they like time to make decisions? Will they be happy to leave you to take the lead, or will they want ownership of the initiative?

Networking

Many people working in organisations belong to one or more interest groups who meet to discuss, debate and exchange information on issues that concern the members. By playing an active role in these networks, people can extend their influence. Networks provide access to information that can help with making a case, to people with experience of successful influencing, and to other resources. There are different types of networks:

Professional networks. Members are from the same profession. Professional networks may attempt to influence employers and organisations to reconsider their policies or to develop new policies for the future. Professional networks institute criteria for professional practice and are active in the professional development of their members.

Elitist networks. Members of an elitist group can join by invitation only. The network operates by personal contact and personal introduction. Members of such networks may have considerable power and influence, often through their position in organisations.

Pressure groups. Members wish to pursue certain objectives, which may be environmental, social or political. In order to enter a particular network it may be necessary to identify the gatekeepers who control entry, and other people who are influential in the network and could act as a sponsor for someone seeking to join. Having entered a network it is important to support the values and established ways of working. Later, having been accepted, it may be possible to challenge accepted practices.

Making deals and negotiating

Making deals is common practice in most organisations. Individuals or groups agree to support a proposal in return for agreement on something that benefits them. In order to make deals successfully, it pays to know the person with whom you are dealing, paying careful attention to their values and intentions and what you could realistically expect from them.

Negotiation is the art of creating agreement on a specific issue between two or more parties with different views. Successful negotiation takes place when there is a desire to solve problems and the parties genuinely commit to going through a number of steps. There are many guides on how to improve your negotiation skills. While these are mainly written for the business community, the skills are also relevant to health promotion. See, for example, Hawver (2007).

ON BEING POLITICAL

A final point is about political behaviour, which refers to finding out about who holds power, and working to use this information to change a situation. When is it acceptable and when is it unethical?

Being political can be considered devious and manipulative. Some people may view it with suspicion and will therefore not be easily influenced by such behaviour. To manipulate covertly, or coerce, lie or deliberately withhold information that affects others is unethical and unprofessional. But to ignore the politics within organisations is unwise, because it results in failure to make a realistic appraisal of situations, and failure to make the best of the opportunities for positive health promotion. Furthermore, it is possible to be political without losing professional integrity: for example, by ensuring deals are made as the outcome of open negotiations, and that relationships should be based on genuineness, trust, goodwill and mutual respect. Case study 16.1 offers an example of the politics of influence in practice.

DEVELOPING AND IMPLEMENTING POLICIES

There are numerous kinds of health promotion policies. Many are about health issues that relate to workplaces or other settings such as schools, communities and hospitals. Other policies can be about health issues in a range of contexts, such as a national policy on teenage pregnancies, which would cover action across many different settings (Department for Children, Schools and Families 2008). For some health issues, such as alcohol in the workplace, it is common practice to have a policy (http://www.alcoholpolicy.net).

POLICIES ON PROMOTING HEALTH IN WORKPLACES

The benefits of health promotion at work are well established and reviews of the literature identify the major benefits as a decrease in absenteeism and staff turnover, and an increase in productivity and morale (Fleming 2007). The European Network for Workplace Health Promotion (http://www.enwhp.org) has a range of publications that will support policy development that encourages employers and trade unions to take on a wider concept of health at work, including giving priority to issues such as smoking, alcohol and stress. The World Health Organization (WHO) also has a number of guidelines on supporting workplace policy development on issues such as mental health (for example, WHO 2005).

In the UK in 2008, the cross-government Work, Health and Wellbeing programme published *Improving Health and Work: Changing Lives* (http://www.workingforhealth.gov.uk). It was the government's response to *Working for a Healthier Tomorrow* (Black 2008) and follows the launch in 2005 of the Work, Health and Wellbeing Programme, which is

CASE STUDY 16.1 THE POLITICS OF INFLUENCE – HEALTH AND SAFETY AT WORK

Bob is an environmental health officer working for Midshire City Council. His aim is to improve the implementation of the health and safety at work policy of the council. He makes a list of the *helping* forces and the *hindering* forces:

Helping:

- the existing safety officers
- existing codes of practice, for example sight checks for VDU operators
- a councillor who is a health lecturer at the university
- a human resources officer interested in improving the working environment for staff
- an existing commitment to appoint an occupational health nurse.

Hindering:

- the cost of any improvements (the council has severe financial constraints)
- staff time to attend health and safety training
- problems with recruiting an occupational health nurse
- deficiencies in the structure of council buildings (poor ventilation, open-plan offices, lack of showers for those staff wishing to take physical exercise during the day)
- lack of councillors' commitment to improve health and safety conditions for staff
- lack of access to council buildings for disabled people.

He identifies the stakeholders as:

- the staff themselves
- the trade unions
- departmental managers, senior and chief officers
- the councillors
- the public health specialist and the health promotion specialist from the local PCT.

He further identifies key stakeholders as:

- officers in the department of engineering because they enforce building regulations
- council members on the health committee
- the director of personnel.

He then identifies ways of increasing the helping forces and decreasing the hindering forces. Through making an ally of the interested human resources officer he is able to increase the commitment of the director of human resources, who is also a chief officer. One short-term outcome is that an occupational health nurse is recruited. Another outcome is a plan agreed by the human resources department and the trade unions for training staff in health and safety.

By joining a local network of people interested in health promotion he is able to find out what is going on elsewhere, and this gives him some useful ideas, including sources of help in stress management training which he incorporates into the training plan.

He makes a deal with the engineering department by agreeing to assist with monitoring construction sites of new buildings in order to prevent accidents on the site. In return, they agree to assist with a plan for improving soundproofing and modifications to open-plan offices. Their commitment grows after a report shows that accidents on construction sites are reduced. He discusses with them the issue of raising with council members the plan for modifying council buildings.

Finally, he makes an ally of the councillor at the university by offering to provide an input to some of the courses. This councillor is on the health committee and provides him with useful advice on how to approach the committee and how to prepare documents for its consideration.

---

sponsored by five government partners: the Department for Work and Pensions, the Department of Health, the Health and Safety Executive, the Scottish Government and the Welsh Assembly Government. Work, Health and Wellbeing is an initiative to protect and improve the health and wellbeing of working age people. It encourages workplace wellness policies through such tools as The Business HealthCheck.

In the UK, the Health and Safety Executive is also a source of information on all statutory policies

governing health and safety in the workplace (http://www.hse.gov.uk).

POLICIES ON PROMOTING HEALTH IN HOSPITALS

Health Promoting Hospitals is a WHO initiative, designed to improve health and environmental conditions for both staff and patients by reviewing and implementing a range of health promoting policies (http://www.euro.who.int). Many hospitals have taken up the idea of being a health promoting hospital, but it can be difficult in practice to inform and involve everyone in an institution as large and complex as a hospital (Whitehead 2004, Groene 2005).

PROMOTING HEALTH IN URBAN SETTINGS: HEALTHY CITIES

The WHO's Healthy Cities initiative promotes comprehensive and systematic policy and planning with a special emphasis on health inequalities and urban poverty, the needs of vulnerable groups, participatory governance and the social, economic and environmental determinants of health. It also strives to include health considerations in economic, regeneration and urban development efforts. It aims to work from the bottom up, not from the top down, and to involve collaborative work between local government, health authorities, local businesses, community organisations and, of course, individual citizens (http://www.euro.who. int; see also Lawrence & Fudge 2007).

See Chapter 15 for principles of bottom-up working.

The Health for All (UK) Network is a coordinating body for action on Healthy Cities within the UK (http://independent.livjm.ac.uk). The Healthy Cities work in Belfast is a good example of what is being achieved (http://www.belfasthealthycities. com).

POLICIES ON PROMOTING HEALTH IN SCHOOLS

The European Network of Health Promoting Schools (ENHPS), now known as Schools for Health In Europe (http://www.schoolsforhealth.eu), sets out to show that schools can be powerful agents for change through the adoption of whole-school approaches. This means that the school promotes health not only by curriculum policies which includes sufficient time for social, personal and health education for the pupils, but also by wider school policies that ensure that the school promotes a sense of positive self-esteem and the health and wellbeing of teachers and other staff, parents and the wider community who have contact with the school. An evaluation found there was evidence that the policies implemented as a result of the health promoting school initiative have some influence on various domains of health for the school community (Mükoma & Flisher 2004).

See Chapter 4, section on local authorities, for more about health promotion in educational institutions.

The UK government's commitment to the whole-school approach to health is strong, as can be seen from their support of the Healthy Schools programme, which has become one of the country's most widely embraced initiatives in schools.

Health promotion in the education sector also covers higher education settings, such as universities (Dooris 2002, Dooris & Martin 2002).

POLICIES ON PROMOTING HEALTH IN PRISONS

The WHO coordinates the Health in Prisons Project (HIPP) (http://www.euro.who.int) to promote health in prisons, and is working to develop an award scheme for health promoting prisons. See also Department of Health (2002) for the UK policy on health in prisons.

For a useful overview of the effectiveness of health promotion using a settings approach and related policies see Dooris (2009).

GUIDELINES ON DEVELOPING AND IMPLEMENTING A POLICY

Many health promoters have a role in developing and implementing polices in specific settings such as those discussed above. An example is the workplace alcohol policy outlined in Exercise 16.1. The process of developing and implementing a health promotion policy involves four aspects: preparation, implementation, education and training, and evaluation (adapted from Simnett & Chiles 1989 and Sheffield City Council Health and Consumer Services 1989).

1. Preparation of the policy

The formulation of a policy by any organisation is a corporate matter, so the usual starting point is to convene a working group. This group:

- Clarifies its terms of reference and elects a Chair.
- Identifies the need for a policy.

EXERCISE 16.1   A workplace alcohol policy

Westshire NHS Hospital Trust is encouraged by a national sensible drinking initiative to develop a policy on alcohol for its workforce.

A senior health promotion specialist working with Westshire Trust convenes a working group to develop a policy, which includes representatives of human resources officers, general management, consultant psychiatrists, trade unions and the local voluntary organisation on alcohol.

The working group meets four times, and produces a draft policy. The policy specifies that the trust sees sensible drinking as everyone's responsibility and that all employees will receive basic information about sensible drinking. It also covers the trust's responsibility to develop an environment conducive to self-referral by anyone with an alcohol problem, early identification of alcohol-related problems and the provision of expert confidential help. It looks at the provision of alcohol on trust premises, and specifies that nonalcoholic drinks should be provided as an alternative at all social functions where alcohol is served, and that alcohol consumption should be discouraged at nonsocial functions.

This draft policy goes to the trust board. It receives a lukewarm reception, and there is much concern that it will interfere with personnel policies on dealing with people who drink on duty. There is also discussion and disagreement about what constitutes a social and a nonsocial function, and resistance to the idea of curtailing social drinking, such as selling alcohol at the employees' bar and serving it at working lunches, publicity events such as the opening of new clinics and leaving parties.

Nevertheless, it is passed for consultation, and comes back to the board for final approval. The board members are still unenthusiastic, and one major change they make alters the working group's recommendations on implementation. These were that many different staff groups had a key role, including human resources, health promotion, general management and the training department. This is changed so that responsibility for implementation rests entirely with the trust Director of Human Resources. The alcohol policy is finally approved formally by the trust board.

In the meantime, the trust has been engaged in a major strategic review that has affected many of its services, and there follows a long period of substantial organisational change. Two years after the alcohol policy was approved, it had still not been implemented. There had been no education of the workforce about sensible drinking and no change in the way alcohol was served and sold on trust premises.

Looking at the stages for developing and implementing a workplace policy in the section above, and the section on the politics of influence, consider these questions:

- What steps were taken that facilitated policy development?
- What else could have been done?
- Why did the policy receive such a lukewarm reception by the trust board? Could anything have been done to prevent this?
- Why was the policy never implemented? Could anything have been done to ensure that the implementation stage actually happened?
- Are there any other significant points to note about the lessons learnt from this example?

- Identifies the committee, department or senior person who has overall responsibility for taking the policy forward.
- Identifies key personnel to consult with and convince of the need for a policy.
- Establishes a timescale for policy development.
- Prepares a draft policy and consults widely.
- Prepares the final draft policy for approval.

In the case of a workplace policy, it is important to involve trade unions. This can be achieved either by including trade union representatives on the working group or by setting up an effective framework for consultation and negotiation. This may be crucial in persuading the workforce to look positively on the new policy.

It is also important that an identified senior member of staff or manager, with political influence, acts as a champion for the policy. This person will be crucial in getting the commitment of other managers to the policy.

2. Implementation of the policy

This starts with planning, which will include:

- Setting aims and objectives.
- Setting up a system for monitoring and evaluation.

- Identifying resources and defining key implementation tasks.
- Defining the role of key personnel.
- Developing an action plan.

Key personnel should be encouraged to participate actively in identifying their roles and in discussing boundaries and overlap in roles, so that the potential for conflict and confusion is reduced. For example, managers have the primary responsibility for ensuring that their staff are fully conversant with workplace policies and understand what is expected of them. Nevertheless, the trade unions also have a role in informing the workforce of the policy. These sources of information hopefully will be complementary and spell out the same, not contradictory, messages. The open discussion of these issues will help to increase commitment to making the policy work.

Any policy that is not the subject of regular review risks becoming obsolete. So the working group must reconvene at intervals to consider issues such as the following:

- Does the workforce know about and understand the policy?
- Have attitudes changed to the health issue covered by the policy? If so, how? How do staff feel about the policy?
- Has the behaviour of individual staff changed? Does this include changes in working practices and/or individual lifestyles?
- Are staff getting the help they need?
- Are managers and trade unions supporting the policy?
- Are indicators showing that the policy is making progress towards the attainment of its aims and objectives? For example, in the case of a workplace policy, have absenteeism and sickness reduced? Or have accident rates decreased? Has work performance improved? Is morale better?
- How can we improve the effectiveness of the policy?

3. Education and training

This is a continuous process, not a one-off event. Wherever possible it should be integrated into existing provision for professional and managerial staff development. The purposes of education and training include the following:

- Securing the commitment of management (such as elected members, chief officers and senior management in the case of a local authority).
- Obtaining the commitment of the whole workforce or group at which the policy is aimed (such as the prison population or the staff of a business).
- Providing those responsible for implementing the policy with the necessary skills.
- Overcoming prejudices, discrimination and stereotyping where relevant (for example, in policies on alcohol and HIV/AIDS).
- Encouraging and assisting the workforce, or the particular groups of people the policy is concerned with, to make choices and individual lifestyle changes.

4. Evaluation

This should include evaluation of both process and outcomes. It will require the collection of information, both baseline and ongoing.

See Chapter 5, section on planning evaluation methods for further suggestions.

CAMPAIGNING

You, or clients with whom you work, may feel strongly about changing policy or practice about a health issue, and decide that the way forward is to mount a campaign.

Policy campaigns can range from short-lived local campaigns with the objective of making a single change to long-term national campaigns. Examples of a national pressure group campaigning for policy change is Action on Smoking and Health (ASH), which is a campaigning public health charity that works to eliminate the harm caused by tobacco. ASH has a list of policy issues on their website http://www.ash.org.uk, which includes inequalities in health.

Some pressure groups (such as Shelter) may provide direct services as well as acting as a pressure group.

PRINCIPLES OF CAMPAIGNING FOR POLICY CHANGE

Some important principles to keep in mind if you are setting up a policy campaign (originally adapted from Wilson 1984) are:

- **Be persistent:** success requires persistent effort, so you must be committed and prepared to put in a lot of time and energy over a long period.
- **Be professional:** give care and attention to details (such as well-written campaign materials with the name of the campaign clearly evident), and ensure that activities such as keeping records are undertaken properly.
- **Keep a sense of perspective:** your campaign may be vitally important to you, but being perceived as fanatical will do your cause no good.
- **Reflect your ideals:** it is no good, for example, campaigning for changes to equal opportunities policy if your own organisation does not have good access for people with disabilities.
- **Be positive:** Shelter is called the National Campaign for the Homeless, not the Campaign against Bad Housing.
- **Join with others:** rival pressure groups campaigning on similar (or even identical) issues waste a lot of time, effort and other resources. If someone is already campaigning on your issue, join them rather than setting up a rival organisation. Or if there is more than one organisation working on similar issues, form a coalition.
- **Involve as many people as possible:** this not only harnesses support but also informs people about what is wrong and what needs to change.

PLANNING A POLICY CAMPAIGN

When you plan a policy campaign, it helps to go through the same planning process as you would with any other kind of health promotion activity.

See also Chapter 5 for help with planning that applies to planning a campaign.

- Identify your aims clearly.
- Decide the best way of achieving them (public meetings? press coverage? lobbying MPs and local councillors? a petition?).

- Identify your resources (do you need to fundraise?).
- Clarify how you will know if your aim is achieved (set milestones and specific outcomes?).
- Set an action plan of who is going to do what and when.

PRACTICE POINTS

- Recognise that you and all health promoters have a role in influencing policy at national, local and at the organizational level.
- Influencing policy requires careful planning and timing. You need to know how national and local health promotion policy is created, developed and changed, and how you can have a voice by commenting on proposals and plans.
- Know the rights and standards you can expect from NHS services, and comment on those which you and your clients receive.
- Challenge health damaging policy by working with others, using your vote and by collective action.
- Identify how you could be more effective in influencing policy through reviewing your skills in planning, networking, negotiating and joint working.
- Start policy change by identifying key stakeholders and looking at issues from each of their viewpoints; use techniques such as force field analysis to establish how to move forward.
- When campaigning on health issues, pay attention to careful planning and be persistent, professional and positive; involve as many other people as possible.
- Keep the ethical aspects of activities in mind when campaigning, lobbying and working towards changing health policy and practice; work with other people to build up trust and mutual respect.

References

Black C 2008 Working for a healthier tomorrow. London, The Stationery Office.

Care Quality Commission 2009 Voices into action. London, The Stationery Office.

Cialdinin RB 2007 Influence: the psychology of persuasion, 2nd edn. New York, HarperBusiness.

Cialdini RB 2008 Influence: science and practice, 5th edn. Oxford, Pearson Education.

Department for Children, Schools and Families 2008 Teenage parents: who cares? A guide to commissioning and delivering maternity services for young parents, 2nd edn. Nottingham, DCSF.

Department of Health 2000a National service framework for coronary heart disease. London, The Stationery Office.

Department of Health 2000b The NHS plan. A plan for investment. A plan for reform. London, The Stationery Office.

Department of Health 2002 Health promoting prisons: a shared approach. London, The Stationery Office.

Department of Health 2008 The coronary heart disease national service framework: building on excellence, maintaining progress – Progress report for 2008. London, The Stationery office.

Department of Health 2009 The NHS constitution: the NHS belongs to us all. London, The Stationery Office.

Dooris M 2002 The health promoting university: opportunities, challenges and future developments. Promotion & Education Supplement 1: 20–24.

Dooris M 2009 Holistic and sustainable health improvement: the contribution of the settings-based approach to health promotion. Perspective in Public Health 129(1): 29–36.

Dooris M, Martin E 2002 The health promoting university – from idea to implementation. Promotion & Education Supplement 1: 16–19.

Duncan B 2002 Health policy in the European Union: how it's made and how to influence it. British Medical Journal 324: 1027–1030.

Fleming P 2007 Workplaces as setting for public health development. In: Scriven A, Garman G 2007 Public health: social context and action. Maidenhead, Open University Press.

Groene O 2005 Evaluating the progress of health promoting hospitals' initiative. A WHO perspective.

Health Promotion International 20(2): 205–207.

Hawver DA 2007 How to improve your negotiation skills. India, Vision Books

Health Promotion Agency of Northern Ireland 2009 A healthy legacy. 20 years of the Health Promotion Agency for Northern Ireland. Belfast, HPANI.

House of Commons Health Committee 2009a NHS Next stage review: first report of session 2008–09: volume I report, together with formal minutes. London, The Stationery Office.

House of Commons Health Committee 2009b NHS Next stage review: first report of session 2008–09: volume II oral and written evidence. London, The Stationery Office.

Lawrence R, Fudge C 2007 Healthy Cities: key principles for professional practice. In: Scriven A, Garman G 2007 Public health: social context and action. Maidenhead, Open University Press.

Leathard A 2003 Policy overview. In: Leathard A (ed.) Interprofessional collaboration: from policy to practice in health and social care. Sussex, Brunner Routledge.

Mükoma W, Flisher AJ 2004 Evaluations of health promoting schools: a review of nine studies. Health Promotion International 19(3): 357–368.

Scriven A 2007 Healthy public policies: rhetoric or reality. In: Scriven A, Garman G 2007 Public health: social context and action. Maidenhead, Open University Press.

Sheffield City Council Health and Consumer Services 1989 Guidelines for local authorities on the development, implementation and evaluation of an alcohol policy for their staff. London, Health Education Authority.

Simnett I, Chiles M 1989 A practical guide to developing and implementing alcohol policies. Bristol, Frenchay Health Authority.

Social Exclusion Unit 2001 A new commitment to neighbourhood renewal. national strategy action plan. London, The Stationery Office.

Whitehead D 2004 The European Health Promoting Hospitals HPH project: how far on? Health Promotion International 19(2): 259–267.

Wilson D 1984 Pressure: the A to Z of campaigning in Britain. London, Heinemann.

World Health Organization 2005 Mental health policy and programmes in the workplace. Geneva, WHO.

Websites

http://www.alcoholpolicy.net/workplace

http://apho.org.uk/resource/item.aspx?RID=44154

http://www.ash.org.uk

http://www.belfasthealthycities.com

http://www.communities.gov.uk

http://www.cqc.org.uk

http://www.enwhp.org

http://www.euro.who.int/healthpromohosp

http://www.euro.who.int/Healthy-cities

http://www.euro.who.int/prisons

http://www.hse.gov.uk

http://independent.livjm.ac.uk/healthforall

http://www.nationalleadershipnetwork.org

http://www.nice.org.uk

http://www.pals.nhs.uk

http://www.rsph.org.uk

http://www.schoolsforhealth.eu

http://www.un.org/esa/sustdev/documents/agenda21

http://www.un.org/millenniumgoals

http://www.workingforhealth.gov.uk/Government-Response

Glossary

This glossary contains explanations of terms and abbreviations used in this book, and in health promotion and public health generally. Refer to the Index to find where the terms are used and also explained in more detail in the text.

Words in *italics* appear in this list as separate entries.

Advocacy: Representing the interests of people who cannot speak up for themselves because of illness, disability or other disadvantage.

Agenda 21: A worldwide movement to address environmental concerns for the 21st century, focusing on *sustainable development*.

Aim: Broad statement of what you are trying to achieve (e.g. in a health programme or activity).

Audit: Systematic examination of a service in order to check and improve its quality.

Care trust: NHS organisation that provides *health and social care* services, formed by the merger of local authority social care services with NHS primary and community health services.

Commissioning: In the context of commissioning health services, this means deciding what health services and programmes are needed to improve the health status of the local population and ensuring that they are provided.

Communicable disease: Diseases that can be transmitted from one person to another; often called infectious or contagious diseases.

Community action: Activity carried out by people under their own control in order to improve their collective conditions. It may involve campaigning, negotiating with or challenging authorities and those with power.

Community development: Working with people to identify their concerns, and support them in collective action for the good of the community as a whole.

Community health project: A programme of work organised by an agency or a local organisation with the aim of improving health by some combination of community activity, self-help, *community action* and/or *community development*.

Community health services/community services: Health services provided in people's homes or from premises in the community such as GP surgeries, health centres, clinics and small community hospitals (as distinct from services provided in major hospitals).

Community health work: This is *community work* with a focus on health concerns, but generally health is defined broadly to include social and economic aspects, so that community health work may encompass almost as broad a range of activities as community work that does not have a specific health remit.

Community strategy: Local plan led by local authorities with the aim of improving economic, social and environmental wellbeing.

Community work: Working with community groups and organisations to overcome the community's problems and improve people's quality of life. Community work aims to enhance the sense of solidarity and competence in the community.

Comparative need: Comparison between similar groups of people, some in receipt of something such as a service and some not. Those who are not are then defined as being in comparative need. (See also *expressed need, felt need* and *norma-tive need*.)

Competencies: The combination of knowledge, attitudes and skills needed to do a particular job.

Coronary heart disease (CHD). Heart disease caused by poor circulation of blood to the heart muscle because the blood vessels have become blocked. This may show up as a heart attack or chest pain (angina).

Cost–benefit analysis: The process of comparing the benefits with the costs (e.g. of a health programme or activity).

Cost-effectiveness analysis: Comparing the costs and outcomes of alternative activities to achieve the same goal (e.g. comparing the cost of a telephone helpline with nicotine replacement therapy to achieve the goal of successfully helping people to stop smoking).

Cross-sectoral: Working across the boundaries of different *sectors*, e.g. health services working together with businesses and voluntary organisations. Sometimes also called intersectoral.

Demography: The study of the statistics about a population, such as birth, death and age profile.

Educational objectives: What an educator would like clients to know, feel and do as a result of the education.

Effectiveness: The extent to which a programme, activity, service or treatment achieves the result it aimed for (e.g. the effectiveness of a health promotion programme would mean the extent to which it had achieved objectives such a specified positive change in the population's health).

Efficiency: A term applied to a programme or activity to denote how good the *process* (as distinct from the *outcome*) is in terms of, for example, value for money or use of time; it is about how results are achieved compared with other ways of achieving them.

Epidemiology: The study of the distribution, determinants and control of disease in populations.

Ethnicity: Racial origin or cultural background.

Ethnic minority: Group differentiated from the main population of a community by racial origin or cultural background.

Evaluation: The process of assessing what has been achieved (the *outcome*) and how it has been achieved (the *process*).

Evidence-based practice: Based on reliable evidence that something works. For example, evidence-based health promotion means health promotion projects or programmes based on sound research that shows they are likely to be successful in achieving their aims

Expressed need: What people say they need; expressed requests or demands. (See also *comparative need, felt need* and *normative need*.)

Facilitation/facilitator: The process of making/a person who makes something more easily achieved. For example, a group facilitator will help a group of people to get to know each other and discuss things together, but will not be the dominant leader.

Felt need: Need that people feel; what they want. This is not necessarily what they say they need. (See also *comparative need, expressed need* and *normative need*.)

Green Paper: A government policy document issued for consultation. Becomes a *White Paper* when it is finalised and formally agreed as government policy.

Health 21: A policy framework published by the *World Health Organization* in 1999, which set out 21 targets for the European region in the 21st century.

Health action zone: Area of high health need selected by government for special funding and health programmes.

Health and social care services: A wide range of services to meet people's health and social needs. Health care tends to mean services provided by the NHS, and social care usually refers to services provided by local authorities, especially social services departments. In many instances services are provided by both. They may also be provided by the *voluntary sector*.

Health authority: The statutory NHS organisation responsible for health services for a defined population until abolished in 2002, when its responsibilities were largely taken on (in England) by *primary care trusts* and *care trusts*.

Health education: Planned opportunities for people to learn about health, and to undertake voluntary changes in their behaviour.

Health For All: A movement started in the 1980s by the *World Health Organization*. It included *health targets* and stressed basic principles of promoting positive health through health promotion and disease prevention; reducing *inequalities in health*; community participation; cooperation between health authorities, local authorities and others with an impact on health; and a focus on *primary care* as the main basis of the healthcare system.

Health gain: A measurable improvement in health status, in an individual or a population, attributable to earlier intervention.

Health gap: The difference between the overall health of the more wealthy and more deprived communities in a population.

Health impact assessment (HIA): Systematic process of estimating the effects of a specified action – a programme, policy or project – on the health of a defined population. For example, what difference a new transport policy would have on the health of the population affected by it.

Health promotion: The process of enabling people to increase control over, and to improve, their health.

Health-related behaviour: Things people habitually do in their daily life that affect their health. Usually refers to issues such as whether they smoke, whether they take exercise, what they eat, their sexual behaviour, how much alcohol they drink, drug use. Sometimes simply called 'health behaviour'.

Health target: A quantified, measurable improvement in health status, by a given date, which achieves a health objective. It provides a yardstick against which progress can be monitored.

Healthy Cities: A *World Health Organization* initiative started in 1987 to improve health in urban areas. Involves collaborative work between local government, health services, local businesses, community organisations and citizens. The *Health for All* (UK) Network is the coordinating body for action on Healthy Cities within the UK.

Healthy living centres: Centres or networks of activity that aim to promote good health, developed by partnerships with local participation. Funded from the National Lottery.

Healthy Universities: *World Health Organization* initiative to promote health in university settings.

High-risk approach: Public health approach that prioritises people particularly at risk of ill health. (Compare with *whole-population approach*.)

Holistic: In the health context (as in 'holistic approach to health') this means taking into account all aspects of a person – physical, mental, emotional, social – as well as their social, economic and physical environment. (As distinct from an approach which focuses only on, for example, the physical functioning of the body.)

Impact: A term sometimes used to describe short-term *outcomes*. For example, the impact of a programme to encourage women to attend for a breast cancer screening test (mammogram) might be assessed in terms of how many women attended; the long-term outcome could be a change in the rate of women who died of breast cancer.

Incidence: The number of new episodes of illness arising in a population over a specified period of time.

Inequalities in health: The gap between the health of different population groups, such as better-off and more deprived communities, or people with different ethnic backgrounds.

Input: The resources that go into a programme or activity, including money, time, staff and materials.

Lifestyle: The particular way of life of a person or group, often referring to *health-related behaviour* such as smoking, drinking, diet and exercise.

Local strategic partnership (LSP): Local NHS, local authority and other agencies working together to develop and implement local strategy for *neighbourhood renewal*.

Low birthweight: The weight of a baby at birth of less than 2500 grams. High rates of low birthweight babies in a population indicate poor health overall.

Monitoring: The process of regularly reviewing achievements and progress towards goals.

Morbidity/morbidity rate: Illness/incidence of illness in a population in a given period.

Mortality/mortality rate: Death/incidence of death in a population in a given period.

Multidisciplinary: Involving people from different professions (disciplines) and backgrounds.

National Healthy Schools Standard (NHSS): Government standard introduced in 1998 as a joint venture between the Department for Education and Skills and the Department of Health. Aims to develop health promoting schools through programmes of social, personal and health education for the pupils, the way the school is run; and the health and wellbeing of staff, parents and the wider community who have contact with the school.

National Institute for Health and Clinical Excellence (NICE): National body that provides patients, health professionals and the public with authoritative, robust and reliable guidance on best practice in relation to public health drugs, treatments and services across the NHS.

National occupational standards: Nationally agreed statements of best practice about what people are expected to do in their jobs.

National service framework (NSF): National document that sets out the pattern and level of service (standards) which should be provided for a major care area or disease group, such as mental health or heart disease.

National strategies for health: Government strategies to improve the health of national populations.

Neighbourhood renewal strategy: Strategy developed by local agencies with a coordinated approach to tackle the social and economic conditions in the most deprived local authority areas.

Network: A group of people who exchange information, contacts and experience for mutual benefit.

New Deal for Communities: Government funding for deprived communities to support plans that bring together local people, community and voluntary organisations, public agencies and local businesses in an attempt to make improvements in health, employment, education and the physical environment.

New public health: An approach to public health that emerged in the 1980s. It shifted emphasis from a *lifestyle* approach focused on people's individual health behaviour to a new focus on political and social action to address underlying issues that affect health (such as poverty, employment, discrimination and the environment people live in).

NHS Direct: A national NHS telephone helpline staffed by specially trained nurses.

NHS trust: An independent body within the NHS that provides health services in hospitals. Some NHS trusts provide specialised services, such as ambulance services or mental health services.

Nongovernmental organisation (NGO): Organisation that is independent of government control.

Normative need: Need defined by an expert or professional according to that person's or profession's standards. (See also *comparative need, felt need* and *expressed need.*)

Objective: Applied to a health programme or activity, this means the desired end state (or result, or *outcome*) to be achieved within a specified time period. Objectives are usually more specific and detailed than *aims.*

Opportunity costs: Potential benefits, which will not be realised if one thing is done instead of another. For example, if there is only enough time and money for one health programme (A or B), and it is spent on A, the opportunity costs are the potential benefits of spending on B that will be forgone.

Ottawa charter: A document launched in 1986 at an international *World Health Organization* conference in Ottawa, Canada, which identified key themes for health promotion practice.

Outcome: The end product of a health programme or activity, expressed in whatever terms are appropriate (e.g. changes in people's attitudes or knowledge, changes in health policy, changes in the uptake of services or changes in the rate of illness).

Patient advice and liaison services (PALS): Established from April 2002 within NHS trusts to help patients, families and carers to resolve problems or air concerns. Replaced Community health councils.

Performance management: Systematic management practices and monitoring systems, which support people so that they can achieve their work objectives.

Policy: A broad statement of the principles of how to proceed in relation to a specific issue, such as a national policy on transport, a local authority policy on housing or a policy on how to deal with alcohol issues in a workplace.

Premature death: Death under 65 years of age. High rates of premature death in a population indicate poor health overall.

Prevalence: Measure of how much illness there is in a population at a particular point in time or over a specified period.

Primary care: Services that are people's first point of contact with the NHS, such as services provided by GPs, practice nurses, district nurses and health visitors. (As distinct from *secondary care,* provided in hospitals.)

Primary care trust (PCT): An NHS body whose main tasks are to assess local health needs, develop and provide *primary care* services and commission *secondary care* services from hospitals and specialised services run by *NHS trusts.* PCTs are run by a board whose members include GPs, nurses, representatives from local authority social services and the lay public.

Primary healthcare team: Health workers, usually based at a GP surgery or health centre, who provide *community health services*. They include GPs, district nurses, practice nurses and health visitors.

Primary health education: *Health education* directed at healthy people, aiming to prevent ill health arising in the first place.

Primary prevention: Stopping ill health arising in the first place. For example, eating a healthy diet, not smoking and taking enough exercise are factors in the primary prevention of heart disease.

Private sector: A collective term for business and commercial organisations. (See also *sector*.)

Process: All the implementation stages of a health programme or activity that happen between *input* and *outcome*.

Project: A one-off, time-limited programme of work with clearly identified start and finish times, aims and objectives.

Public health: Preventing disease, prolonging life and promoting health through work focused on the population as a whole.

Public sector: A collective term for organisations that are controlled by the state and publicly funded, such as the NHS, local authorities, police, fire, probation and prison services. Often also called statutory sector/services because they are governed by laws (statutes). (See also *sector*.)

Qualitative: Concerned with quality – how good or bad something is according to specified criteria, usually expressed as a description in words rather than numbers. For example, qualitative data about the outcome of a breast screening programme could include users' descriptions of how they felt about it: whether they found it painful, embarrassing, well-organised, etc. (compare with *quantitative*).

Quality: How good something (such as health service) is when judged against a number of criteria.

Quality Protects: Services for children in need, including vulnerable children in local authority care.

Quality standard: An agreed level of performance negotiated within available resources.

Quantitative: Concerned with measurable quantity, usually expressed in numbers. For example, quantitative data about the outcome of a breast screening programme could include the percentage of the women invited who actually attended, the percentage called back for further assessment, and (ultimately) the decrease in rates of illness and death from breast cancer (compare with *qualitative*).

Resources: A term often used in health education and health promotion to mean educational and/or publicity materials such as leaflets, posters, displays and videos.

Risk factor: An attribute, such as a habit (e.g. smoking) or exposure to an environmental hazard, that increases the likelihood of developing an illness.

Saving Lives: Our Healthier Nation: *National strategy for health* in England, published in 1999, which sets out priority areas (cancer, heart disease and stroke, accidents, mental health) and sets national targets.

Screening: The application of a special test for everyone at risk of a particular disease to detect whether the disease is present at an early stage. It is used for diseases where early detection makes treatment more successful.

Secondary care: Specialised healthcare services provided by hospital inpatient and outpatient services.

Secondary health education: *Health education* directed at people who are already ill, to prevent ill health moving to a chronic or irreversible stage, and to restore people to their former state of health. Often involves educating patients about their condition and what to do about it.

Secondary prevention: Intervention during the early stages of a disease to prevent further damage.

Sector: Organisations are often categorised into three types: *public sector* (such as the NHS and local authorities), *private sector* (business and commerce) and *voluntary sector* (charities, not-for-profit and *voluntary organisations*).

Self-empowerment: Ability to have control over your own life.

Self-esteem: How good you feel about yourself; your opinion of yourself.

Social capital: Investment in the social fabric of society, so that communities have characteristics such as high levels of trust and supportive networks for the exchange of information, ideas and practical help.

Social inclusion/exclusion: A sense of belonging to/feeling alienated from the community in which a person lives.

Social marketing: The systematic application of marketing, along with other concepts and techniques, to achieve specific behavioral goals for a social good.

Stages of change: A cycle of stages a person usually goes through when changing a health-related behaviour, such as stopping smoking. Stages are: (1) not yet thinking about it; (2) thinking about changing; (3) being ready to change; (4) action – making changes; (5) maintaining change; then either maintaining the changed behaviour permanently or (6) relapsing – often then repeating the cycle by thinking about changing again (2).

Statutory organisations/agencies: *Public sector* organisations or agencies such as local authorities and NHS organisations.

Statutory sector: Another term for the *public sector*.

Strategy: A broad plan of action that specifies what is to be achieved, how and by when; it provides a framework for more detailed planning.

Sure Start: Government schemes in areas of high health need, which aim to support parents and children under 4 years.

Sustainable development: Development that meets the needs of the present without damaging the health or environment of future generations.

Target group: The people who are intended to benefit from a public health or health promotion activity.

Targets: Quantified and measurable achievements to aim for, by specified dates, which provide yardsticks against which progress can be monitored. (See also *health target*.)

Tertiary health education: *Health education* directed at people whose ill health has not been, or could not be, prevented and who cannot be completely cured. Concerned with educating about how to make the most of the remaining potential for healthy living, and how to avoid unnecessary hardships, restrictions and compli-

cations (e.g. in rehabilitation programmes following a stroke).

Victim-blaming: Blaming people for their own ill health when it is rooted in their social and/or economic circumstances. For example, blaming people for contracting lung cancer ('it's their own fault') because they smoke, but ignoring the reasons for smoking – which could include lack of education, no support available to stop smoking, or smoking used as a way of coping with stresses such as poverty, poor housing, single parenthood or unemployment.

Voluntary organisations: Not-for-profit organisations, ranging from large national ones to small groups of local people, run by volunteers but possibly employing paid staff. Small local voluntary organisations are often called community groups.

Voluntary sector: A collective term for *voluntary organisations*, community groups and charities. (See also *sector*.)

Walk-in centre: NHS service offering advice, information and treatment for health problems from specially trained nurses, with no appointment necessary.

White Paper: Government policy, often accompanied by legislation. Usually follows a *Green Paper*.

Whole-population approach: Public health approach that focuses on a whole community rather than on individuals who are identified as being in particular need. (Compare with *high-risk approach*.)

World Health Organization (WHO): An intergovernmental organisation within the United Nations system whose purpose is to help all people attain the highest possible level of health through public health programmes. Its headquarters are in Geneva, Switzerland.

Index